MEDICAL TERMINOLOGY

*The Language of
Health Care*

MEDICAL TERMINOLOGY

The Language of Health Care

MARJORIE CANFIELD WILLIS, CMA-AC
Program Director
Medical Assisting / Medical Transcription Programs
Orange Coast College
Costa Mesa, California

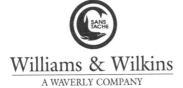

Williams & Wilkins
A WAVERLY COMPANY

BALTIMORE • PHILADELPHIA • LONDON • PARIS • BANGKOK
HONG KONG • MUNICH • SYDNEY • TOKYO • WROCLAW

Editor: John P. Butler
Managing Editor: Victoria M. Vaughn
Development Editor: Tom Lochhaas
Production Coordinators: Carol Eckhart, Anne Stewart Seitz
Copy Editor: Therese Grundl
Designer: Norman W. Och
Illustration Planner: Lorraine C. Wrzosek
Cover Designer: Rita Baker-Schmidt
Typesetter: Mario Fernández
Manufacturing: R. R. Donnelley & Sons, Co.
Color Separator: Publicity Engravers, Inc.

Williams & Wilkins
351 West Camden Street
Baltimore, Maryland 21201-2436 USA

Rose Tree Corporate Center
1400 North Providence Road
Building II, Suite 5025
Media, Pennsylvania 19063-2043 USA

Accurate indications, adverse reactions and dosage schedules for drugs are provided in this book, but it is possible that they may change. The reader is urged to review the package information data of the manufacturers of the medications mentioned.

Printed in the United States of America

First Edition,

Library of Congress Cataloging-in-Publication Data

Willis, Marjorie Canfield.
    Medical terminology: the language of health care / Marjorie Canfield Willis
        p.   cm.
    Includes bibliographical references and index.
    ISBN 0-683-09055-0
    1. Medicine—Terminology. I. Title.
    [DNLM: 1. Nomenclature. W 15 W735m 1996]
R123.W476 1996
610'.14—dc20
DNLM/DLC
for Library of Congress   95-40256
                                                                    CIP

The author and publishers have made every effort to trace the copyright holders for borrowed material. If they have inadvertently overlooked any, they will be pleased to make the necessary arrangements at the first opportunity.

To purchase additional copies of this book, call our customer service department at **(800) 638-0672** or fax orders to **(800) 447-8438**. For other book services, including chapter reprints and large quantity sales, ask for the Special Sales department.

Canadian customers should call **(800) 268-4178**, or fax **(905) 470-6780**. For other calls originating outside of the United States, please call **(410) 528-4223** or fax **(410) 528-8550**

Visit Williams & Wilkins on the Internet: http://www.wwilkins.com or contact our customer service department at **custserv@wwilkins.com**. Williams & Wilkins customer service representatives are available from 8:30 a.m. to 6:00 pm, EST, Monday through Friday, for telephone access.

97 98 99
3 4 5 6 7 8 9 10

To the allied health students
of Orange Coast College:

May you grow in knowledge and skill
and always consider your patients
as important as your procedures.

PREFACE

This text is designed to provide a framework for building a medical vocabulary using an applied approach. Emphasis is on understanding basic medical terms and how they are used in documenting and reporting patient care procedures. Practical applications are provided by exercises and medical record analyses in each chapter. The goal is to develop a basic "working" knowledge of the language of health care to serve as a basis for individual expansion.

Text Overview

Chapter 1 identifies the need for personal commitment that is required to develop a basic knowledge of medical language. Included are methods of time management, techniques for making use of the senses to reinforce memory, and preparation and utilization of flash cards.

Chapter 2 starts with the origin of medical language, then introduces basic term components (prefixes, suffixes, and a selected number of combining forms) illustrating how these structures are combined to form medical terms. Rules of pronunciation, spelling, and formation of singular and plural forms are included. Medical word components covered in this chapter are used repeatedly throughout the book.

Chapter 3 examines the evolution of the physician in medicine and identifies fields of medical practice, including scopes of practice and the expansion of allied health professions.

Chapter 4 establishes the basis for the application of learning medical terms covered throughout the text by introducing common forms, formats, abbreviations, symbols, and methods of documenting patient care. This enables the student to understand basic communication between professionals, including physician's orders and prescriptions. The content of this chapter is reinforced in medical record analyses in succeeding chapters.

Periodic review of chapters 2 and 4 is essential for successful use of this book. Term components first encountered in these chapters are revisited in subsequent chapters to reinforce memory of common term components.

Chapters 5–17 cover terms related to the body systems. In each chapter, basic anatomical terms are outlined, additional combining forms related to the system are identified, and common terms and abbreviations related to symptoms, diagnoses, tests, procedures, surgeries, and therapies are identified. Practice exercises at the end of each chapter are designed to reinforce the memory of basic term components by repetitive word structure analysis. Answers to practice exercises are in Appendix D.

Another feature of chapters 5–17 is the medical record analysis. Each analysis requires reading a particular medical record and answering questions specific to each. Knowledge of Chapter 4 is a prerequisite for understanding questions presented in the medical record analyses. Answers to questions in the medical record analyses are in the instructor's guide.

Other Features

Ancient artifacts (AA) provide historical information about the origins of selected medical terms. More than 50 ancient artifacts are sprinkled throughout the text in the margins.

The *color atlas* is placed before Chapters 5–17 to serve as a handy, color-rich visual reference when learning terms related to the body systems. Each plate links health care technology to the anatomy.

Appendix A summarizes medical term components (prefixes, suffixes, and combining forms) in two lists: (*a*) term component to English definition and (*b*) English definition to term component. Appendix B is a glossary of abbreviations and symbols. Appendix C lists commonly prescribed drugs, including therapeutic classifications. Appendix D contains answers to the practice exercises (answers to questions in the medical record analyses are in the instructor's guide).

Audiotapes are available through Williams & Wilkins to reinforce pronunciation of all key terms covered in this text. Also available from Williams & Wilkins is the *Medical Terminology: The Language of Health Care* CD-ROM. This multimedia course contains all the material in the book and also provides the additional capability of tracking student progress through pre- and posttesting, chapter review exercises, additional medical record analyses, spelling exercises, and human voice pronounciations.

ACKNOWLEDGMENTS

I am very fortunate to enjoy a wide circle of support from medical care facilities, providers and suppliers, and allied health graduates working in the field. They have been my link to all that is current and vital to the needs of students. I extend to them my heartfelt thanks for their contributions and hope that the quality of this text will serve as a tribute to their individual input.

Through all the years of development of this textbook, which was born of the need to teach medical terminology to the allied health students at Orange Coast College, my colleagues have stood by me in continued support, offering their thoughts and expertise, always with the best interests of our students in mind. I especially acknowledge those who gave of their time to review text materials:

Daniel Adelmann, RRT
Kevin Ballinger, R.EEG/EPT
K. Joan Clasby, RDMS, ARRT
Daniel Farrell, RRT, CRTT, CPFT
Linda Harloe, MT (ASCP)
Lorraine Henry, CRT, ARRT, (RT-M), CMA-C
Lynn Keene, MS
Linda Pullano, CRT, ARRT
Ann Zanelli, RN

I am grateful for the many reviewers chosen by Williams & Wilkins who examined my work and gave thoughtful feedback. In addition, I am thankful for the review of selected chapters by Jeffrey I. Barke, M.D., Raymond J. Merchant, M.D., John M. Parkinson, M.D., Harry B. Peled, M.D., Miguel P. Prietto, M.D., Richard R. Reed, M.D., and Richard D. Underwood, M.D. I also thank Mary Ann Ruff King and Joyce Murphy for their expertise in preparing the medical records included in this book. A special thanks also goes to Leslie Gartner, Ph.D., for checking accuracy of anatomical drawings.

During development and production, the text has had the loving handling of the Williams & Wilkins publishing staff. The names of key individuals are listed on the copyright page, but there are many others who have guided me through the incredible process to publication. I thank them all.

I want to recognize J/B Woolsey Associates, Todd Smith in particular, for the outstanding illustrations drawn for this text. Also, the credits at the end of this text list individuals and companies who have supplied the many photographs that enrich this book. Their generosity and enthusiastic support are greatly appreciated.

Last, but not least, I thank my family for their love and support.

M.C.W.

The author and publisher acknowledge the contributions of the following reviewers for their valuable comments and suggestions.

Arleen Bates
Vicki Rose
ETON
Port Orchard, Washington

Pamela Bayliss, MS, PT
Tidewater Community College
Virginia Beach, Virginia

Sharon Blesie, CMA
National Education Center
West Des Moines, Iowa

John E. Buynak, RN
Berks Technical Institute
Wyomissing, Pennsylvania

Kathryn C. Cauble
Bunker Hill Community College
Boston, Massachusetts

Ruth Darton, CMA
National Education Center
San Bernardino, California

Barbara F. Ensley, RN, CMA-C, MS
Haywood Community College
Clyde, North Carolina

Catherine M. Gierman, RN, BA, CMA
Northwestern Business College
Chicago, Illinois

Anthony Giletto, RN, BSc, MT
National Education Center (Thompson
Institute)
Philadelphia, Pennsylvania

Margie Golding
Itawamba Community College
Tupelo, Mississippi

Michele Green
State University of New York
Alfred, New York

Marsha Hemby, RN, CMA
Pitt Community College
Greenville, North Carolina

Julie Hosley, RN, CMA
Carteret Community College
Morehead City, North Carolina

Jeanne Howard, AAS, CMA
El Paso Community College
El Paso, Texas

Sue A. Hunt, MA, RN, CMA
Middlesex Community College
Wakefield, Massachusetts

Virginia Johnson, CMA
Lakeland Medical-Dental Academy
Minneapolis, Minnesota

Benna Kisin, CMT
DIAL & DICTATE
Southfield, Michigan

Estelle G. Landry, BS, MS
Hesser College
Manchester, New Hampshire

Catherine C. McCandless, MA
Cypress College
Cypress, California

Joyce Nakano, BA, CMA-A
Pasadena City College
Pasadena, California

Carol Faye Peterson, CMA-C
Albany Technical Institute
Albany, Georgia

Jo Ann C. Rowell
Anne Arundel Community College
Arnold, Maryland

Marcia Schirle, MLT(AMT)
Professional Careers Institute
Madison Heights, Michigan

Nancy Schlapman, RN
University of Wisconsin
Oshkosh, Wisconsin

Bob Villines, BSMT, MA, CLS(NCA)
Nashville College
Madison, Tennessee

CONTENTS

Building a Medical Vocabulary: Getting Started

OBJECTIVES

After completion of this chapter you will be able to

1. Make a personal commitment to learn medical terminology

2. Describe methods of study time management

3. Explain the value of positive thinking in the learning process

4. Choose a relaxing environment in which to study

5. Explain how a healthy diet and regular exercise are beneficial to learning

6. Use all senses to reinforce memory

7. Prepare and use flash cards

8. List suggested study tips

Personal Aspects of Successful Learning

To begin learning medical terminology, organize your study time and examine methods for efficient memorization. Consider the following personal aspects of successful learning.

Commitment

Personal commitment is key to developing a solid knowledge of medical language. A strong pledge and lots of practice are necessary to memorize the basic building blocks of medical terms. Make that promise now!

Time Management

Effective time management is essential. Other activities will always compete with the time available for study. Once committed to your goal, you must outline a reasonable plan for completion. Follow the study path this text and your instructor provide, and incorporate the necessary study time into your personal schedule.

Set aside *prime time* for study. Prime time is time during the day or evening when you feel most alert and at your finest, and it is when learning is best accomplished. Identify your personal prime time, and try your best to allot a concentrated block of it for memory work.

The most common time management problem is procrastination—putting tasks off until later. If you suffer from this affliction, you will need to act to curb this ineffective habit pattern and keep yourself on target. When you catch yourself procrastinating, focus immediately on the positive aspects of your commitment and the learning goals you have set. Try easing your way in by dividing studies into small segments you can reasonably complete. Take time to notice what you have accomplished, and reward yourself periodically for a job well done! Focus on your goals and the many rewards of accomplishment (Fig. 1.1).

Attitude

Positive thinking is vital for effective learning. Feeling confident stems from positive thoughts. Negative thoughts always lead to defeat. Replace all negative thoughts with "can do" affirmatives that make confident thoughts a habit. A positive approach will help you to stay balanced when you encounter the inevitable hurdles and problems of life. Concentrate on what is "good"!

Relaxation

Mental relaxation is indispensable for successful learning. The tension resulting from fear of failure or any other cause makes learning difficult or impossible. Give yourself a comfortable, relaxing atmosphere for studying. Consider listening to music you enjoy and find relaxing while studying.

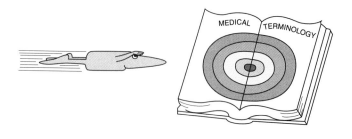

Figure 1.1.

Fitness

Regular, moderate exercise has been proven to reduce stress. Include it in your overall plan for successful learning. A healthy diet also provides the "fuel power" necessary for mental stamina.

Use Your Good Senses

When you are learning, your brain reinforces and retains facts as a result of interaction with the senses. The senses form mental images that are the basis for thought. We *see* (visual sense), we *hear* (auditory sense), we *feel* (kinesthetic sense), and, to a lesser degree, we *taste* (gustatory sense) and *smell* (olfactory sense).

An effective memory depends on intricate processes that recall mental images of sights, sounds, feelings, tastes, and smells. For this reason, try to include as many senses as possible in the process of reinforcing learning. Remember the three basics:

SEE IT   For visual reinforcement

SAY IT   For auditory reinforcement

WRITE IT   For kinesthetic reinforcement

Flash Cards for Prefixes, Suffixes, and Combining Forms

Make a 3 × 5 card for each prefix, suffix, and combining form listed in Chapter 2. Write each component on the front and its meaning on the back. Include a sample word or a drawing depicting the component to reinforce your visual sense (Fig. 1.2).

Use cards with different colors for each category, e.g., prefixes on blue cards, suffixes on green cards, and combining forms on pink cards. You can use pens of different colors for special emphasis, such as the prefix (blue card) in blue ink and the meaning on the reverse in red ink. Choose colors that are most pleasing to your visual and kinesthetic senses.

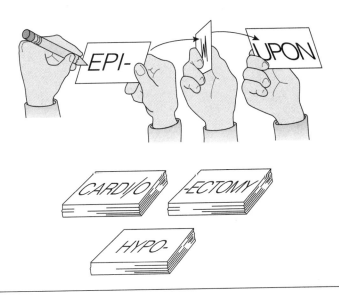

Figure 1.2. Preparing flash cards.

Also, within a category you can make distinctions; e.g., use green cards for all suffixes, but use different colors when writing meanings to indicate the types of suffixes [symptomatic suffixes (blue ink), diagnostic suffixes (green ink), operative/surgical suffixes (red ink), and general suffixes (black ink)]. These are just suggestions. Be as creative as you wish, and use colors that you find most pleasing or eyecatching.

Organizing Flash Cards

Punch a hole in the top of each flash card, and loop each card through a key chain or ring holder to make a "rotary file." This method keeps groups of cards together and prevents them from becoming lost or scattered. Within this file, you can group associated cards for components related to color, size, position, direction, etc.

Frugal Flash Card

Preparing flash cards for each prefix, suffix, and combining form in Chapter 2 is well worth your effort and will pay off in memory reinforcement. Continue to make flash cards for each combining form added in Chapters 5–17.

Also include abbreviations, symbols, and terms found throughout the text; however, if your stack of flash cards has become cumbersome, you may want to try the frugal flash card, so named because it consolidates paper and is inexpensive.

Fold a piece of 8½ × 11" lined paper in half lengthwise. Write the word component, symbol, or term on the first line of the first column and its definition on the same line in the second column. Skip a line and write the next word component, symbol, or term with its definition on the same line in the second column. Continue listing terms with corresponding definitions until you reach the bottom. Then fold the paper at the lengthwise crease so that the word component, symbol, or term is listed on one side and the definition appears on the same line on the other side. This lets you flip from one side to the other, "flashing" and reinforcing the meanings of the terms. Use the other side of the paper in the same way (Fig. 1.3).

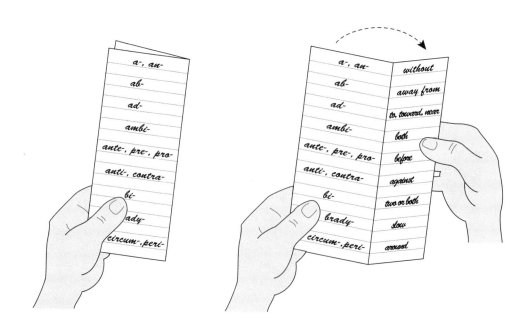

Figure 1.3. Using the frugal flash card.

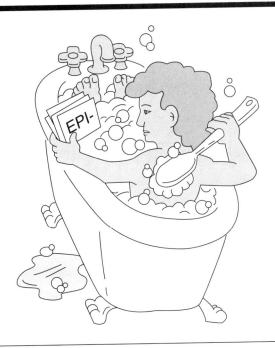

Figure 1.4. Snatching moments.

Snatching Moments!

Carry your flash cards with you at all times. During most days there are times when you can snatch a moment to use your flash cards. You will feel less stress when waiting in a line or for an appointment if you know that you can use that time for study (Fig. 1.4).

Remember to use your good senses:

SEE IT   Employ your visual sense by making and repeatedly reviewing flash cards

SAY IT   Pronounce each component out loud three times as you flash each card to reinforce your auditory sense

WRITE IT   Make each flash card by hand using pleasant colored paper and ink to satisfy your kinesthetic sense

Other Study Tips

Draw pictures of word components for reinforcement. Often the most absurd associations can help you to remember. It does not matter if they make sense to no one but you (Fig. 1.5)!

Listen to audiotapes your instructor provides.

Make up songs and rhythms to help remember facts. Take a song with which you are familiar, such as "Row, row, row, your boat . . .," and insert words with definitions that are in tune with the song. Make up rhymes that help to differentiate meanings. For example, peri- (the prefix meaning around) is often confused with para- (the prefix meaning alongside of). Use the two components in a sentence to compare their meanings: I sat "para" Sarah on the merry-"peri"-go-around.

Find a study "buddy" or group from class. Compare notes, study techniques, quiz each other, and enjoy healthy competition.

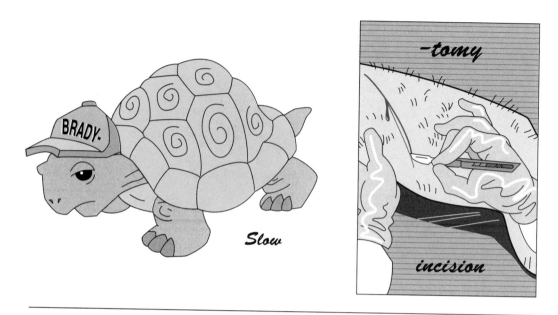

Figure 1.5. Draw pictures of word components for reinforcement.

Give yourself a memory drill by listing word components, symbols, or terms on one side of a paper and then filling in the definitions from memory. Write corrections in red ink. List the incorrectly defined components on a separate paper and repeat the drill. Repeat this process until you have identified a list of those most continually found incorrect. Spend additional time on those troublesome terms.

Let your imagination be your guide. Be creative and make learning fun!

PRACTICE EXERCISES

1. Name the key component to successfully build a basic medical vocabulary.

   _____

2. Identify your personal prime time. _____ _____

3. Identify at least three methods for confronting procrastination.

   _____ _____

   _____ _____

   _____

   _____

4. How can a positive attitude help you with learning?_____

   _____

   _____

5. Give an example of a positive affirmation _____

   _____

6. List at least three ways you can provide a relaxed environment in which to study.

   _____

   _____

   _____

   _____

7. How can a healthy diet and regular exercise help you learn?_____

   _____

   _____

8. List the three basic sensory rules for memorizing facts._____

   _____

   _____

9. Describe a method of preparing flash cards:_____

_____

_____

_____

10. Identify at least three other study tips described in Chapter 1.

_____

_____

_____

11. Prepare flash cards for all prefixes, suffixes, and combining forms listed in Chapter 2.

Basic Term Components

OBJECTIVES

After completion of this chapter you will be able to

1. Describe the origin of medical language

2. Analyze the component parts of a medical term

3. List basic prefixes, suffixes, and combining forms

4. Use basic prefixes, suffixes, and combining forms to build medical terms

5. Explain common rules for proper medical term formation, pronunciation, and spelling

ETYMOLOGY. The Greek root etymon refers to that which is true or genuine. Etymology is the study of the origin and development of words from the source language, original meaning, and history of usage.

Most medical terms stem from Greek or Latin origins. These date to the founding of modern medicine by the Greeks and the influence of Latin when it was the universal language in the Western world. Other languages, such as German and French, have also influenced medical terms, and many new terms are derived from English, which is considered the universal language. Most terms related to diagnosis and surgery have Greek origin, and most anatomical terms can be traced to Latin.

Once you understand the basic medical term structure and know the common prefixes, suffixes, and combining forms, you can learn most medical terms by analyzing each component. Those mysterious words, which are almost frightening at first, will soon no longer be a concern. You will analyze each term with your newly acquired knowledge and the help of a good medical dictionary.

This chapter lists common prefixes and suffixes and many common combining forms. More combining forms will be added to your vocabulary as you learn terms related to the body systems. You will also learn basic rules for proper medical term formation, pronunciation, and spelling.

Make flash cards now for all the basic structures in Chapter 2 (see Chapter 1, "Flash Cards for Prefixes, Suffixes, and Combining Forms"). The key to success in building a medical vocabulary is memorizing these basic structures. If you do that, your work will pay big dividends.

Term Components

Most medical terms have three components: root, suffix, and prefix.

Root and Suffix

Each term is formed by combining at least one root, the foundation of the word, and a suffix, the ending that modifies and gives essential meaning to the root. For example,

$$\text{lip} \ / \ \text{emia}$$

Root	Suffix
fat	blood condition

Lip (fat), the root, is the subject. It is modified by the suffix (emia) to indicate a condition of fat in the blood. Note that each component is dependent on the other to express meaning. No component can stand alone.

Prefix

The prefix is a word structure at the beginning of a term that further modifies the root or roots. For example,

$$\text{hyper} \ / \ \text{lip} \ / \ \text{emia}$$

Prefix	Root	Suffix
excessive	fat	blood condition

The addition of the prefix, hyper, modifies the root to denote excessive fat in the blood.

Additional Roots

Often a medical term is formed of two or more roots. For example,

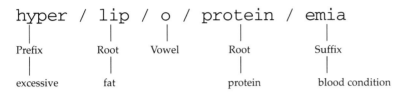

In this term, the additional root, protein, further defines the word to indicate an excessive amount of fat and protein in the blood.

Combining Vowels and Combining Forms

When a medical term has more than one root, each is joined by a vowel, usually an o. As shown in the term hyper/lip/o/protein/emia, the o links the two roots and fosters easier pronunciation. This vowel is known as a *combining vowel*; o is the most common combining vowel (i is the second most common) and is used so frequently to join root to root or root to suffix that it is routinely attached to the root and presented as a *combining form*:

lip   root

lip/o   combining form (root with combining vowel attached)

Required Activity

Using the guidelines found in Chapter 1, prepare flash cards for all of prefixes, suffixes, and combining forms in Chapter 2. Memorize them in preparation for analysis of medical term formations, spelling considerations, and rules of pronunciation.

Quick Review

Complete the following sentences:

1. Most medical terms have three basic parts: the _____, _____, and _____.

2. The root is the _____ of the term.

3. The _____ is the word ending that modifies and gives essential meaning to the root.

4. The _____ is a word structure at the beginning of a term that further modifies the root.

5. Often a medical term is formed of _____ or more roots.

6. When a medical term has more than one root, it is joined together by a _____ (usually an _____).

7. A combining form is a_____ with a _____ attached.

Quick Review Answers

1. root, suffix, prefix
2. foundation or subject
3. suffix
4. prefix
5. two
6. combining vowel, o
7. root, vowel

Rules for Forming and Spelling Medical Terms

Memorizing and spelling basic medical word components are the first steps for learning how to form medical terms. The next step is to construct the words using the following rules:

a. A combining vowel is used to join root to root as well as root to any suffix beginning with a consonant:

```
electr  +   cardi  +  gram
  |           |          |
 Root        Root      Suffix
  |           |          |
electric    heart      record
```

electr/o/cardi/o/gram (electrical record of the heart)

b. A combining vowel is *not* used before a suffix that begins with a vowel:

```
vas   +  ectomy
 |          |
Root      Suffix
 |          |
vessel    excision
```

vas/ectomy (excision of a vessel)

c. If the root ends in a vowel and the suffix begins with the same vowel, drop the final vowel from the root and do not use a combining vowel:

```
cardi  +  itis
  |         |
 Root     Suffix
  |         |
heart    inflammation
```

card itis

card/itis (inflammation of heart)

d. Most often, a combining vowel is inserted between two roots even when the second root begins with a vowel:

```
cardi  +  esophag  +  eal
  |          |          |
 Root       Root      Suffix
  |          |          |
heart    esophagus  pertaining to
```

cardi/o/esophageal (pertaining to heart and esophagus)

e. Occasionally, when a prefix ends in a vowel and the root begins with a vowel, the final vowel is dropped from the prefix:

```
par a  +  e nter  +  al
 |          |         |
Prefix     Root     Suffix
 |          |         |
alongside of  intestine  pertaining to
```

```
par e nter al
```

```
par/enter/al
```
(pertaining to alongside of the intestine)

Breaking down and defining the components in a term often clues you to its meaning. Frequently, however, you must consult a medical dictionary to obtain a precise definition. Take a moment to look up parenteral, so you understand the complete meaning.

Note: there are many exceptions to these rules. Follow the basic guidelines, but be prepared to accept exceptions as you encounter them. Rely on your medical dictionary for additional guidance.

Defining Medical Terms through Word Structure Analysis

You can usually define a term by interpreting the suffix first, then the prefix (if present), then the succeeding root or roots. For example,

```
peri  +  card  +  itis
 |          |         |
Prefix     Root     Suffix
 |          |         |
around     heart   inflammation
```

```
peri/card/itis
```
(inflammation around the heart)

You sense the basic meaning of this term by understanding its components; however, the dictionary clarifies that the term refers to inflammation of the pericardium, the sac that encloses the heart.

Quick Review

a. A combining vowel is used to join root to root as well as root to any suffix beginning with a consonant.
b. A combining vowel is not used before a suffix that begins with a vowel.
c. If the root ends in a vowel and the suffix begins with the same vowel, drop the final vowel from the root and do not use a combining vowel.
d. Most often, a combining vowel is inserted between two roots even when the second root begins with a vowel.
e. Occasionally, when a prefix ends in a vowel and the root begins with a vowel, the final vowel is dropped from the prefix.

Identify which of the rules listed above were applied when forming the following terms:

1. angi + ectasis = angi/ectasis _____

2. hemat + logy = hemato/logy _____

3. oste + ectomy = ost/ectomy _____

4. electr + encephal + gram = electro/encephalo/gram _____

5. para + umbilic + al = par/umbilic/al _____

6. vas + ectomy = vas/ectomy _____

7. arteri + itis = arter/itis _____

8. gastr + enter + cele = gastro/entero/cele _____

9. gastr + tomy = gastro/tomy _____

10. hypo + ox + ia = hyp/ox/ia _____

Quick Review Answers

1. b	5. e, b	9. a
2. a	6. b	10. e, b
3. c	7. c	
4. d, a	8. d, a	

Formation of Medical Terms

All medical terms build from the root. Prefixes and suffixes are attached to the root to modify its meaning. Often two or more roots are linked before being modified. The following are examples of the various patterns of medical term formation using the root cardi (heart) as a base. Note the rules used for forming each term.

Root/Suffix
    cardi/ac
    heart / pertaining to
    (pertaining to the heart)

Prefix/Root/Suffix
    epi/card/ium
    upon / heart / tissue
    (tissue upon the heart, i.e., external lining of the heart)

Prefix/Prefix/Root/Suffix
    sub/endo/cardi/al
    beneath/within / heart / pertaining to
    (pertaining to beneath and within the heart)

Root/Combining vowel/Suffix
    cardi/o/logy
    heart / study of
    (study of the heart)

Root/Combining vowel/Root/Suffix
    cardi/o/pulmon/ary
    heart / lung / pertaining to
    (pertaining to the heart and lungs)

Root/Combining vowel/Suffix (symptomatic)

cardi/o/dynia

heart   /   pain

(pain in the heart)

Root/Combining vowel/Suffix (diagnostic)

cardi/o/rrhexis

heart   /   rupture

(a rupture of the heart)

Root/Combining vowel/Suffix (operative)

cardi/o/rrhaphy

heart   /   suture

(a suture of the heart)

Quick Review

Analyze the following terms by separating each component, and then define the individual elements:

1. gastric _____

2. epigastric _____

3. gastrocardiac _____

4. epigastralgia _____

5. gastroscopy _____

6. epigastrocele _____

7. gastrotomy_____

8. epigastrorrhaphy _____

Quick Review Answers

1. gastr/ic   pertaining to the stomach

2. epi/gastr/ic   pertaining to upon the stomach

3. gastr/o/cardi/ac   pertaining to the stomach and heart

4. epi/gastr/algia   pain upon the stomach

5. gastr/o/scopy   examination of the stomach

6. epi/gastr/o/cele   pouching or hernia upon the stomach

7. gastr/o/tomy   incision in the stomach

8. epi/gastr/o/rrhaphy   suture upon the stomach

Spelling Medical Terms

Correct spelling of medical terms is crucial for communication among health care professionals. Careless spelling causes misunderstandings that can have serious consequences. The following are some of the pitfalls to avoid.

1. Some words sound exactly the same but are spelled differently and have different meanings. Context is the clue to spelling. For example,

    ileum (part of the intestine)

    ilium (part of the hip bone)

    sitology (study of food)

    cytology (study of cells)

2. Other words sound similar but are spelled differently and have different meanings. For example,

    abduction (to draw away from)

    adduction (to draw toward)

    hematoma (blood tumor)

    hepatoma (liver tumor)

    aphagia (inability to swallow)

    aphasia (inability to speak)

3. When letters are silent in a term, they risk being omitted when spelling the word. For example,

    pt has a "t" sound

    nephro<u>pt</u>osis

    ph has an "f" sound

    <u>ph</u>armacy

    ps has an "s" sound

    <u>ps</u>ychology

4. Some words have more than one accepted spelling. For example,

orthopedic

orthopaedic (British)

leukocyte

leucocyte

5. Some combining forms have the same meaning but different origins that compete for usage. For example, there are three combining forms that mean uterus:

hyster/o (Greek)
metr/o   (Greek)
uter/o   (Latin)

Acceptable Term Formations

As you learn medical terms, you can have fun experimenting with creating words, such as glyco (sweet) + cardio (heart) = sweetheart! However, in the real medical world, the word is formed when the term is coined. Often there seems no reason why a particular word form became acceptable. That is why you should check your medical dictionary when in doubt of the spelling, formation, or precise meaning.

Rules of Pronunciation

When you first learn to pronounce medical terms, the task can seem insurmountable. The first time you open your mouth to say a term is a tense moment for those who want to get it right! The best preparation is to study the basic rules of pronunciation, repeat the words after your instructor has said them, listen to audiotapes when available, and try to keep the company of others who use medical language. There is nothing like the validation you get from the fact that no one laughed or snarled at you when you said something "medical" for the very first time! Your confidence will build with every word you use.

Shortcuts to Pronunciation

Consonant	Example
c (before a, o, u) = k	cavity colon cure
c (before e, i) = s	cephalic cirrhosis
ch = k	cholesterol
g (before a, o, u) = g	gallstone gonad gurney

continued

Consonant	Example
g (before e, i) = j	generic giant
ph = f	phase
pn = n	pneumonia
ps = s	psychology
pt = t	ptosis pterygium
rh **= r** **rrh**	 rhythm hemorrhoid
x = z (as first letter)	xerosis

Phonetic spelling for pronunciation of most medical terms in this text is in parentheses below the term (beginning with Chapter 3). The phonetic system used is basic and has only a few standard rules. The macron and breve are the two diacritical marks used. The macron (⁻) is placed over vowels that have a long sound:

$\bar{a}$ day
$\bar{e}$ be
$\bar{i}$ kite
$\bar{o}$ no
$\bar{u}$ unit

The breve (˘) is placed over vowels that have a short sound:

$\breve{a}$ alone
$\breve{e}$ ever
$\breve{i}$ pit
$\breve{o}$ ton
$\breve{u}$ sun

The primary accent (´) is placed after the syllable that is stressed when saying the word. Monosyllables do not have a stress mark. Other syllables are separated by hyphens.

Singular and Plural Forms

Most often plurals are formed by adding s or es to the end of a singular form. The following are common exceptions.

Singular		Plural	
Ending	**Example**	**Ending**	**Example**
-a	vertebra	**-ae**	vertebrae
-is	diagnosis	**-es**	diagnoses

continued

Singular		Plural	
Ending	Example	Ending	Example
-ma	condyloma	**-mata**	condylomata
-on	phenomenon	**-a**	phenomena
-um	bacterium	**-a**	bacteria
-us[a]	fungus	**-i**	fungi
-ax	thorax	**-aces**	thoraces
-ex	apex	**-ices**	apices
-ix	appendix	**-ices**	appendices
-y	myopathy	**-ies**	myopathies

[a]Exceptions: viruses and sinuses.

Common Prefixes

The following list of common prefixes is in alphabetical order except for grouped prefixes with the same meaning. For example, ante, pre, and pro mean "before" and are listed together in alphabetical order under ante.

Prefix	Meaning	Example
a-	without	aphonia (*without* voice or speech)
an-		anaerobic (pertaining to *without* air)
ab-	away from	abnormal (pertaining to *away from* normal)
ad-	to, toward, or near	adhesion (*to* stick to)
ambi-	both	ambidextrous (dexterity in *both* hands)
ante-	before	antepartum (*before* labor)
pre-		premature (*before* ripe)
pro-		prognosis [*before* knowing (prediction of course and outcome of a disease)]
anti-	against or opposed to	anticoagulant (*against* clotting)
contra-		contraception (*opposed* to becoming pregnant)
bi-	two or both	bilateral (pertaining to *two or both* sides)
brady-	slow	bradycardia (condition of *slow* heart)
circum-	around	circumvascular (pertaining to *around* a vessel)
peri-		periosteum (pertaining to *around* bone)

continued

Prefix	Meaning	Example
con-	together or with	congenital (pertaining to being born *with*)
sym-		symbiosis (presence of life *together*)
syn-		syndactylism (webbing *together* of toes or fingers)
de-	from, down, or not	decapitate [separation of the head (caput) *from* the body]
dia-	across or through	dialysis [dissolution *across* or *through* (a membrane)]
trans-		transmission (to send *across* or *through*)
dis-	separate from or apart	dislocation (to place *apart*)
dys-	painful, difficult, or faulty	dysphonia [condition of *difficult* voice or sound (hoarseness)]
e-	out or away	edentia (condition of teeth *out*)
ec-		eccentric (pertaining to *away* from center)
ex-		excise (to cut *out*)
ecto-	outside	ectopic (pertaining to a place *outside*)
exo-		exocrine (denoting secretion *outside*)
extra-		extravascular (pertaining to *outside* vessel)
en-	within	encapsulate (*within* little box)
endo-		endoscope (instrument for examination *within*)
intra-		intradermal (pertaining to *within* skin)
epi-	upon	epidermal (pertaining to *upon* the skin)
eu-	good or normal	eugenic (pertaining to *good* production)
hemi-	half	hemicephalic (pertaining to *half* of the head)
semi-		semilunar (pertaining to *half* moon)
hyper-	above or excessive	hyperlipemia (*excessive* fat in blood)
hypo-	below or deficient	hypothermia (condition of *below* normal temperature)
infra-	below or under	infraumbilical (pertaining to *below* the navel)
sub-		sublingual (pertaining to *under* the tongue)

continued

Prefix	Meaning	Example
inter-	between	intercostal (pertaining to *between* ribs)
meso-	middle	mesomorphic (pertaining to *middle* form)
meta-	beyond, after, or change	metastasis [*beyond* stopping or standing (spread of disease from one part of the body to another)]
		metamorphosis (condition of *change* in form)
micro-	small	microlith (*small* stone)
mono-	one	monochromatic (pertaining to *one* color)
uni-		unilateral (pertaining to *one* side)
neo-	new	neoplasia [a *new* (abnormal) formation]
pachy-	thick	pachycephaly (pertaining to *thick* head)
pan-	all	panacea (a cure-*all*)
para-	alongside of or abnormal	paramedic (pertaining to *alongside of* medicine)
		paranoia (condition of *abnormal* thinking)
poly-	many	polyphobia (condition of *many* fears)
multi-		multicellular (pertaining to *many* cells)
post-	after or behind	postoperative [*after* operation (surgery)]
re-	again or back	reactivate (to make active *again*)
retro-	backward or behind	retrograde (going *backward*)
super-	above or excessive	supernumerary [*excessive* numbers (too many to count)]
supra-		suprarenal (pertaining to *above* the kidney)
tachy-	fast	tachycardia (a condition of *fast* heart)
tri-	three	triangle (*three* angles)
ultra-	beyond or excessive	ultrasonic (pertaining to *beyond* sound)

Common Combining Forms

Following are selected combining forms (roots with combining vowels attached) to give you a start toward building medical terms. Additional combining forms are introduced at the beginning of Chapters 5–17 on body systems.

Appendix A contains a summary list of combining forms.

CANCER. Cancer is Latin for crab. The word is derived from the Greek word karkinos that was used by Hippocrates and other early writers and also means crab. Some authorities say the word was used because it describes the appearance of the disease; just as the crab's feet extend in all directions from its body, so can the disease extend in the human. Other authorities relate the term to the obstinacy of a crab in pursuing prey.

Combining Forms

Combining Form	Meaning	Example
abdomin/o	abdomen	abdominal (pertaining to *abdomen*)
lapar/o		laparotomy (incision into the *abdomen*)
acr/o	extremity or topmost	acrodynia (pain in an *extremity*)
		acrophobia [exaggerated fear of *topmost* places (heights)]
aden/o	gland	adenoma (*gland* tumor)
aer/o	air or gas	aerobic (pertaining to *air*)
angi/o	vessel	angioplasty (surgical repair of a blood *vessel*)
vas/o		vasectomy (excision of a *vessel*)
carcin/o	cancer	carcinogenic (pertaining to production of *cancer*)
cardi/o	heart	cardiologist (one who specializes in treatment of the *heart*)
cephal/o	head	cephalic (pertaining to the *head*)
cyan/o	blue	cyanotic (pertaining to *blue*)
cyt/o	cell	cytology (study of *cell*)
dextr/o	right or on the right side	dextrocardia (condition of the heart *on the right side*)
erythr/o	red	erythrocyte (*red* cell)
fibr/o	fiber	fibroma (*fiber* tumor)
gastr/o	stomach	gastric (pertaining to the *stomach*)
hem/o **hemat/o**	blood	hematology (study of *blood*)
hydr/o	water	hydrophobia (exaggerated fear of *water*)
leuk/o **leuc/o**	white	leukocyte (*white* cell)
lip/o	fat	lipoid (resembling *fat*)
lith/o	stone or calculus	lithiasis (presence of a *stone*)
macr/o	large or long	macrocyte (*large* cell)
melan/o	black	melanoma (*black* tumor)
morph/o	form	morphology (study of *form*)
necr/o	death	necrocytosis (condition of cell *death*)
olig/o	few or deficient	oligospermia (condition of *deficient* sperm)

continued

Combining Form	Meaning	Example
or/o	mouth	oral (pertaining to the *mouth*)
orth/o	straight, normal, or correct	orthostatic (pertaining to standing *straight*)
path/o	disease	pathology (study of *disease*)
ped/o	child or foot	pediatrics (treatment of *child*)
		pedal (pertaining to the *foot*)
phob/o	exaggerated fear or sensitivity	hydrophobia (*exaggerated fear* of water)
		photophobia (*sensitivity* to light)
phon/o	voice or speech	phonic (pertaining to *voice* or *speech*)
pod/o	foot	podiatry (treatment of the *foot*)
psych/o	mind	psychology (study of the *mind*)
py/o	pus	pyopoiesis (formation of *pus*)
scler/o	hard	sclerosis (a condition of *hardness*)
sinistr/o	left or on the left side	sinistropedal (pertaining to *left* foot)
son/o	sound	sonometer (an instrument to measure *sound*)
sten/o	narrow	stenosis (a condition of *narrow*)
tox/o	poison	toxemia (*poison* in blood)
toxic/o		toxicology (study of *poison*)
troph/o	nourishment or development	trophocyte (a cell that provides *nourishment*)
		hypertrophy (condition of excessive *development*)
ur/o	urine	urology (study of *urine*)

TOXIN. The Greek root toxicon means arrow poison and is derived from the word for the archer's bow. The Greeks often used darts and arrows coated with a poisonous substance.

Common Suffixes

Suffixes are endings that modify the root. They give the root essential meaning by forming a noun, verb, or adjective.

There are two types of suffixes: simple and compound. Simple suffixes form basic terms. For example, ic (pertaining to), a simple suffix, combined with the root gastr (stomach) forms the term gastric (pertaining to the stomach). Compound suffixes are formed by a combination of basic term components. For example, the root tom (to cut) combined with the simple suffix y (denoting a process of) forms the compound suffix tomy (incision); the compound suffix ectomy (excision or removal) is formed by a combination of the prefix ec (out) with the root tom (to cut) and the simple suffix y (a process of).

Compound suffixes are added to the roots to provide a specific meaning. For example, hyster (a root meaning uterus) combined with ectomy forms hysterectomy (excision of the uterus). Noting the differences between simple and compound suffixes will help you analyze medical terms.

Suffixes in this text are divided into four categories:

• Symptomatic suffixes, which describe the evidence of illness
• Diagnostic suffixes, which provide the name of a medical condition
• Operative suffixes, which describe a surgical treatment
• General suffixes, which have general application

Commonly used suffixes follow in alphabetical order except for groups with the same meaning.

Appendix A contains a summary list of suffixes.

Suffix	Meaning	Example

Symptomatic Suffixes (word endings that describe evidence of illness)

Suffix	Meaning	Example
-algia	pain	cephalalgia [*pain* in the head (headache)]
-dynia		cephalodynia [*pain* in the head (headache)]
-genic	origin or production	pathogenic (pertaining to *production* of disease)
-genesis		pathogenesis (*origin* of disease)
-lysis	breaking down or dissolution	hemolysis (*breakdown* of blood)
-megaly	enlargement	hepatomegaly (*enlargement* of the liver)
-oid	resembling	lipoid (*resembling* fat)
-penia	abnormal reduction	leukopenia [*abnormal reduction* of white (blood cells)]
-rrhea	discharge	amenorrhea (absence of menstrual *discharge*)
-spasm	involuntary contraction	vasospasm (*involuntary contraction* of a blood vessel)

Diagnostic Suffixes (word endings that describe a condition or disease)

Suffix	Meaning	Example
-cele	pouching or hernia	gastrocele (*pouching* of the stomach)
-ectasis	expansion or dilation	angiectasis (*expansion* or *dilation* of a blood vessel)
-emia	blood condition	hyperlipemia (excessive fat *blood condition*)

continued

Suffix	Meaning	Example
-iasis	formation of or presence of	lithiasis (*formation* or *presence* of a stone or stones)
-itis	inflammation	appendicitis (*inflammation* of the appendix)
-malacia	softening	osteomalacia (*softening* of bone)
-oma	tumor	carcinoma (cancer *tumor*)
-osis	condition or increase	sclerosis (*condition* of hard) leukocytosis (*increase* of white cells)
-phil	attraction for	pneumophilia (condition that has an *attraction* for the lungs)
-philia		pedophilia (abnormal adult *attraction* for children)
-plasia	formation	dysplasia (faulty *formation*)
-ptosis	falling or downward displacement	gastroptosis (*downward* displacement of the stomach)
-rrhage **-rrhagia**	to burst forth	hemorrhage (*to burst forth* blood)
-rrhexis	rupture	cardiorrhexis (*rupture* of the heart)

Operative Suffixes [word endings that describe a surgical (operative) treatment]

Suffix	Meaning	Example
-centesis	puncture for aspiration	abdominocentesis (*puncture for aspiration* of the abdomen)
-desis	binding	arthrodesis (*binding* of a joint)
-ectomy	excision (removal)	appendectomy (*excision* or *removal* of the appendix)
-pexy	suspension or fixation	gastropexy [*fixation* of the stomach (to the abdominal wall)]
-plasty	surgical repair or reconstruction	rhinoplasty (*surgical repair* of the nose)
-rrhaphy	suture	osteorrhaphy (*suture* of bone)
-tomy	incision	laparotomy (*incision* into the abdomen)
-stomy	creation of an opening	colostomy (*creation of an opening* in the colon)
-tripsy	crushing	lithotripsy (*crushing* of stone)

continued

Suffix	Meaning	Example

General Suffixes (suffixes that have general applications)

Noun Endings (suffixes that form a noun when combined with a root)

Suffix	Meaning	Example
-e	noun marker	erythrocyte (a red blood cell)
-ia	condition of	pneumonia (*condition of* the lung)
-ism		embolism (*condition of* a traveling clot)
-ium	structure or tissue	epigastrium [*structure* upon the stomach (region in the abdomen)]
		pericardium [*tissue* around the heart (sac enclosing the heart)]
-y	condition or process of	adenopathy (*condition of* gland disease)

Adjective Endings (suffixes that mean "pertaining to" and form an adjective when combined with a root)

Suffix	Meaning	Example
-ac		cardiac (*pertaining to* the heart)
-al		pedal (*pertaining to* the foot)
-ar		glandular (*pertaining to* a gland)
-ary		pulmonary (*pertaining to* the lung)
-eal		esophageal (*pertaining to* the esophagus)
-ic		toxic (*pertaining to* poison)
-ous		fibrous (*pertaining to* fiber)
-tic		cyanotic (*pertaining to* blue)

Diminutive Endings (suffixes meaning "small")

Suffix	Meaning	Example
-icle		ventricle (*small* belly or pouch)
-ole		bronchiole (*small* airway)
-ula		macula (*small* spot)
-ule		pustule (*small* pimple)

Other General Suffixes

Suffix	Meaning	Example
-gram	record	sonogram (*record* of sound)
-graph	instrument for recording	sonograph (*instrument for recording* sound)
-graphy	process of recording	sonography (*process of recording* sound)
-iatrics	treatment	pediatrics (*treatment* of children)
-iatry		psychiatry (*treatment* of the mind)

continued

Suffix	Meaning	Example
-logy	study of	cytology (*study of* cells)
-logist	one who specializes in the study or treatment of	oncologist (*one who specializes in the study or treatment of* tumors, i.e., cancer)
		audiologist (*one who specializes in the study or treatment of* hearing)
-ist	one who specializes in	optometrist (*one who specializes in* measuring the eye)
-meter	instrument for measuring	spirometer (*instrument for measuring* breathing)
-metry	process of measuring	spirometry (*process of measuring* breathing)
-poiesis	formation	hemopoiesis (*formation* of blood)
-scope	instrument for examination	endoscope (*instrument for examination* within)
-scopy	examination	endoscopy (*examination* within)
-stasis	stop or stand	hemostasis (*stop* blood)
		orthostasis (*stand* straight)

Note: some word components serve as a combining form or a suffix depending on how the term is constructed. The following are examples.

Combining Form	Compound Suffix	Meaning
path/o	-pathy (path/o + y)	disease
phil/o	-philia (phil/o + ia)	attraction for
plas/o	-plasia (plas/o + ia)	formation
troph/o	-trophy (troph/o + y)	nourishment or development

PRACTICE EXERCISES

For the following terms, separate prefixes, combining forms, and suffixes. Then define the term.

1. laparotomy _____

2. cephalalgia _____

3. neoplasia _____

4. hydrophilia _____

5. pathopsychology _____

6. interfibral _____

7. pyogenesis _____

8. pachycephaly _____

9. ultrasonography _____

10. melanocytoma _____

11. gastropexy _____

12. exocardia _____

13. cephalometry _____

14. periadenitis _____

15. pancytopenia _____

16. endotoxemia _____

17. carcinoma _____

18. intragastric _____

19. cyanosis _____

20. metamorphosis _____

21. abdominocentesis _____

22. erythropoiesis _____

23. lithotripsy _____

24. euphonia _____

25. hemodialysis _____

26. hypertrophic _____

27. cytorrhexis _____

28. vasospasm _____

29. podiatry _____

30. leukorrhea _____

31. tachycardia _____

32. polyphobia _____

33. dysphonic _____

34. hemigastrectomy _____

35. fibroid _____

36. gastroptosis _____

37. angiomegaly _____

38. ectogenic _____

39. macrocephalous _____

40. adenomalacia _____

41. cardiograph _____

42. epigastrocele _____

43. hypolipiasis _____

44. urologist _____

45. subscleral _____

46. gastrostomy _____

47. necroscopy _____

48. acrodynia _____

49. pediatrics _____

50. preoral _____

51. microscope _____

52. oliguria _____

53. gastrorrhaphy _____

54. aerometer _____

55. orthopedic _____

56. syndesis _____

57. angiectasis _____

58. podalgia _____

59. sonar _____

60. epigastrium _____

Complete the following terms by adding the appropriate prefix:

61. _____ nasal = *above* the nose

62. _____ jointed = *separate from* joint

63. _____ produce = make *again*

64. _____ operative = *before* surgery

65. _____ partum = *after* labor

66. _____ hydrated = *not* watered

67. _____ morphic = pertaining to *one* form

68. _____ dermal = *across or through* the skin

69. _____ acute = *excessively* severe

70. _____ umbilical = *below or under* the navel

71. _____ normal = *half* normal

72. _____ halation = breathe *out*

73. _____ version = to turn *backward*

74. _____ cranial = *outside* the skull

75. _____ medic = *alongside* of the doctor

76. _____ flexion = bend *before*

77. _____ phonia = *difficult* voice

78. _____ duction = to turn *away from*

79. _____ phylaxis = to guard *before*

80. _____ arthritis = inflammation of *many* joints

81. _____ cardia = *slow* heart

82. _____ vascular = *around* a blood vessel

83. _____ indicated = *against or opposed to* being indicated

84. _____ duction = to turn *toward or near*

85. _____ genital = born *with*

86. _____ cardial = *behind* the heart

87. _____ aerobic = pertaining to life *without* air

88. _____ sexual = pertaining to *both* sexes

89. _____ genic = *against* origin

90. _____ physis = growing *together*

91. _____ cellular = pertaining to *without* cells

Combine the following components to form a correctly spelled term:

92. poly + neur/o + algia _____

93. acr/o + –megaly _____

94. gastr/o + enter/o + stomy _____

95. erythr/o + cyt/o + penia _____

96. angi/o + ectasis _____

97. abdomin/o + centesis _____

98. post + cardi/o + al _____

99. cephal/o + dynia _____

100. endo + arteri/o + itis _____

101. micro + ot/o + ia _____

102–113. *Circle the 12 operative terms in the following list:*

lumpectomy	neuroblastoma	morphology
neurology	vesicocele	meningocele
ileostomy	cardiocentesis	toxicology
arteriorrhexis	splenomegaly	gastroscopy
necrolysis	hepatotomy	hysteropexy
erythropoiesis	spirometry	cytopenia
angiectasis	lithotripsy	arthrodesis
pericardiectomy	splenorrhexis	rhinorrhea
nephroptosis	colostomy	herniorrhaphy
rhinorrhea	dysmenorrhea	lithiasis
thoracostomy	cervicoplasty	osteomalacia

Write the plural of the following:

114. endoscopy _____

115. fungus _____

116. speculum _____

117. ampulla _____

118. bacterium _____

119. stoma _____

Write the singular of the following:

120. psychoses _____

121. phenomena _____

122. maculae _____

123. condylomata _____

124. indices _____

125. bronchi _____

3 Fields of Medical Practice

OBJECTIVES

After completion of this chapter you will be able to

1. Trace the evolution of medicine

2. Identify the purpose of the American Board of Medical Specialists

3. Define diplomate and fellow

4. Describe the scope of medical practice for the medical specialties recognized by the American Board of Medical Specialists

5. Identify other medical practitioners with the title of doctor and list their scope of practice

6. List titles of other health professionals

The Evolution of Medicine

Today's practice of medicine evolved from the customs of ancient times. Care for the *patient* (one who suffers) was often given by priests who gave homage to mythological gods and performed rituals designed to appease those gods to rid the body of disease.

Hippocrates, the ancient Greek physician who lived about 400 B.C., is known as the "Father of Medicine." He was the first to attempt to separate medicine from myth, and his writings include the first rational documentation of disease. He also wrote the Hippocratic Oath, which was the standard of medical ethics for physicians in his day and is the basis of modern ethical codes (Fig. 3.1).

Curiosity about the body and the causes of disease led to the study of anatomy and physiology and the art of healing practiced by medieval physicians. Scientific progress led to the development of surgery, pharmacy, pathology, and other aspects of medicine. Hospitals were built to care for the sick and dying, and universities were established to study disease (Fig. 3.2).

Medieval methods have evolved into the modern sophisticated health care system that provides comprehensive care. Physicians have branched out into many specialties of medicine and have been joined by a team of other health care professionals with highly developed training and skills.

The Physician

Today, health care is delivered by a complicated system involving many types of professionals. The most prominent professional meeting the medical needs of the patient is the physician, also called a medical doctor (Fig. 3.3).

The doctor of medicine (M.D.) degree is earned by successfully completing medical school. To practice medicine, however, the graduate with an M.D. must be licensed. The license to practice medicine is granted after the applicant passes a specified medical

HIPPOCRATES. Born on the island of Cos about 400 B.C. and known as the founder of medicine, this Greek physician created the art and science of medicine and removed it from the realm of superstition and magic. Our medical terminology really begins with Hippocrates because he was the first to write terms.

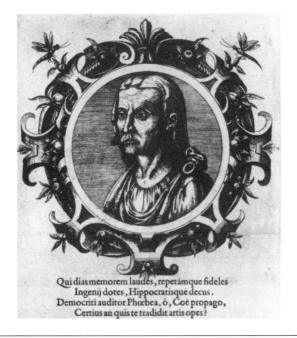

Figure 3.1. Hippocrates.

HOSPITAL. Hospital is derived from the Latin word meaning guest house. The words hospital, hospice, host, hostel, and hotel have the same origin but now have different meanings. It is unknown where special institutions for sick people originated. The Romans had military hospitals by 100 A.D. Christian hospitals seem to have originated from the tradition of a guest house for travelers. In 6th century France, an institution for the sick was called hostel Dieu (God's hotel). Most hospitals were run by religious orders whose members devoted themselves to the care of the sick. In the 19th century, hospitals became centers for treating disease for all classes of society, and they operated for both profit and nonprofit.

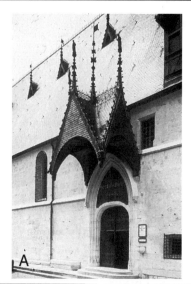

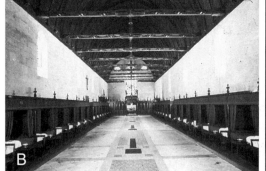

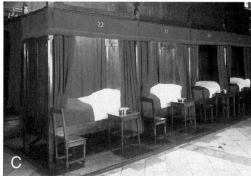

Figure 3.2. Three photographs of Hostel-Dieu, Beaune France, medieval hospital founded in 1443; it is now a museum. **A.** Entrance. **B.** Grand salle ("great room"—combination hospital ward and church). **C.** Bedsides.

licensing examination and meets any other requirements established by the medical board in the state where the applicant wants to practice.

The doctor of osteopathic medicine (D.O.) is a medical practitioner similar to an M.D. but with a traditional emphasis on the role of the musculoskeletal system in maintaining function and balance in the body. Osteopathic physicians are trained at osteopathic colleges and are often affiliated with osteopathic hospitals. The licensing requirements for the osteopath are also similar to the M.D. and are established by medical boards in each state.

American Board of Medical Specialists

The licensed physician in the past was often both physician and surgeon. Today, with the rapid expansion of technology and the greater knowledge required to be proficient in treating patients, physicians have entered various nonsurgical and surgical specialty areas.

With increasing medical specialties, standards and monitoring of specialty practices were required. The American Board of Medical Specialists (ABMS) was founded in 1933 for this purpose. The 23 individual specialty boards recognized by ABMS have established criteria for specific training after medical school (3–7 years depending on the specialty). After the specialty training (called a residency or fellowship), the physician gains eligibili-

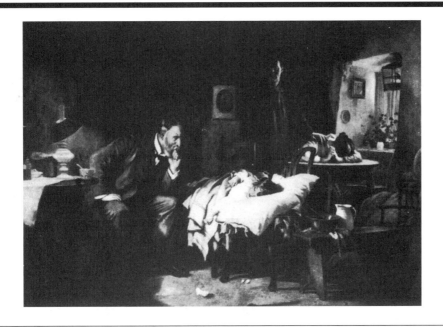

Figure 3.3. Luke Fildes' *The Doctor.*

PHYSICIAN. Physician is derived from a Greek word for natural or according to the laws of nature. In ancient Greece natural science, which included biology and medicine, was concerned with speculation about the origin and existence of things. Physic, in the sense of drug, especially a laxative made from herbs and natural sources, has the same origin. The teaching of medicine came under the general heading of physicus, and practitioners were called physicians.

ty to take the specified board examination. A physician who has completed specialty requirements and passed the board examination is designated "board certified" and referred to as a "diplomate" (e.g., Joan Jones M.D., diplomate of the American Board of Family Practice). The boards' standards extend beyond the usual requirement for licensure.

Other organizations, such as the American College of Physicians (ACP) and the American College of Surgeons (ACS), recognize members who have met set published criteria for standards of distinction. These include fellow of the American College of Surgeons (F.A.C.S.) and fellow of the American College of Physicians (F.A.C.P.) (Fig. 3.4).

Approved specialty boards of the United States follow:

American Board of Allergy and Immunology
American Board of Anesthesiology
American Board of Colon and Rectal Surgery
American Board of Dermatology
American Board of Emergency Medicine
American Board of Family Practice
American Board of Internal Medicine
American Board of Neurological Surgery
American Board of Nuclear Medicine
American Board of Obstetrics and Gynecology
American Board of Ophthalmology
American Board of Orthopaedic Surgery
American Board of Otolaryngology
American Board of Pathology
American Board of Pediatrics
American Board of Physical Medicine and Rehabilitation
American Board of Plastic Surgery
American Board of Preventive Medicine
American Board of Psychiatry and Neurology
American Board of Radiology
American Board of Surgery

CADUCEUS. The word for the staff of Mercury, an emblem in Greek mythology represented by two serpents twined around a staff, is the most common symbol of the medical profession. From earliest history, serpents have been symbols of wisdom and health and objects of worship. They appear as regular shrine equipment and were involved in ancient healing rituals. The significance of the caduceus for the medical profession is said to lie in the fact that the serpent symbolizes healing—some say because of its long life, others because the annual shedding of its skin suggests a renewal of youth and health, others because of its keen eyesight. The earliest representation of serpent and staff was the staff of Aesculapius, the god of medicine, which shows a single serpent twining around the staff (Fig. 3.5).

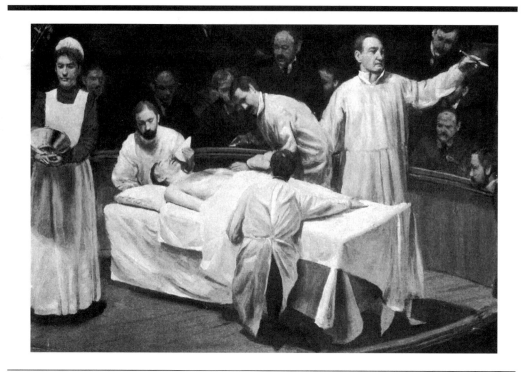

Figure 3.4. The early days of surgery and anesthesiology.

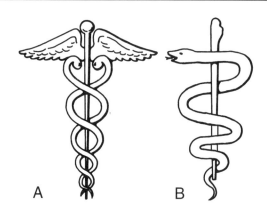

Figure 3.5. The caduceus. **A.** Staff of Mercury. **B.** Staff of Aesculapius.

American Board of Thoracic Surgery
American Board of Urology

Each specialty or subspecialty has its own scope of practice as follows. All earn the M.D. or D.O. degree.

Specialty Fields of Medical Practice of Physicians

Specialty and Specialist	Scope of Practice
allergy and immunology al'er-jē im'y ū-nol' ō-jē **allergist/immunologist**	treatment of allergy and contagious disease (immun/o = safe)
anesthesiology an'es-thē-zē-ol' ō-jē **anesthesiologist**	administration and management of anesthesia during surgery (an = without; esthesi/o = sensation)
cardiology kar-de-ol'ō-jē **cardiologist**	nonsurgical treatment of heart and vascular diseases (cardi/o = heart)
cardiovascular surgery kar'dē-ō-vas'kyu-lăr **cardiovascular surgeon**	surgical treatment of the heart and vascular disease (vascul/o = vessel)
colon and rectal surgery **proctologist** prok-tol'ō-jist	surgical treatment of colon and rectal disorders (proct/o = rectum)
dermatology der-mă-tol'ō-jē **dermatologist**	treatment of diseases of the skin (dermat/o = skin)
emergency medicine **emergency physician**	treatment of the acutely ill or injured
endocrinology en'dō-kri-nol' ō-jē **endocrinologist**	treatment of diseases of the endocrine glands (e.g., diabetes, obesity, thyroid dysfunction) (endo = within; crin/o = to secrete)
family practice **family practitioner** prak-tish'ŭ-ner	general practice treatment of medical and minor surgical ailments
gastroenterology gas'trō-en-ter-ol' ō-jē **gastroenterologist**	nonsurgical treatment of the digestive system (gastr/o = stomach; enter/o = intestine)
gerontology jār-on-tol' ō-jē **(geriatrics)** **gerontologist**	diagnosis and treatment of diseases affecting the elderly (geron = old man; geras = old age)
hematology hē-mă-tol' ō-jē **hematologist**	treatment of blood disorders (hemat/o = blood)
internal medicine **internist**	diagnosis and treatment of diseases of internal organs in adults
nephrology ne-frol'ō-jē **nephrologist**	treatment of kidney disorders (nephr/o = kidney)
neurology nū-rol'ō-jē **neurologist**	nonsurgical treatment of the nervous system (neur/o = nerve)

ANESTHESIA. Anesthesia is a condition in which there is an absence of sensation [an (without)/esthesio (sensation)/ia (condition)]. The inhalation of various vapors to produce a sort of intoxication or stupification is an ancient practice. By the 14th century, methods of inducing sleep for surgical operations included the inhalation of hemlock, mandrake, and lettuce. Other attempts to produce anesthesia included the use of snow and ice. Interest in chemistry at the end of the 18th century resulted in the investigation of various chemicals that could be used for inhalation anesthesia. Early anesthetics included nitrous oxide, ether, and chloroform.

continued

SURGEON. The Greek word chirurgeon (chiro, the hand; urgeon, to work) refers to one who works with the hands. The earliest conception of surgery was that diseases of an external nature were suitable for treatment by manual operations, as opposed to internal conditions that were treated with drugs, etc. The name surgeon has been in English since the 14th century. There was no distinction between barbers and surgeons until 1745 when the barbers and surgeons of London were separated and given individual charters.

Specialty and Specialist	Scope of Practice
neurological surgery **neurosurgeon**	surgical treatment of diseases of the nervous system
nuclear medicine **nuclear medicine physician**	use of radioactive substances to diagnose and treat disease
obstetrics and gynecology (OB/GYN)	
obstetrics ob-stet′riks	care and treatment of mother and fetus throughout pregnancy, childbirth, and immediate postpartum period
obstetrician ob-stĕ-trish′ŭn	[obstetr/o = midwife (one who aides in delivery of a baby)]
gynecology gī-nĕ-kol′ō-jē **gynecologist**	treatment of disorders of the female reproductive and urinary system (gynec/o = woman)
oncology ong-kol′ ō-jē **oncologist**	treatment of tumors and cancers (onc/o = tumor, mass)
ophthalmology of-thal-mol′ ō-je **ophthalmologist**	medical and surgical treatment of the eye (ophthalm/o = eye)
orthopaedic surgery ōr-thō-pē′dik **orthopaedic surgeon, orthopedist**	medical and surgical treatment of the musculoskeletal system including bones, joints, muscles, etc. (orth/o = straight; ped/o = foot)
otolaryngology ō′tō-lar-ing-gol′ ō-jē	medical and surgical treatment of diseases and disorders of the ear, nose, throat, and adjoining structures of head and neck (ot/o = ear; rhin/o = nose; laryng/o = voice box)
otorhinolaryngologist o′tō-rī′nō-lar-ing-gol′ ō-jist **ENT (ear, nose, throat) physician**	
pathology pa-thol′ ō-jē	study of disease emphasizing examination of tissue for diagnosis (e.g., biopsy, autopsy)
pathologist	(path/o = disease)
pediatrics pē-dē-at′riks **pediatrician**	treatment of well and sick children (ped/o = child)
physical medicine and rehabilitation	treatment of patients suffering from neuromusculoskeletal disorders caused by illness or injury (e.g., stroke, spinal cord injury) (physi/o = physical)
physiatrist fiz-ī′ă-trist	

continued

Specialty and Specialist	Scope of Practice
plastic surgery	surgery for restoration, repair, or reconstruction of body structures (e.g., body contouring, skin grafting, etc.)
plastic surgeon	(plas/o = formation; -plasty = surgical repair or reconstruction)
preventive medicine	medical care that focuses on prevention of disease and health maintenance (subspecialties include public health and occupational medicine)
psychiatry sī-kī′ǎ-trē **psychiatrist**	diagnosis, treatment, and prevention of mental, emotional, and behavioral disorders (psych/o = mind)
radiology rā-dē-ol′ō-jē **radiologist**	use of x-rays to diagnose and treat disease (radi/o = x-ray)
rheumatology rū-mǎ-tol′-ō-jē **rheumatologist**	treatment of arthritis and related disorders (rheumat/o = flux or watery flow)
surgery **surgeon**	treatment of diseases and trauma requiring an operation
thoracic surgery thō-ras′ik **thoracic surgeon**	treatment of diseases and trauma requiring an operation within the chest (e.g., heart and lungs) (thorac/o = chest)
urology yū-rol′ō-jē **urologist**	surgical and nonsurgical treatment of the male urinary and reproductive system and the female urinary system (ur/o = urine)

Other Fields of Medical Practice

Many other medical specialists are called doctors even though they do not have an M.D. or D.O. degree. They have graduated from a college of podiatry, chiropractic, optometry, or dentistry and are licensed to practice. Because they commonly provide health care services in hospitals and/or medical clinics, you need a basic knowledge of their scope of practice.

Degree	Field of Practice	Scope of Practice
D.C. (doctor of chiropractic medicine)	chiropractic medicine	treatment centered on manipulation of the spine to maintain function and balance in the body
	chiropractor	(chir/o = hand; prattein = to do)
D.D.S. (doctor of dental surgery)	oral surgery	treatment of dental disorders requiring surgery
	oral surgeon	(or/o = mouth) (dent/i = tooth)

continued

Degree	Field of Practice	Scope of Practice
D.P.M. (doctor of podiatric medicine)	podiatry	diagnosis and treatment (including surgery) of disorders of the foot
	podiatrist	(pod/o = foot)
O.D. (doctor of optometry)	optometry	examination of eyes to test vision and adapt lenses to preserve or improve vision
	optometrist	(opt/o = eye)
Ph.D. (doctor of philosophy)	psychology	counsel of patients with mental or emotional disorders
	psychologist	(psych/o = mind)

Other Health Care Professions

As the result of the major advances in health care technology, various licensed and nonlicensed allied health professionals with specialized training and skill have emerged to the meet the increasing needs of the population. They are integral to today's health care team. The following is a list of professions for which formal training is available.

acupuncturist
anesthesiologist assistant
audiologist
cardiovascular technologist
cytotechnologist
dental assistant
dental hygienist
dental lab technologist
diagnostic medical sonographer
dialysis technician
dietetic technologist
dietician
electrocardiographic technologist
electroencephalographic technologist
electroneurodiagnostic technologist
emergency medical technician
fitness therapist
geriatric home aide
health information manager
histologic technologist
home health aide
massage therapist
medical assistant
medical coding specialist
medical illustrator
medical laboratory technician
medical record administrator
medical record technician
medical technologist
medical transcriptionist
medical unit coordinator (unit clerk/ secretary or ward clerk/secretary)
music therapist
nephrology technician
nuclear medicine technologist
nurse, licensed vocational or practical

nurse, registered
nurse anesthetist
nurse assistant
nurse midwife
nurse practitioner
nutrition care technologist
occupational therapist
occupational therapy assistant
operating room technician
ophthalmic medical technician/ technologist
optician
paramedic
perfusionist
pharmacist
pharmacologist
pharmacy technician/assistant
phlebotomist
physical therapist
physical therapist assistant
physician assistant
prosthetist
psychiatric technician
radiation therapy technologist
radiologic technologist/radiographer
recreational therapist
rehabilitation technologist
respiratory therapist
specialist in blood bank technology
speech pathologist
speech therapist
surgeon assistant
surgical technologist
veterinarian
veterinary assistant

PRACTICE EXERCISES

For the following terms, draw a line or lines to separate prefixes, combining forms, and suffixes. Then define the term.

1. oncology _____

2. immunologist _____

3. otorhinolaryngology _____

4. optometry _____

5. proctologist _____

6. gynecology _____

7. pathology _____

8. orthopedic _____

9. urologist _____

10. pediatric _____

11. neurology _____

12. psychologist _____

13. osteopathy _____

14. ophthalmology _____

15. obstetric _____

16. anesthesiology _____

17. cardiology _____

18. dermatology _____

19. gerontology _____

20. endocrinologist _____

21. nephrologist _____

22. gastroenterology_____

23. hematologist _____

24. chiropractic _____

25. geriatric _____

Match the following specialists or specialties with the definition:

26. emergency physician _____   a. treats internal organs in adults

27. neurosurgeon _____   b. treats foot disorders

28. physiatrist _____   c. provides emotional counsel

29. radiologist _____   d. performs dental surgery

30. plastic surgeon _____   e. operates on heart and lungs

31. rheumatologist _____   f. interprets x-rays

32. thoracic surgeon _____   g. nonsurgical care of brain and spinal cord

33. podiatrist _____   h. treats disease of the mind

34. oral surgeon _____   i. cares for acutely ill

35. psychiatrist _____   j. general practice

36. neurology _____   k. performs brain surgery

37. nuclear medicine _____   l. uses radioactive substances

38. internist _____   m. performs reconstructive surgical repairs

39. family practice _____   n. treats arthritis

40. psychologist _____   o. rehabilitation specialist

Write the full medical term for the following abbreviations:

41. OB/GYN _____

42. D.D.S. _____

43. ENT _____

44. ABMS _____

45. O.D. _____

46. F.A.C.S. _____

47. ACP _____

48. D.C. _____

49. D.P.M. _____

50. D.O. _____

51–53. *From the following list, identify the three specialists who perform surgery:*

gynecologist

allergist

internist

cardiologist

otorhinolaryngologist

rheumatologist

gerontologist

gastroenterologist

nephrologist

endocrinologist

urologist

Match the type of school with the degree it grants:

54. dental _____   a. Ph.D.

55. graduate _____   b. O.D.

56. podiatric _____   c. D.D.S.

57. medical _____   d. D.O.

58. chiropractic _____   e. D.P.M.

59. optometric _____   f. D.C.

60. osteopathic _____   g. M.D.

The Medical Record

OBJECTIVES

After completion of this chapter you will be able to

1. List the common forms used in documenting the care of a patient

2. Define basic terms used in documenting a history and physical

3. Define commonly used medical record abbreviations

4. Explain the concepts used in a problem oriented medical record

5. Define common terms related to disease

6. Define common pharmacological terms

7. Define the symbols used in documenting a physician's order

8. Explain the terms used in documenting a medical history and physical record

CHART. The word originates from the Latin *charta*, a kind of paper made from papyrus. *Charta* came to mean any leaf or thin sheet of fine paper on which graphic illustrations were made. In medicine, the chart most often refers to patient record documentations.

Common Records Used in Documenting Care of a Patient

To put your knowledge of medical terminology to practical use, you need to see how this language is used in everyday communication about patients. Learning the common abbreviations, symbols, forms, and formats used in recording patient care will help you comprehend medical record documentation.

History and Physical

The record that serves as a cornerstone for patient care is the *history and physical*. It documents the patient's medical history and findings from the physical examination. It is usually the first document generated when a patient presents for care, most often recorded at the time of a new patient visit, or as part of a consultation (Fig. 4.1).

Subjective information is obtained from the patient and documented in the patient *history*, starting with the *chief complaint* (the reason for seeking care) along with the *history of present illness* (indicating duration and severity of the complaint) and any other symptoms that the patient is experiencing. Information about the patient's past *medical history*, *family history*, *social history*, and *occupational history* is then noted. The history is complete after documenting the patient's answers to questions related to the *review of systems*, which is intended to uncover any other significant evidence of disease.

Once subjective data have been recorded, the provider begins a physical examination to obtain *objective information*, facts that can be seen or detected by testing. Signs, or objective evidence of disease, are documented, and selected diagnostic tests are performed or ordered when further evaluation is necessary.

The *impression*, *diagnosis*, or *assessment* is made after evaluation of all subjective and objective data including the results of the physical examination and diagnostic test findings. R/O (rule out) is the abbreviation used to indicate a differential diagnosis when two or more possible diagnoses are in question. Further tests are then necessary to rule out or eliminate these possibilities and verify the final diagnosis.

Final notations include the provider's *plan*, also called a *recommendation* or *disposition*, which outlines strategies designed to remedy the patient's condition.

Further documentations in the form of *progress notes* are made as care continues.

Most often, physicians are required to dictate a current history and physical before admitting a patient to the hospital. When the patient is to have surgery, this report is often called a "preoperative" history and physical.

Following are common terms and abbreviations used in documenting a history and physical examination.

H & P   **History and Physical**
documentation of patient history and physical examination findings

SUBJECTIVE INFORMATION—information obtained from the patient including his or her personal perceptions

Hx   **History**
record of subjective information regarding the patient's personal medical history including past injuries, illnesses, operations, defects, and habits

CC   chief complaint

c/o   complains of
patient's description of what brought him or her to the doctor or hospital; it is usually brief and is often documented in the

patient's own words indicated within quotes (e.g., CC: left lower back pain; patient states, "I feel like I swallowed a stick and it got stuck in my back")

PI   present illness

HPI   history of present illness
amplification of the chief complaint recording details of the duration and severity of the condition (e.g., PI: the patient has had left lower back pain for the past 2 weeks since slipping on a rug and landing on her left side; the pain worsens after sitting upright for any extended period but gradually subsides after lying in a supine position)

Sx   symptom
subjective evidence (from the patient) that indicates an abnormality

PH   past history

PMH   past medical history
a record of information about the patient's past illnesses starting with childhood, including surgical operations, injuries, physical defects, medications, and allergies

UCHD   usual childhood diseases
an abbreviation used to note that the patient had the "usual" or commonly contracted illnesses during childhood (e.g., measles, chickenpox, or mumps)

NKA   no known allergies

NKDA   no known drug allergies

FH   family history
state of health of immediate family members

A & W   alive and well
L & W   living and well
(e.g., father, age 92, L & W; mother, age 91, died, stroke)

SH   social history
a record of the patient's recreational interests, hobbies, and use of tobacco and drugs including alcohol (e.g., SH: plays tennis twice/wk; tobacco—none; alcohol—drinks 1–2 beers per day)

OH   occupational history
record of work habits that may involve work-related risks (e.g., OH: the patient has been employed as a coal mine engineer for the past 16 years)

ROS   review of systems

SR   systems review
a documentation of the patient's response to questions organized by a head-to-toe review of the function of all body systems (note: this review allows evaluation of other symptoms that may not have been mentioned)

OBJECTIVE INFORMATION—facts and observations noted

PE Px	**Physical Examination** documentation of a physical examination of a patient, including notations of positive and negative objective findings	

HEENT   head, eyes, ears, nose, throat

PERRLA   pupils equal, round, and reactive to light and accommodation

WNL   within normal limits

Dx   diagnosis

IMP   impression

A   assessment
identification of a disease or condition after evaluation of the patient's history, symptoms, signs, and results of laboratory tests and diagnostic procedures

R/O   rule out
[used to indicate a *differential diagnosis* when two or more possible diagnoses are suspect (note: each possible diagnosis is outlined and then either verified or eliminated after further testing is performed, e.g., diagnosis: R/O pancreatitis, R/O gastroenteritis; this documentation indicates that either of these two diagnoses is suspected and that further testing is required to eliminate one)]

PLAN, RECOMMENDATION, DISPOSITION—outline of the treatment plan designed to remedy the patient's condition, which includes instructions to the patient, orders for medications, diagnostic tests, or therapies

Problem Oriented Medical Record

The problem oriented medical record (POMR) is a method of record keeping introduced in the 1960s. It is a highly organized approach that encourages a precise method of documenting the logical thought processes of health care professionals. Data are organized so that information can be accessed readily at a glance, with a focus on the patient's health problem. The use of POMR and its adaptations has grown in many areas of medicine. The approach is often used in medical schools, hospitals, clinics, and private practices (Fig. 4.2).

The central concept is a medical record in which all information is linked to specific problems. The record has four sections:

- *Database*   patient's history, physical examinations, and diagnostic test results; from the database, the problem is identified and a plan is developed to address it.

- *Problem list*   directory of the patient's problems; each problem is listed and often assigned a number; problems include

        1. a specific diagnosis
        2. a sign or symptom
        3. an abnormal diagnostic test result
        4. any other problem that may influence health or well-being

CENTRAL MEDICAL GROUP, INC.

Department of Internal Medicine

201 Medical Center Drive • Central City, US 90000-1234 • PHONE: (012) 125-8888 • FAX: (012) 125-3434

PATIENT: COHEN, SARA E.

DATE: April 8, 199x

HISTORY

CHIEF COMPLAINT: Epigastric distress

HISTORY OF PRESENT ILLNESS: This 33-year-old Caucasian female comes in because of excessive burping, epigastric distress and nausea for several weeks. Coffee makes it worse. She complains that it is worse at night when lying down. She gets an acid-like taste in her mouth. She has tried antacids, to no avail.

PAST MEDICAL HISTORY: The patient states that she had the usual childhood diseases. She has had no serious medical illnesses and has been involved in no accidents. Family History: There is some diabetes on her mother's side. Her mother is 52 and has hypertension. Her father, age 56, is living and well. She has a sister who is anemic and a brother who has ulcers. Social History: The patient discontinued smoking ten years ago. Drinks alcohol socially. Allergies: NKDA. Current Medications: Medications at this time consist of Entex, Guaifed, birth control pills, iron and vitamin supplements.

REVIEW OF SYSTEMS: HEENT: Chronic sinusitis. She sees an ENT specialist and an allergist. Respiratory: Negative. Cardiac: Occasional flutters. Gastrointestinal: As stated above. Genitourinary: Occasional infections. Pap smear is up-to-date and negative. She has had no mammogram at this point. Neuromuscular: Negative.

PHYSICAL EXAMINATION

GENERAL APPEARANCE: Reveals a well-developed, well-nourished female in no acute distress.

VITAL SIGNS: Blood Pressure: 120/80. Pulse: 76 and regular.

HEENT: Head normocephalic. Eyes: Pupils are equal, round, and reactive to light and accommodation. Fundi are benign. Ears, nose and throat are negative. NECK: No thyromegaly. No carotid bruits.

CHEST: Clear to percussion and auscultation. BREASTS: Reveal no masses. HEART: Normal sinus rhythm. No murmurs.

ABDOMEN: Liver, spleen and kidneys could not be felt. Femorals pulsate well, no bruits.

EXTREMITIES: No edema. Pulses are good and equal.

PELVIC & RECTAL EXAMS: Deferred to gynecologist.

NEUROLOGIC EXAM: Physiologic.

IMPRESSION: 1. PROBABLE PEPTIC ULCER DISEASE WITH GASTROESOPHAGEAL REFLUX.
2. POSSIBLE GALLBLADDER DISEASE.

PLAN: Patient started on Pepcid 40 mg, 1 at night. She is given Gaviscon tablets so she can carry them with her. Schedule routine lab work and upper GI series. If negative, schedule ultrasound of the gallbladder.

D. Everley, M.D.

DE:mc
D: 4/8/9x
T: 4/9/9x

Figure 4.1. History and physical for patient complaining of epigastric distress.

CENTRAL MEDICAL GROUP, INC.

Department of Otorhinolaryngology

201 Medical Center Drive • Central City, US 90000-1234 • PHONE: (012) 125-8888 • FAX: (012) 125-3434

Patient: Perron, Carleen   DATE: February 17, 199x

Referring Physician: C. Camarillo, M.D.

CONSULTATION

REASON FOR CONSULTATION: This 28-year-old white female presents with a one week history of upper respiratory infection (URI), sinusitis, and some periorbital headaches in recent weeks. She also has expectorated yellow-green mucus occasionally and has had a history of tonsillitis.

MEDICATIONS: None. **ALLERGIES:** No known allergies (NKA). **SURGERIES:** None. **HOSPITALIZATIONS:** None.

PAST MEDICAL HISTORY/REVIEW OF SYSTEMS: Cardiopulmonary: There is no history of angina, dyspnea, hemoptysis, emphysema, asthma, chronic obstructive pulmonary disease (COPD), hypertension, or heart murmurs. Cardiovascular: There is no history of high blood pressure. Renal: There is no history of dysuria, polyuria, nocturia, hematuria, or cystoliths. Gastrointestinal: There is no history of gallbladder disease, hepatitis, pancreatitis, or colitis. Musculoskeletal: There is no history of arthritis. Endocrine: There is no history of diabetes. Hematologic: There is no history of anemia, blood transfusion, or easy bruising. Gynecological: The patient states her menses are regular, and the start of her last menstrual cycle occurred 15 days ago.

FAMILY HISTORY: The patient states her maternal grandmother has diabetes.

SOCIAL HISTORY: The patient is single and has no children. She denies smoking tobacco. She denies drinking alcoholic beverages. She denies taking drugs.

CHILDHOOD DISEASES: The patient has had the usual childhood diseases.

OTOLARYNGOLOGIC EXAMINATION: Otoscopy: Tympanic membranes (TMs) are dull and slightly congested. Sinuses: There is maxillary fullness. Rhinoscopic examination reveals mild nasoseptal deviation (NSD). Pharynx: There is moderate inflammation; no exudates. Oropharynx: No masses. Nasopharynx: No masses. Larynx: Clear. Neck: Supple. Cervical Adenopathy: There is mild adenopathy.

IMPRESSION:
1. MAXILLARY SINUSITIS.
2. PHARYNGITIS.
3. CHRONIC TONSILLITIS.

DISPOSITION:
1. Warm salt water gargle (WSWG).
2. Ery-Tab 333, #24, 1 t.i.d. p.c.
3. Robitussin.
4. Return to office (RTO) in one week.

P. Rodden MD
PATRICK RODDEN, M.D.

JR:ti
D: 2/17/9x
T: 2/18/9x

Figure 4.1. *Continued.* History and physical documented as part of a consultation for patient with upper respiratory infection.

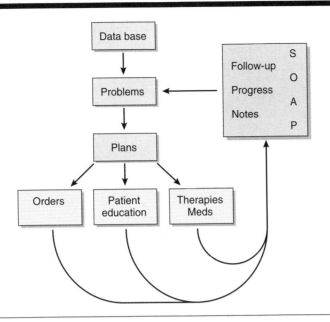

Figure 4.2. Problem oriented medical record (POMR) diagram.

Once identified, each problem is evaluated, and a plan for treating it is written. When a problem is resolved, a notation is made to show its resolution, but the problem remains on the summary list. The original problem list is maintained in the record so that personnel can easily orient themselves to the patient's prior medical history.

• *Initial plan* strategy employed to resolve each problem is listed. There are three subdivisions:

1. *Diagnostic plan* orders are given for specific diagnostic testing to confirm suspicions
2. *Therapeutic plan* goals for therapy are specified
3. *Patient education* instructions communicated to the patient are notated

• *Progress notes* documentations of the progress concerning each problem are organized using the SOAP format (Fig. 4.3).

S—subjective that which the patient describes

O—objective observable information (e.g., test results, blood pressure readings, etc.)

A—assessment patient's progress and evaluation of the effectiveness of the plan (note: any new problem identified is added to the problem list, and a separate plan for its treatment is recorded)

P—plan decision to proceed or alter the plan strategy

The SOAP method of documenting a patient's progress appears to be the most popular adaptation to the entire system, and it is commonly utilized with or without assigning a number to the problem.

CENTRAL MEDICAL GROUP, INC.
Department of Internal Medicine

201 Medical Center Drive • Central City, US 90000-1234 • PHONE: (012) 125-8888 • FAX: (012) 125-3434

PROGRESS NOTES

PATIENT: COHEN, SARA E.

DATE: April 11, 199x

CC: Epigastric distress

S: The patient returns for reports. She states that she has only marginal relief from Pepcid and Gaviscon.

O: Her GI showed minimal gastroesophageal reflux and the rest of her studies, except for a slightly high cholesterol, were normal.

A: 1) MINIMAL GASTROESOPHAGEAL REFLUX
2) MILD HYPERCHOLESTEROLEMIA

P: Discontinue Pepcid and Gaviscon. Start Reglan 10 mg 1 q.i.d. The patient is advised to lower the intake of fat in her diet. RTO in one month for a recheck.

D. Everley, M.D.

Figure 4.3. POMR progress notes using SOAP format. CC: epigastric distress.

CENTRAL MEDICAL GROUP, INC.

Department of Otorhinolaryngology

201 Medical Center Drive • Central City, US 90000-1234 • PHONE: (012) 125-8888 • FAX: (012) 125-3434

PROGRESS NOTES

Patient: PERRON, CARLEEN

03/30/9x

S: The patient presents with a sore throat x 2 weeks.

O: Sinus exam: Maxillary and frontal congestion. Hypopharynx/adenoids: No inflammation.

A: Recurrent pharyngitis/sinusitis x 2 weeks.

P: 1)   Ceftin 250 mg, #21, 1 t.i.d. p.o. p.c.

       2)   Entex LA, #30, 1 b.i.d. p.o.

       3)   Warm salt water gargle.

P Rodden MD
PATRICK RODDEN, M.D.

05/25/9x

S: Recurrent sore throat every month.

O: Recurrent tonsillitis, cryptic tonsillitis. Sinus exam: Maxillary and frontal congestion. Neck: Supple; no masses. Hypopharynx/Adenoids: No inflammation. Paranasal Sinus X-ray: Bilateral frontal and maxillary sinusitis.

A: Recurrent tonsillitis, 8-10 times per year. Chronic maxillary and frontal sinusitis.

P: 1)   Tonsillectomy discussed with the patient. The risks of general and local anesthesia, as well as the surgical procedure, were discussed with the patient. The consent form was signed.

       2)   An admitting order was given to the patient for CBC, UA, and BCP-7 to be done one day prior to being admitted.

       3)   Ceftin 250 mg, #21, 1 t.i.d. p.o. p.c.

       4)   Entex LA, #30, 1 b.i.d. p.o.

       5)   Beconase nasal inhaler, 2 sprays each nostril b.i.d.

       6)   Warm salt water gargle.

P Rodden MD
PATRICK RODDEN, M.D.

Figure 4.3. *Continued.* CC: upper respiratory infection.

Hospital Records

The *history and physical* is usually the first document entered into the patient's hospital record on admission. *Physician's orders* list the directives for care prescribed by the doctor attending the patient. The *nurse's notes* and *physician's progress notes* chronicle the care throughout the patient's stay, and *ancillary reports* note the various procedures and therapies including *diagnostic tests* and *pathology reports*. In a difficult case, a specialist may be called in by the attending physician, and a *consultation report* is filed. If a surgical remedy is indicated, a narrative *operative report* is required of the primary surgeon. The anesthesiologist, who is in charge of life support during surgery, must file the *anesthesiologist's report*. The final document, which is recorded at the time of discharge from the hospital, is the *discharge summary*.

The following are descriptions of common forms used in documenting the care of a hospital patient.

history and physical	documentation of the patient's recent medical history and results of physical examination—required before hospital admission (Fig. 4.4)
consent form	document signed by the patient or legal guardian giving permission for medical or surgical care
informed consent	consent of a patient after being informed of the risks and benefits of a procedure and alternatives—often required by law when a reasonable risk is involved (e.g., surgery)
physician's orders	a record of all orders directed by the attending physician (Fig. 4.5)
diagnostic tests/ laboratory reports	records of results of various tests and procedures used in evaluating and treating a patient (e.g., laboratory tests, x-rays) (Fig. 4.6)
nurse's notes	documentation of patient care by the nursing staff (note: flow sheets and graphs are often used to display recordings of vital signs and other monitored procedures) (Fig. 4.7)
physician's progress notes	physician's daily account of patient's response to treatment including results of tests, assessment, and future treatment plans (Fig. 4.8)
ancillary reports	miscellaneous records of procedures or therapies provided during a patient's care (e.g., physical therapy or respiratory therapy)
consultation report	report filed by a specialist asked by the attending physician to evaluate a difficult case; note: a patient may also see another physician in consultation as an outpatient (in a medical office or clinic)
operative report (op report)	surgeon's detailed account of the operation including the method of incision, technique, instruments used, types of suture, method of closure, and the patient's responses during the procedure and at the time of transfer to recovery (Fig. 4.9)

pathology report	report of the findings of a pathologist after the study of tissue (e.g., biopsy) (Fig. 4.10)
anesthesiologist's report	anesthesiologist's or anesthetist's report of the details of anesthesia during surgery including the drugs used, dose and time given, and records indicating monitoring of the patient's vital status throughout the procedure
discharge summary, clinical resume, clinical summary	three terms that describe an outline summary of the patient's hospital care including date of admission, diagnosis, course of treatment, final diagnosis, and date of discharge (Fig. 4.11)

The sample medical records in Figures 4.4–4.11 chronicle the hospital care of Carleen Perron, a 28-year-old woman who was seen in consultation by Dr. Patrick Rodden, an ENT specialist, who recommended a surgical remedy for the repeated infections she has had over the past six months.

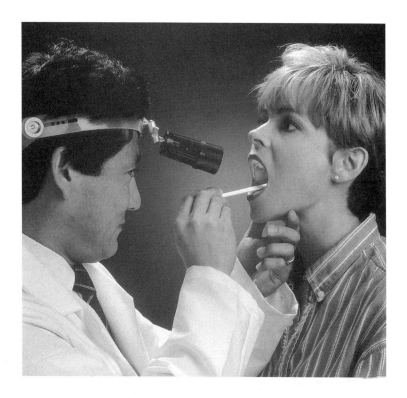

CENTRAL MEDICAL CENTER

211 Medical Center Drive • Central City, US 90000-1234 • PHONE: (012) 125-6784 • FAX: (012) 125-9999

PREOPERATIVE HISTORY AND PHYSICAL

HISTORY

DATE OF ADMISSION: June 3, 199x.

HISTORY OF PRESENT ILLNESS:
The patient is a 28-year-old white female with a chief complaint of frequent, recurrent, suppurative tonsillitis. She has had some eight infections over the last six months and is admitted at this time for elective tonsillectomy. The surgery has been discussed with the patient and family, including risks and complications. The patient's internist is C. Camarillo, M.D.

MEDICATIONS: None.

ALLERGIES: None known.

PAST SURGICAL HISTORY: None.

PAST MEDICAL HISTORY: UCHD (usual childhood diseases).

REVIEW OF SYSTEMS: CARDIOVASCULAR: No high blood pressure, heart murmurs, or shortness of breath. PULMONARY: No chronic lung disease; no asthma. GASTRO-INTESTINAL: No hepatitis. RENAL HISTORY: Negative for infections. ENDOCRINE: No diabetes or thyroid disease. MUSCULOSKELETAL: Negative for arthritis. HEMATOLOGIC: No history of anemia or bleeding tendencies.

FAMILY HISTORY: Grandmother has history of diabetes.

GYNECOLOGICAL HISTORY: Regular menses.

SOCIAL HISTORY: The patient is a nonsmoker. Alcohol use was denied, and drug use was denied.

(continued)

P. Rodden MD
PATRICK RODDEN, M.D.

JR:bst

D: 6/1/9x
T: 6/2/9x

HISTORY AND PHYSICAL Page 1	PT. NAME: PERRON, CARLEEN ID NO: 672894017 ROOM NO: ATT. PHYS: PATRICK RODDEN, M.D.

Figure 4.4. Preoperative history and physical. A documentation of a patient's presurgical history and physical, dictated and transcribed for the hospital record before admission.

CENTRAL MEDICAL CENTER

211 Medical Center Drive • Central City, US 90000-1234 • PHONE: (012) 125-6784 • FAX: (012) 125-9999

PREOPERATIVE HISTORY AND PHYSICAL

PHYSICAL EXAMINATION

VITAL SIGNS: Afebrile, alert, oriented, normotensive. Blood Pressure: 124/80. Pulse: 84. Respirations: 18.

HEENT: PERRLA (pupils equal, round, and reactive to light and accommodation). Tympanic membranes are clear. Light reflex is present. No sinus tenderness on percussion. Oropharynx: Clear. Hypertrophic tonsils. No exudates. Nasopharynx: No masses. Larynx: Clear.

NECK: Supple; no masses or tenderness. No cervical adenopathy.

LUNGS: Clear to percussion and auscultation.

HEART: Rate: 84 and regular; normal sinus rhythm; no murmurs or gallops.

RECTOPELVIC: Deferred.

EXTREMITIES: No peripheral edema. No ecchymoses.

NEUROLOGICAL: Physiologically intact.

IMPRESSION: Chronic, recurrent tonsillitis. The patient is admitted for an elective tonsillectomy.

P. Rodden MD
PATRICK RODDEN, M.D.

JR:bst
D: 6/1/9x
T: 6/2/9x

HISTORY AND PHYSICAL PAGE 2	PT. NAME: PERRON, CARLEEN ID NO: 672894017 ROOM NO: ATT. PHYS: PATRICK RODDEN, M.D.

Figure 4.4. *Continued.*

CENTRAL MEDICAL CENTER

211 Medical Center Drive • Central City, US 90000-1234 • PHONE: (012) 125-6784 • FAX: (012) 125-9999

PHYSICIAN'S ORDERS FOR:	PAGE
PRESURGICAL ADMITTING ORDERS	1 OF 1

A THERAPEUTICALLY EQUIVALENT PRODUCT, WHICH HAS BEEN APPROVED BY THE PHARMACY AND THERAPEUTICS COMMITTEE OF THE MEDICAL STAFF, MAY BE DISPENSED AND ADMINISTERED UNLESS OTHERWISE SPECIFIED. PHYSICIAN: CROSS OUT ANY ORDERS WHICH DO NOT APPLY.

DOCTOR: PLEASE STATE PERTINENT CLINICAL INFORMATION WHEN ORDERING RADIOLOGY PROCEDURES.

DATE	TIME	[XX] Same Day Surgery (Admit to Observation if overnight stay req'd)	[ ] Regular Inpatient Admission
06/02/9x			

ADMIT DATE: _____ JUNE 3, 199x _____

ADMIT TO: [ ] Surgical Admit Unit _____ or [ ] _____
                                  (date)   (specific unit)   (date)

PATIENT'S NAME: PERRON, CARLEEN _____ ALLERGIES: ___ NKA ___

DIET: NPO   SURGEON: PATRICK RODDEN, M.D. _____

SURGERY CONSENT TO READ: TONSILLECTOMY _____

DATE AND TIME OF SURGERY: JUNE 3, 199x at 9 a.m. _____

DATE TESTS TO BE DONE: JUNE 2, 199x _____

TESTS: (Check box for desired tests)

    [ ] HGB   [XX] CBC   [XX] BCP-7   [ ] PT
    [ ] HCT   [XX] UA   [ ] BCP-20   [ ] PTT
    [ ] Other _____
    [ ] Group, Type, and Screen
    [ ] Prepare: _____ units Autologous Red Blood Cells (packed cells)
    [ ] Crossmatch: _____ units Directed Red Blood Cells (packed cells)
            _____ units Red Blood Cells (packed cells)
    [ ] EKG
    [ ] CHEST FILM Reason for x-ray; R/O active cardiopulmonary disease
    [ ] OTHER X-RAY _____
            Reason for x-ray: _____

OTHER:

MEDICATIONS: Pre-Meds by Anesthesia

P Rodden MD

Physician's Signature

PERRON, CARLEEN   6/3/9x
DOB 07/20/9x   F284
672894017
Rodden, Patrick MD

PHYSICIAN'S ORDERS

Figure 4.5. Presurgical admitting orders. A form completed by the admitting physician that is forwarded to the hospital before the date of surgery.

CENTRAL MEDICAL CENTER

211 Medical Center Drive • Central City, US 90000-1234 • PHONE: (012) 125-6784 • FAX: (012) 125-9999

DOCTOR: PLEASE STATE PERTINENT CLINICAL INFORMATION WHEN ORDERING RADIOLOGY PROCEDURES

WRITE WITH BALLPOINT INK PEN; PRESS HARD

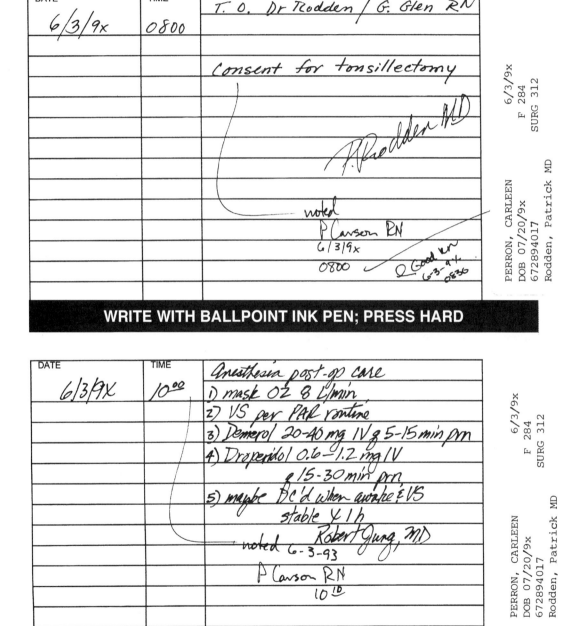

WRITE WITH BALLPOINT INK PEN; PRESS HARD

PHYSICIAN'S ORDERS

Figure 4.5. *Continued.* Physician's orders. Orders written by the anesthesiologist and surgeon and noted by the nursing staff during the patient's surgical care.

CENTRAL MEDICAL CENTER

211 Medical Center Drive • Central City, US 90000-1234 • PHONE: (012) 125-6784 • FAX: (012) 125-9999

DOCTOR: PLEASE STATE PERTINENT CLINICAL INFORMATION WHEN ORDERING RADIOLOGY PROCEDURES

WRITE WITH BALLPOINT INK PEN; PRESS HARD

DATE	TIME	
6-3-9x	10 ⁰⁰	POST-OP
		1) V.S q ÷ h x 4 then q 2 h x 4, then q 4 h
		2) bed rest ē BRP when alert
		3) continue IV's 80 cc/hr 5°/₁₀ D/. 2 NS until taking fluids well
		4) tylenol elixir ē cod ††† tsp q 4 h po prn pain
		5) Demerol 50 mg) IM q 4 h Vistaril 50 mg) prn severe pain
		6) Ice ¢ liquids at bedside ¢ encourage P Rodden MD
		noted W. Cliff. R.N. 6-3-9x 1130

(text at bottom right of block) Mⱼ 6/3/9x 11 45

WRITE WITH BALLPOINT INK PEN; PRESS HARD

Note (right margin, vertical): 6/3/9x F 284 SURG 312 PERRON, CARLEEN DOB 07/20/9x 67289017 Rodden, Patrick MD

DATE	TIME	
6-3-9x	12 ³⁰	1) full liquids requiring soft diet
		2) admit
		3) Dalmane 15 mg po q hs prn sleep MRx1 prn P Rodden M
		noted W. Cliff R.N. 12:30

(text at bottom right of block) Mⱼ 6/3/9x 12 30

Note (right margin, vertical): 6/3/9x F 284 SURG 312 PERRON, CARLEEN DOB 07/20/9x 67289017 Rodden, Patrick MD

PHYSICIAN'S ORDERS

Figure 4.5. *Continued.*

CENTRAL MEDICAL CENTER

211 Medical Center Drive • Central City, US 90000-1234 • PHONE: (012) 125-6784 • FAX: (012) 125-9999

DOCTOR: PLEASE STATE PERTINENT CLINICAL INFORMATION WHEN ORDERING RADIOLOGY PROCEDURES

WRITE WITH BALLPOINT INK PEN; PRESS HARD

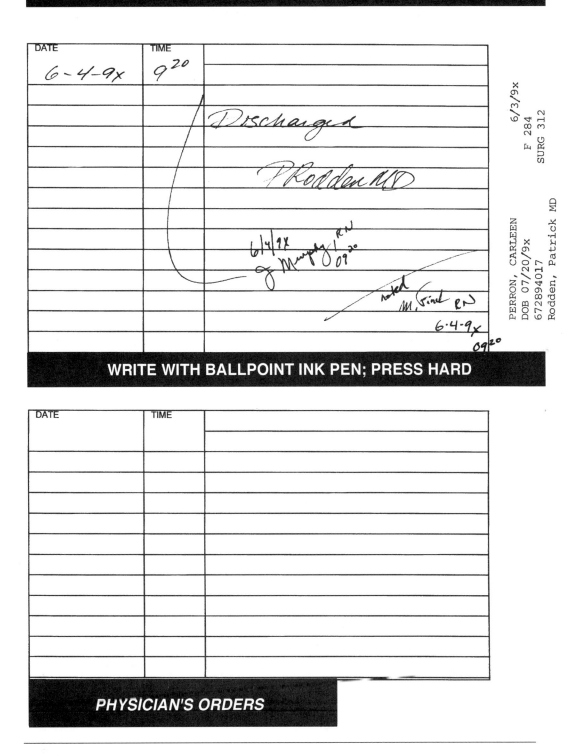

WRITE WITH BALLPOINT INK PEN; PRESS HARD

PHYSICIAN'S ORDERS

Figure 4.5. *Continued.*

CENTRAL MEDICAL CENTER

211 Medical Center Drive • Central City, US 90000-1234 • PHONE: (012) 125-6784 • FAX: (012) 125-9999

LABORATORY REPORT

June 2, 199x 3 p.m.

Collect: 6/2/9x at 1500 (BLOOD)   28Y F - PERRON, CARLEEN
Service: 6/2/9x at 1450   PATRICK RODDEN, M.D.

CHEMISTRY

141	SODIUM	(135 - 145)	MMOL/L
3.7	POTASSIUM	(3.5 - 5.0)	MMOL/L
109	CHLORIDE	(100 - 110)	MMOL/L
29	CARBON DIOXIDE	(24 - 32)	MMOL/L
88	GLUCOSE	(65 - 110)	MG/DL
0.8	CREATININE	(0.4 - 1.5)	MG/DL
14	BUN	(7 - 22)	MG/DL

HEMATOLOGY

	<<CBC>>		
11.8*	WBC	(4.8 - 10.8)	1000/CUMM
4.1*	RBC	(4.20 - 5.40)	MIL/CUMM
12.9	HGB	(12.0 - 16.0)	G/DL
37.7	HCT	(37.0 - 47.0)	%
91.5	MCV	(80 - 100)	CU MICRON
31.0	MCH	(27 - 31)	MCMCG
34.1	MCHC	(32 - 37)	G/DL
12.8	RDW	(11.5 - 14.5)	RBC INDEX
253	PLT	(150 - 400)	1000/CUMM
20.1	LYM%	(14 - 51)	%
7.5	MONO%	(1 - 11)	%
70.2	NEUTRO%	(35 - 74)	%
1.5	EOS%	(0 - 6)	%
0.7	BASO%	(0 - 2)	%
2.3	LYM#	(1.5 - 4.0)	1000/CUMM
0.8	MONO#	(0.2 - 0.9)	1000/CUMM
7.9*	NEUTRO#	(1.0 - 7.0)	1000/CUMM
0.2	EOS#	(0 - 0.7)	1000/CUMM
0.1	BASO#	(0 - 0.2)	1000/CUMM

(continued)

LABORATORY REPORT   PATIENT: PERRON, CARLEEN   672894017

Figure 4.6. Diagnostic tests/laboratory reports. Reporting forms with results of blood and urine studies ordered before surgery.

CENTRAL MEDICAL CENTER

211 Medical Center Drive • Central City, US 90000-1234 • PHONE: (012) 125-6784 • FAX: (012) 125-9999

LABORATORY REPORT

June 2, 199x 3 p.m.

URINALYSIS

Collect:	6/2/9x at 1500 (URINE)
Service:	6/2/9x at 1450

28Y F - PERRON, CARLEEN
PATRICK RODDEN, M.D.

<<BASIC URINALYSIS>>

	SPECIFIC GRAVITY	(1.005 -	
1.024		1.030)	
HAZY	APPEARANCE		
YELLOW	COLOR		
5.0	PH		
NEGATIVE	PROTEIN		
NEGATIVE	GLUCOSE		GM/DL
NEGATIVE	KETONE		
NORMAL	UROBILINOGEN	(0.1 - 1.0)	MG/DL
NEGATIVE	BLOOD		
NEGATIVE	LEUKOCYTES	(NEGATIVE)	
NEGATIVE	NITRITE	(NEGATIVE)	

<<MICROSCOPIC URINALYSIS>>

NONE	RBC	/HPF
0-3	WBC	/HPF
10-15	EPITHELIAL CELLS	/HPF
NONE	MUCUS	/HPF
3+	BACTERIA	/HPF
NONE	CASTS	/HPF
NONE	CRYSTALS	/HPF

LABORATORY REPORT	**PATIENT: PERRON, CARLEEN**	**672894017**

Figure 4.6. *Continued.*

DATE	TIME	REMARKS
6/3/9x	0615	admitted & oriented to room 312. In no acute distress. VS stable. Afebrile NPO maintained. Condition stable K. Brown RN
6/3/9x	0800	To OR via gurney - awake & oriented accompanied by her mother - condition stable K. Brown RN
6/3/9x	1110	Returned from PAR drowsy but arouses easily Skin warm & dry. Color pink - VS stable - Throat dry unable to take sips of water very well - no nausea - c/o severe sore throat medicated x̄ with IM pain medication with desired effect - mother very supportive & remains @ bedside - Using a bedpan but unable to urinate - IV infusing well K. Brown RN

CENTRAL MEDICAL CENTER
PATIENT'S PROGRESS NOTES
GENERAL CARE & TREATMENT

PT. NAME: PERRON, CARLEEN
ID NO: 672894017
ROOM NO: 312
ATT. PHYS: PATRICK RODDEN, M.D.

Figure 4.7. Nurse's notes. A recording by the nursing staff of the patient's progress made during general care and treatment.

CENTRAL MEDICAL CENTER

211 Medical Center Drive · Central City, US 90000-1234 · PHONE: (012) 125-6784 · FAX: (012) 125-9999

VITAL SIGNS RECORD

DATE: 6-3-9x

NURSE'S INITIALS	TIME	PRESSURE	PULSE	RESP	TEMP	TIME	PRESSURE	PULSE	RESP	TEMP	NURSE'S INITIALS
PAR	11¹⁰	126/76	66	20							
KB	12¹⁰	123/78	59	18	97⁵						
K.B	13¹⁰	115/74	65	16							
K.B	14¹⁰	123/66	64	16							
KB	15¹⁰	123/78	63	16	98						
KB	17¹⁰	109/56	91	16							
KB	19¹⁰	112/62	84	18	99³						

PT. NAME: PERRON, CARLEEN
ID NO: 672894017
ROOM NO: 312
ATT. PHYS: PATRICK RODDEN, M.D.

Figure 4.7. *Continued.* Vital signs record. A chart recording of the patient's vital signs documented by the nursing staff.

DATE	TIME	REMARKS
6/3/9x	10⁰⁵	op note
		Chronic recurrent tonsillitis
		Procedure: tonsillectomy
		Surgeon: P. Rodden MD
		Anesthesiologist: Robert Jang MD
		Procedure tolerated well
		P Rodden MD
6/3/9x	12²⁰	post op check
		VS stable
		c/o pain & poor p o fluid intake
		Will keep pt overnight for observation
		Plan to DC in am
		P Rodden MD
6/4/9x	08⁰⁰	Doing much better – no bleeding
		taking liquids freely
		DC'd on fluids
		Given Rx for tylenol.
		RTO in 48h
		P. Rodden MD

CENTRAL MEDICAL CENTER
PHYSICIAN'S PROGRESS NOTES

PT. NAME: PERRON, CARLEEN
ID NO: 672894017
ROOM NO: 312
ATT. PHYS: PATRICK RODDEN, M.D.

Figure 4.8. Physician's progress notes. Physician's notations of the patient's progress throughout care.

CENTRAL MEDICAL CENTER

211 Medical Center Drive • Central City, US 90000-1234 • PHONE: (012) 125-6784 • FAX: (012) 125-9999

OPERATIVE REPORT

DATE OF OPERATION: June 3, 199x.

PREOPERATIVE DIAGNOSIS: Chronic tonsillitis.

POSTOPERATIVE DIAGNOSIS: Frequent, recurrent tonsillitis.

SURGEON: Patrick Rodden, M.D.

ASSISTANT SURGEON: None

ANESTHESIOLOGIST: Robert Jung, M.D.

ANESTHESIA: General.

SURGERY PERFORMED: Tonsillectomy.

DESCRIPTION OF OPERATION: After general anesthesia induction, with intubation, the McGivor mouth gag and tongue retractor were utilized for exposure of the oropharynx. Local anesthetic consisting of 6 cc of 0.5% Xylocaine with 1:100,000 epinephrine was utilized. Tonsillectomy was carried out using dissection and air technique. The right tonsillectomy electrocoagulation Bovie suction was utilized for hemostasis. Examination of the nasopharynx was normal.

The patient tolerated the procedure well and went to the recovery room in good condition.

P. Rodden MD

PATRICK RODDEN, M.D.

JR:as
D: 6/3/9x
T: 6/4/9x

OPERATIVE REPORT	PT. NAME:	PERRON, CARLEEN
	ID NO:	672894017
	ROOM NO:	312
	ATT. PHYS:	PATRICK RODDEN, M.D.

Figure 4.9. Operative report. Surgeon's account of a surgical procedure.

CENTRAL MEDICAL CENTER

211 Medical Center Drive • Central City, US 90000-1234 • PHONE: (012) 125-6784 • FAX: (012) 125-9999

PATHOLOGY REPORT

PATIENT: PERRON, CARLEEN
                    28 Y (FEMALE)

DATE RECEIVED: June 3, 199x   DATE REPORTED: June 4, 199x

GROSS:

Received are two tonsils each 2.5 cm in greatest diameter.

MICROSCOPIC:

The sections show deep tonsillar crypts associated with follicular lymphoid hyperplasia. No bacterial granules are seen.

DIAGNOSIS:

CHRONIC LYMPHOID HYPERPLASIA OF RIGHT AND LEFT TONSILS.

Mary Needham MD

MARY NEEDHAM, M.D.

MN:gds

D: 6/4/9x
T: 6/5/9x

Figure 4.10. Pathology report.

	MEDICAL RECORDS USE
THAT CONDITION WHICH AFTER STUDY IS DETERMINED TO BE THE REASON FOR ADMISSION TO THE HOSPITAL PRINCIPAL DIAGNOSIS - *Chronic tonsillitis*	474.0
FINAL DIAGNOSIS - NO ABBREVIATIONS	474.0
Same	
SECONDARY DIAGNOSIS:	
COMPLICATIONS AND/OR COMORBIDITY:	
PRINCIPAL OPERATION/PROCEDURES(S)/TREATMENT RENDERED: *Tonsillectomy*	
SECONDARY OPERATIONS/PROCEDURES:	

CONDITION ON DISCHARGE *Stable*

☐ DISCHARGE INSTRUCTIONS   ☐ PRE-PRINTED INSTRUCTIONS GIVEN

MEDICATIONS *Tylenol*
PHYSICAL ACTIVITY *Bed rest*
DIET *full liquid*
FOLLOW-UP *office in 48 h*

DATE OF SUMMARY IF DICTATED:

DATE ADMITTED: *6/3/9X*		DATE DISCHARGED: *6/4/9X*		ATTENDING PHYSICIAN *P. Rodden*		M.D.

06/03/9X

FOR MED. RECORDS USE ONLY	ASSEMBLY *SL*	ANALYSIS *ME/37*	CODED *WX*	KEYED *L*	FINAL CHECK
CONSULTANTS:			AA	1	
			DP	R48	
			SC	1211	

DRG - *059*

CENTRAL MEDICAL CENTER

DIAGNOSIS RECORD/
DISCHARGE SUMMARY

Figure 4.11. Discharge summary. Final report documented at time of discharge that includes the diagnostic record and diagnosis related group (DRG)—the number assigned to the individual hospitalization based on the patient's diagnoses, complications, age, etc. and which translates to a fixed dollar amount payable from a third-party payer (e.g., Medicare).

Medical Record Abbreviations

Following are common medical record abbreviations used in patient care documentations. They represent the "acceptable" terms used extensively throughout this text. Remember that individual medical facilities provide their own list of acceptable terms and abbreviations that may not be used elsewhere. Memorize the terms and abbreviations from this list, and plan on adapting them to the variations you encounter.

Abbreviation	Meaning
Medical Care Facilities	
CCU	coronary (cardiac) care unit
ECU	emergency care unit
ER	emergency room
ICU	intensive care unit
IP	inpatient (a registered bed patient)
OP	outpatient
OR	operating room
PAR	postanesthetic recovery
post-op/postop	postoperative (after surgery)
pre-op/preop	preoperative (before surgery)
RTC	return to clinic
RTO	return to office
Patient Care	
BRP	bathroom privileges
CP	chest pain
DC, D/C	discharge, discontinue
ETOH	ethyl alcohol
Ⓛ	left
Ⓡ	right
pt	patient
RRR	regular rate and rhythm
SOB	shortness of breath
Tr	treatment
Tx	treatment or traction
VS	vital signs
T	temperature
P	pulse
R	respiration

continued

Abbreviation	Meaning
BP	blood pressure
Ht	height
Wt	weight
WDWN	well-developed and well-nourished
y.o.	year old
#	number or pound: if before the numeral it means number (e.g., #2 = number two); if after the numeral it means pound (e.g., 150# = 150 pounds)
♀	female
♂	male
°	degree or hour
↑	increased
↓	decreased
ө	none or negative
⚲	standing
⚵	sitting
○—	lying

Common Medical Record Terms Related to Disease

The following terms related to disease are common in medical records. Learn them as a foundation on which you will build as your vocabulary expands.

Term	Meaning
acute ă-kyūt′	sharp; having severe symptoms and a short course
chronic kron′ik	a condition developing slowly and persisting over time
benign bi-nīn′	mild or noncancerous
malignant mă-lig′nănt	harmful or cancerous
degeneration dē-jen-er-ā′shŭn	gradual deterioration of normal cells and body functions
degenerative disease	any disease in which there is deterioration of structure or function of tissue
diagnosis dī-ag-nō′sis	determination of the presence of a disease based on an evaluation of symptoms, signs, and test findings (results) (dia = through; gnosis = knowing)

continued

FEBRILE. Febrile is derived from the Latin febris, meaning "I am warm." In the ancient world fever was considered a favorable symptom, and the origin of the word is associated with February (the month for cleansing or purifying). Before the clinical thermometer was developed, the method of estimating fever was to lay the hand on the skin.

Term	Meaning
etiology ē-tē-ol'ō-jē	cause of a disease (etio = cause)
exacerbation eg-zas-er-bā'shŭn	increase in severity of a disease with aggravation of symptoms (ex = out; acerbo = harsh)
remission rē-mish'ŭn	a period in which symptoms and signs stop or abate
febrile fe'brĭl	relating to a fever (temperature)
gross	large; visible to naked eye
idiopathic id'ē-ō-path'ik	a condition occurring without a clearly identified cause (idio = one's own)
localized lō'kăl-īzd	limited to a definite area or part
systemic sis-tem'ik	relating to the whole body rather than only a part
malaise mă-lāz'	a feeling of unwellness, often the first indication of illness
marked	significant
equivocal ē-kwĭv'ŏ-kl	vague, questionable
morbidity mor-bid'i-tē	a diseased state; sick
morbidity rate	the number of cases of a disease in a given year; the ratio of sick to well persons in a given population
mortality mor-tal'i-tē	the state of being subject to death
mortality rate	death rate; ratio of total number of deaths to total number in a given population
prognosis prog-nō'sis	foreknowledge; prediction of the likely outcome of a disease based on the general health status of the patient along with knowledge of the usual course of the disease
progressive prō-gres'iv	the advance of a condition as signs and symptoms increase in severity
prophylaxis prō-fi-lak'sis	a process or measure that prevents disease (pro = before; phylassein = to guard)
recurrent rē-kŭr'ent	to occur again; describes a return of symptoms and signs after a period of quiescence (rest or inactivity)

continued

Term	Meaning
sequela sē-kwel′ă	a disorder or condition after, and usually resulting from, a previous disease or injury
sign	a mark; objective evidence of disease that can be seen or verified by an examiner
symptom simp′tŏm	occurrence; subjective evidence of disease that is perceived by the patient and often noted in his or her own words
syndrome sin′drōm	a running together; combination of symptoms and signs that give a distinct clinical picture indicating a particular condition or disease (e.g., menopausal syndrome)
noncontributory	not involved in bringing on the condition or result
unremarkable	not significant or worthy of noting

Pharmaceutical Abbreviations and Symbols

Pharmaceutical abbreviations and symbols are frequently used in documenting patient care. They are found throughout the medical record. Efficient medical record keeping and effective communication among health care workers depend on knowledge of commonly used pharmaceutical abbreviations and symbols.

Units of Measure

The following are common metric and apothecary units of measurement. Consult your medical dictionary for a complete listing of units of measurement and conversion formulas.

METRIC SYSTEM

Metric is the most commonly used system of measurement in health care. It is a decimal system based on the following units.

meter (m)	length	39.37 inches
liter (L)	volume	1.0567 US quarts
gram (g or gm)	weight	15.432 grains

APOTHECARY SYSTEM

The apothecary system is an outdated method of liquid and weight measure used by the earliest chemists and pharmacists. The liquid measure was based on one drop. The weight measure was based on one grain of wheat. Although the small apothecary measures are rarely used, the larger ones (e.g., fluid ounces) are still common.

DRUG. The middle English drogge or drugge is derived from the old French drogue, all meaning drug. Earlier origin is uncertain, possibly either a Teutonic root meaning dry or the Persian droa meaning odor because many drugs had a strong odor. Although the ancients listed the use of various medicines, the term drug did not appear until the end of the medieval period. The word druggist did not appear until the 16th century.

Common Abbreviations and Symbols

Abbreviation	Meaning
Metric	
cc	cubic centimeter (1 cc = 1 ml)
cm	centimeter (2.5 cm = 1 inch)
g or gm	gram
kg	kilogram [one thousand grams (2.2 pounds)]
L	liter
mg	milligram [one-thousandth (0.001) of a gram]
ml, mL	milliliter [one-thousandth (0.001) of a liter]
mm	millimeter [one-thousandth (0.001) of a meter]
cu mm	cubic millimeter
Apothecary	
fl oz	fluid ounce
gr	grain
gt	drop (L. gutta = drop)
gtt	drops
dr	dram (1/8 ounce)
oz	ounce
lb or #	pound (16 ounces)
qt	quart (32 ounces)

Medication Administration

Prescribed medications can be administered to patients in various ways, depending on the indication for the drug and status of the patient. The following is an overview of forms of drugs and routes of administration including abbreviations and symbols.

Drug Form	Route of Administration	
Solid and Semisolid Forms		
tablet (tab)	oral	by mouth [per os (p.o.)]
capsule (cap)	sublingual	under the tongue
	buccal	in the cheek
suppository (suppos)	vaginal	inserted in vagina [per vagina (PV)]
	rectal	inserted in rectum [per rectum (PR)]

continued

Drug Form	Route of Administration	
Liquid Forms		
fluid	inhalation	inhale through nose or mouth [e.g., aerosol (spray) or nebulizer (device used to produce a fine spray or mist)]
parenteral	injection	*intradermal* (ID), within the skin
		intramuscular (IM), within the muscle
		intravenous (IV), within the vein
		subcutaneous (SC or SQ), under the skin (Fig. 4.12)
cream, lotion, ointment	topical	applied to surface of skin
other delivery systems	transdermal	absorption of a drug through unbroken skin
	implant	a drug reservoir imbedded in the body to provide continual infusion of a medication

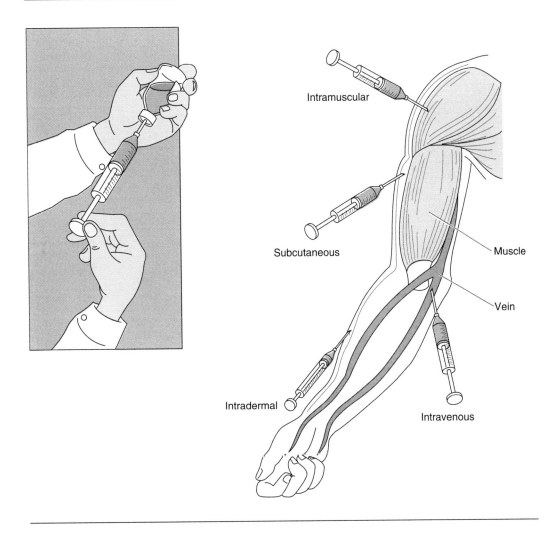

Figure 4.12. Parenteral drug administration.

The Prescription

A prescription is a written direction by a physician for dispensing or administering a medication to a patient. It is an order to supply a named patient with a particular drug of a specific strength and quantity along with specific instructions for administration. The prescription is a legal document that must be written in a specific format (Fig. 4.13).

Drug Names

The *chemical name* is assigned to a drug in the laboratory at the time it is formulated. It is the formula for the drug, which is written exactly according to its chemical structure. The *generic name* is the accepted drug name for the chemical. The *trade* or *brand* is the manufacturer's name for the drug. For example

chemical name	8-chloro-1-methyl-6-phenyl-4H-s-triazolo[4,3-a][1,4]benzodi-azepine
generic name	alprazolam
trade or brand	Xanax (Upjohn Pharmaceutical Co.)

Prescription Abbreviations

Many Latin abbreviations and symbols are commonly used in prescription writing as well as physician's orders. Being familiar with these symbols makes it possible to read a prescription or physician's order.

Common Abbreviations and Symbols

Abbreviation	Meaning	Latin[a]
Time and Frequency		
$\bar{a}$	before	ante
a.c.	before meals	ante cibum

continued

Rx. The Rx symbol found at the beginning of a prescription stands for recipe. The cross on the tail of the Rx incorporates the astrological sign of Jupiter, which has no connection with the word recipe. The sign of Jupiter was placed at the top of a formula to appease the chief Roman god so that the compound might act favorably. The period during the ascendancy of the planet Jupiter was considered a favorable time for the collection of herbs and the preparation of medicines.

CENTRAL MEDICAL GROUP, INC.
Patrick Rodden, M.D.
DEA #: AR 0000000
201 Medical Center Drive
Central City, US 90000-1234

Name of Patient _Carleen Perron_   Date _6/4/9x_

Address _____

Rx   Tylenol c codeine No. 3   #24
Sig: tab i q 4 h p.r.n. pain

_____ M.D.   _Patrick Rodden_ M.D.
SUBSTITUTION PERMITTED   DISPENSE AS WRITTEN

May refill _3_ times

Figure 4.13. Sample prescription.

Abbreviation	Meaning	Latin[a]
a.m.	before noon	ante meridiem
b.i.d.	twice a day	bis in die
d	day	
h	hour	hora
h.s.	at hour of sleep (bedtime)	hora somni
noc.	night	noctis
$\bar{p}$	after	post
p.c.	after meals	post cibum
p.m.	after noon	post meridiem
p.r.n.	as needed	pro re nata
q	every	quaque
q d	every day	quaque die
q h	every hour	quaque hora
q 2 h	every 2 hours	
q.i.d.	four times a day	quater in die
q.o.d.	every other day	quaque altera die
STAT	immediately	statim
t.i.d.	three times a day	ter in die
wk	week	
yr	year	

Miscellaneous

AD	right ear	auris dextra
AS	left ear	auris sinistra
AU	both ears	aures unitas
ad lib.	as desired	ad libitum
amt	amount	
aq	water	aqua
Ⓑ	bilateral	
C	Celsius, centigrade	
$\bar{c}$	with	cum
F	Fahrenheit	
Ⓜ	murmur	
NPO	nothing by mouth	non per os
OD	right eye	oculus dexter
OS	left eye	oculus sinister

DEXTER AND SINISTER. Dexter is Latin for right, and sinister is Latin for left. The origin of these terms, however, is earlier than ancient Rome. Sun worshippers facing the morning sun had the south on their right hand. The Sanskrit word for south is dekkan, allied to dhu, shining; thus the right hand was the south or warm shining hand. The left hand was the north or cold hand. Thus dexterity or right-handedness was skill, whereas sinister was ill-omened. Among the Romans, sinisteritas (left-handedness) meant awkwardness.

continued

Abbreviation	Meaning	Latin[a]
OU	both eyes	oculi unitas
per	by or through	
p.o.	by mouth	per os
PR	through rectum	per rectum
PV	through vagina	per vagina
q.n.s.	quantity not sufficient	
q.s.	quantity sufficient	
Rx	recipe; prescription	
Sig:	label; instruction to the patient	signa
s̄	without	sine
s̄s̄	one-half	semis
w.a.	while awake	
×	times or for [e.g., × 6 (six times), × 2 d (for two days)]	
>	greater than	
<	less than	
ī	one (modified lower-case Roman numeral i)	
īī	two (modified lower-case Roman numeral ii)	
īīī	three (modified lower-case Roman numeral iii)	
īv̄	four (modified lower-case Roman numeral iv)	
I, II, III, IV, V, VI, VII, VIII, IX, X	uppercase Roman numerals 1–10	

[a]Original Latin given when it is deemed helpful.

Recording Date and Time

The date and time are usually required in entries in a medical record. Always include the month, day of the month, and the year (e.g., 12/25/xx); sometimes six digits are required (e.g., 01/08/xx). Often military time is used.

Standard	*Military*	
1:00 a.m.	0100	zero one hundred
2:00 a.m.	0200	zero two hundred
2:15 a.m.	0215	zero two fifteen
3:00 a.m.	0300	zero three hundred
4:00 a.m.	0400	zero four hundred

4:30 a.m.	0430	zero four thirty
5:00 a.m.	0500	zero five hundred
6:00 a.m.	0600	zero six hundred
7:00 a.m.	0700	zero seven hundred
8:00 a.m.	0800	zero eight hundred
9:00 a.m.	0900	zero nine hundred
10:00 a.m.	1000	ten hundred
11:00 a.m.	1100	eleven hundred
12:00 p.m. (noon)	1200	twelve hundred hours
1:00 p.m.	1300	thirteen hundred
2:00 p.m.	1400	fourteen hundred
3:00 p.m.	1500	fifteen hundred
4:00 p.m.	1600	sixteen hundred
5:00 p.m.	1700	seventeen hundred
6:00 p.m.	1800	eighteen hundred
7:00 p.m.	1900	nineteen hundred
8:00 p.m.	2000	twenty hundred
9:00 p.m.	2100	twenty-one hundred
10:00 p.m.	2200	twenty-two hundred
11:00 p.m.	2300	twenty-three hundred
12:00 a.m. (midnight)	2400	twenty-four hundred hours

Regulations and Legal Considerations

Medical record documentations are made by physicians caring for the patient as well as other authorized health care professionals involved with care.

State, federal, and private accrediting agencies (e.g., the Joint Commission on Accreditation of Healthcare Organizations) provide specific guidelines that regulate how medical records are kept, including proper format for all forms, use of appropriate terminology and accepted abbreviations, protocol for personnel having access to records, and responsibilities for documentation.

Corrections

Sometimes mistakes are made when making an entry in a medical record. Careful clarification of the error is essential. If a mistake is made in a handwritten entry, it should be identified by drawing a single line through it, and the correction written in the margin above or immediately after. Include the date, the abbreviation "corr." and the initials of the person making the correction. The use of correction fluid (whiteout) is forbidden!

The medical record often becomes evidence in medical malpractice cases. Obliterations and signs of possible tampering can be construed as trying to withhold information or covering up negligent wrongdoing. Complete and accurate record keeping is your best defense against any possible legal action (Fig. 4.14).

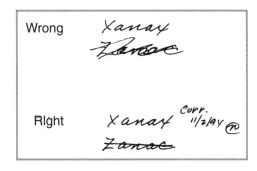

Figure 4.14. Proper correction of a medical record.

PRACTICE EXERCISES

Write the full medical term for the following abbreviations and symbols:

1. CC _____

2. OH _____

3. PR _____

4. BRP _____

5. PAR _____

6. PH _____

7. D/C _____

8. Sig: _____

9. ER _____

10. ICU _____

11. R/O _____

12. NPO _____

13. L&W _____

14. BP _____

15. AU _____

16. Sx _____

17. VS _____

18. ROS _____

19. pt _____

20. OD _____

21. SQ _____

22. H&P _____

23. Tx _____

24. Dx _____

25. PI _____

Match the following terms with their meanings:

26. febrile   _____   a. period in which symptoms stop

27. syndrome   _____   b. probable outcome of a disease

28. chronic   _____   c. name of a disease based on history, examination, and testing

29. remission   _____   d. temperature

30. etiology   _____   e. set of symptoms characteristic of a particular disease or condition

31. malignant   _____   f. increase in severity with aggravation of symptoms

32. prognosis   _____   g. developing slowly over time

33. diagnosis   _____   h. limited to a definite area or part

34. exacerbation   _____   i. cancerous

35. localized   _____   j. the study of the cause of a disease

Match the following definitions with their abbreviations:

36. route of oral medications   _____   a. pre-op

37. place for surgery   _____   b. p. r. n.

38. as desired   _____   c. parenteral

39. subjective, objective, assessment, plan _____   d. p.o.

40. after surgery   _____   e. STAT

41. pound   _____   f. ad lib.

42.	as needed	_____	g. postop
43.	by injection	_____	h. OR
44.	before surgery	_____	i. POMR
45.	immediately	_____	j. #

Write the meaning for the following pharmaceutical phrases:

46. VS q h x 4 h, then q 2 h _____

47. $\dot{T}$ q.i.d. p.c. h.s. _____

48. aspirin (ASA) gr. $\ddot{T}$ $\overline{ss}$ q d _____

49. gr V PR q 4 h p.r.n. temp >101° _____

50. $\dot{T}$ q.o.d. a.m. _____

51. $\ddot{T}$ gtt OU t.i.d. × 7 d _____

52. cap $\ddot{T}$ STAT, then $\dot{T}$ q 6 h _____

Write the standard pharmaceutical abbreviations for the following:

53. one tablet three times a day for seven days _____

54. one suppository in the vagina at bedtime _____

55. 1/2 grain twice a day _____

56. one or two by mouth every three to four hours as needed _____

57. two drops in left ear every three hours _____

58. one capsule two times a day, morning and evening _____

59. two immediately, then one every six hours _____

60. thirty milligrams by mouth at bedtime as needed _____

Give military time for the following:

61. 1:00 a.m. _____

62. 2:30 p.m. _____

63. midnight _____

64. 1:00 p.m. _____

65. 7:00 p.m. _____

Medical Record Analysis

MEDICAL RECORD 4.1

Michael Marsi has had chronic health problems in the last two years and has been seeing Dr. Spaulding, his personal physician, regularly in recent months. Dr. Spaulding uses problem-oriented medical records and writes a new SOAP progress note at each patient visit. Mr. Marsi has come to see Dr. Spaulding today because he feels worse than usual.

Directions

Read Medical Record 4.1 (page 87) for Michael Marsi and answer the following questions. This record is the progress note for today's visit, part of Dr. Spaulding's POMR for Mr. Marsi. Dr. Spaulding handwrote it herself during the patient's visit.

Questions about Medical Record 4.1

Write your answers in the spaces provided.

1. How old is Mr. Marsi? _____

2. Where was the treatment rendered? _____

3. List the three elements of the patient's complaint

   a. _____

   b. _____

   c. _____

4. In your own words, not using medical terminology, briefly summarize Mr. Marsi's history:

   _____

   _____

   _____

5. Which of the following is *not* mentioned at all in this history?

   a. The prescription medication Mr. Marsi takes

   b. Mr. Marsi's smoking habit

   c. Mr. Marsi's activity level at work

   d. Mr. Marsi's consumption of alcohol

6. Dr. Spaulding and Mr. Marsi talked at length about Mr. Marsi's symptoms and how they've changed recently, and then Dr. Spaulding examined him. List three objective findings she noted in this examination.

a. _____

b. _____

c. _____

7. Dr. Spaulding's assessment is that he has _____.

But she also wants to make sure Mr. Marsi does *not* have _____

_____.

8. Dr. Spaulding's treatment plan involves four areas. List the specific plan(s) for each of these.

Diagnostic tests ordered: _____

_____

Instruct patient to change (and how) these personal habits: _____

_____

_____

_____

_____

Drug prescribed (and how much and when): _____

_____

Future diagnostic check and/or action to take: _____

_____

9. When is Dr. Spaulding expecting to see Mr. Marsi again?_____

_____

PROGRESS NOTES

Patient Name: *MARSi, MichAel*

DATE	FINDINGS
2-3-9x	CC: 51 y.o. ♂ c/o dizziness × 3 wk and headaches 5-6 × ↑ wk. Today he woke c̄ numbness in ⓇLeg and hand
	S Hx of ↑BP × 4yrs. Smoker × 20yrs - 1 pkg/d MEDS: Diazide ī g d. ⊕ CP ⊕ SOB occipital headaches ▽ in am mod fat diet 3 beers q noc. NKDA
	O BP 150/100 Ⓛ arm & Ht 68" WT 198# T 98.7° P 76 R 15 Heart - RRR s̄ ⓜ Lungs clear HEENT - WNL
	A Hypertension (HTN) R/O Congestive heart failure (CHF)
	P Chest X-ray and electrocardiogram today ↓ ETOH to ↑ beer q noc DC smoking Rx: Procardia #30 ī P.O. q d. ↑ exercise to 3×/wk for 20-30 min stop if CP, SOB or dizzy ↓ fat and cholesterol in diet re✓ BP ↑ wk RTO sooner if CP, SOB or dizzy
	J.R. Spaulding, MD

COLOR ATLAS

INTRODUCTION

The Language of Health Care

This color atlas provides a visual framework of human anatomy to serve as a clear, concise reference supporting the anatomical terms listed at the beginning of chapters 5–17. Pertinent photographs of common pathologies are highlighted throughout, and common diagnostic images have been selected to illustrate the use of modern technologies. Many illustrations from the atlas are repeated in the chapters but not in the depth or rich color that this section provides. This atlas is purposefully placed before introducing the body systems so that it can be readily available for frequent reference.

Although anatomy is referenced here and anatomical terms are outlined in the beginning of chapters on each body system, note that this text emphasizes related medical terms, not anatomy or physiology. However, because essential elements of anatomy and some physiology are incorporated throughout this text, they may be included in your learning objectives. The choice is up to you or your instructor.

In chapters 1–4 you have examined how medical terms are formed and seen how they are used in health care documentation. In chapters 5–17 each body system will be introduced, and related combining forms and common terms and abbreviations related to symptoms, diagnoses, tests, procedures, surgeries, and therapies will be covered.

Plate 1

Levels of organization

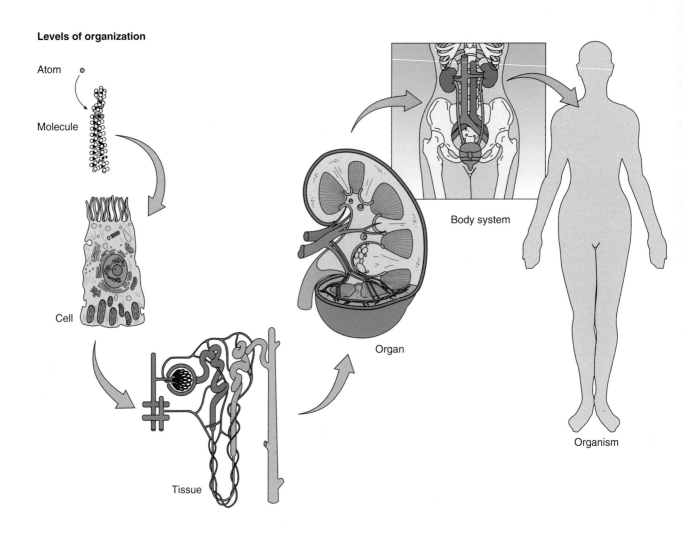

Atom

Molecule

Cell

Tissue

Organ

Body system

Organism

Anatomy of a typical cell

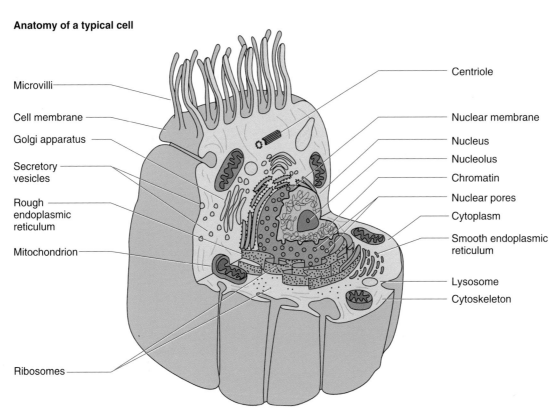

Microvilli

Cell membrane

Golgi apparatus

Secretory vesicles

Rough endoplasmic reticulum

Mitochondrion

Ribosomes

Centriole

Nuclear membrane

Nucleus

Nucleolus

Chromatin

Nuclear pores

Cytoplasm

Smooth endoplasmic reticulum

Lysosome

Cytoskeleton

Plate 2

Body planes

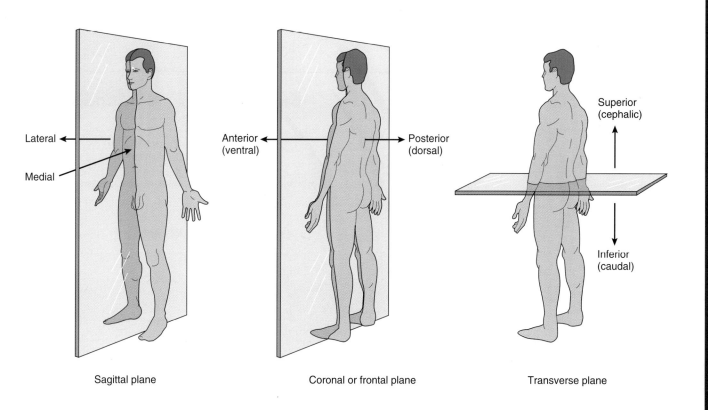

Lateral

Medial

Sagittal plane

Anterior (ventral)

Posterior (dorsal)

Coronal or frontal plane

Superior (cephalic)

Inferior (caudal)

Transverse plane

Body cavities

Thoracic cavity

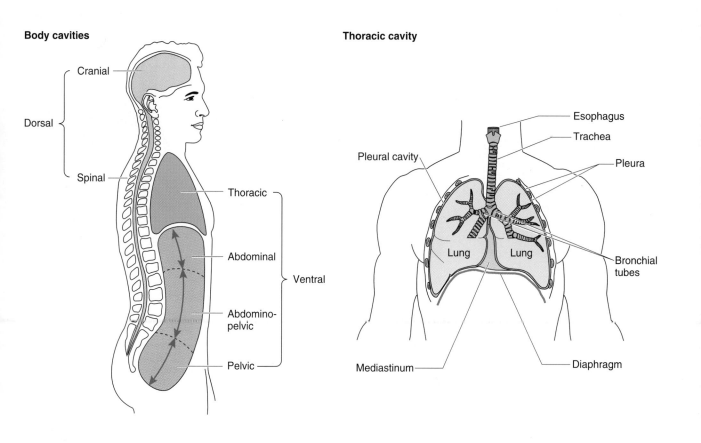

Dorsal

Cranial

Spinal

Thoracic

Abdominal

Ventral

Abdomino-pelvic

Pelvic

Pleural cavity

Esophagus

Trachea

Pleura

Lung

Lung

Bronchial tubes

Mediastinum

Diaphragm

Plate 3

THE SKIN

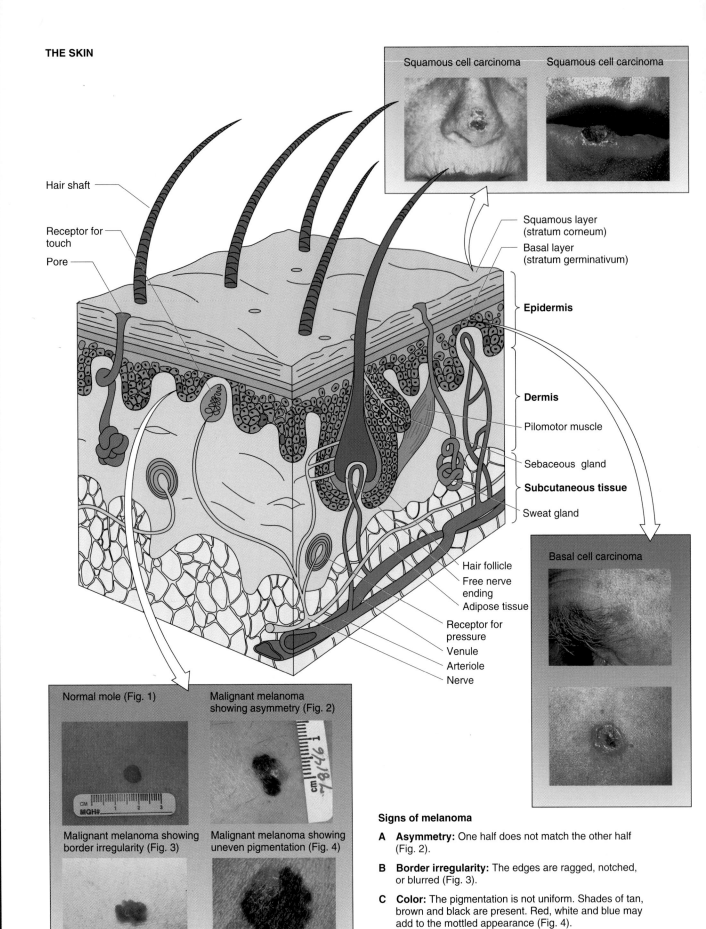

Squamous cell carcinoma   Squamous cell carcinoma

Hair shaft

Receptor for touch

Pore

Squamous layer (stratum corneum)

Basal layer (stratum germinativum)

Epidermis

Dermis

Pilomotor muscle

Sebaceous gland

Subcutaneous tissue

Sweat gland

Hair follicle

Free nerve ending

Adipose tissue

Receptor for pressure

Venule

Arteriole

Nerve

Basal cell carcinoma

Normal mole (Fig. 1)

Malignant melanoma showing asymmetry (Fig. 2)

Malignant melanoma showing border irregularity (Fig. 3)

Malignant melanoma showing uneven pigmentation (Fig. 4)

Signs of melanoma

A **Asymmetry:** One half does not match the other half (Fig. 2).

B **Border irregularity:** The edges are ragged, notched, or blurred (Fig. 3).

C **Color:** The pigmentation is not uniform. Shades of tan, brown and black are present. Red, white and blue may add to the mottled appearance (Fig. 4).

D **Diameter greater than 6 millimeters:** Any sudden or continuing increase in size should be of special concern (not shown).

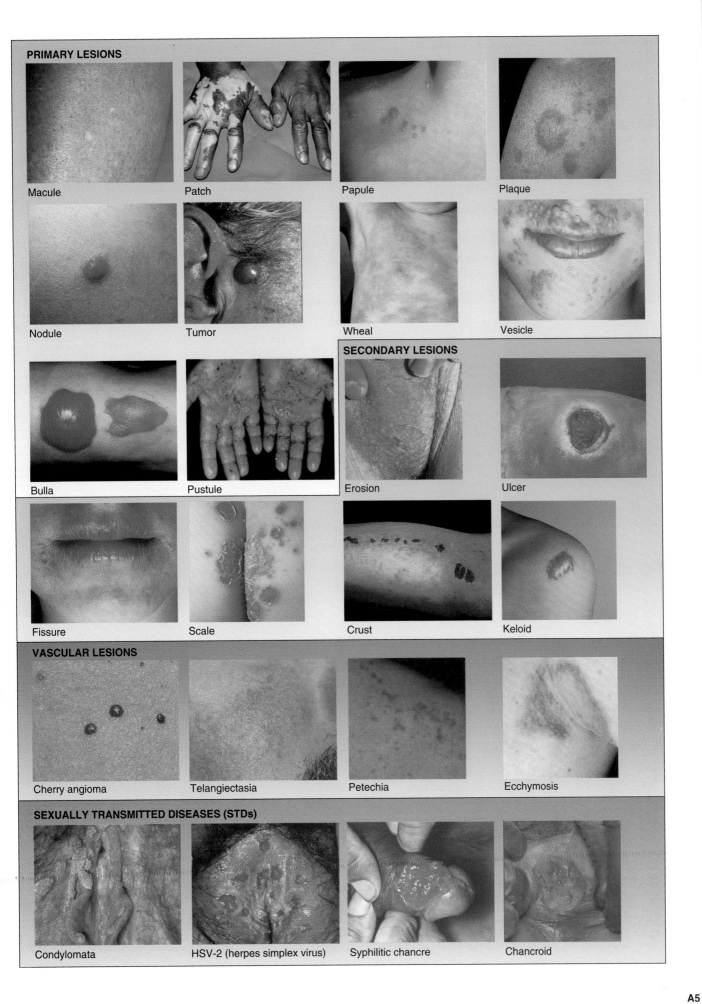

Plate 4

PRIMARY LESIONS

Macule

Patch

Papule

Plaque

Nodule

Tumor

Wheal

Vesicle

Bulla

Pustule

SECONDARY LESIONS

Erosion

Ulcer

Fissure

Scale

Crust

Keloid

VASCULAR LESIONS

Cherry angioma

Telangiectasia

Petechia

Ecchymosis

SEXUALLY TRANSMITTED DISEASES (STDs)

Condylomata

HSV-2 (herpes simplex virus)

Syphilitic chancre

Chancroid

Plate 5

THE SKELETON

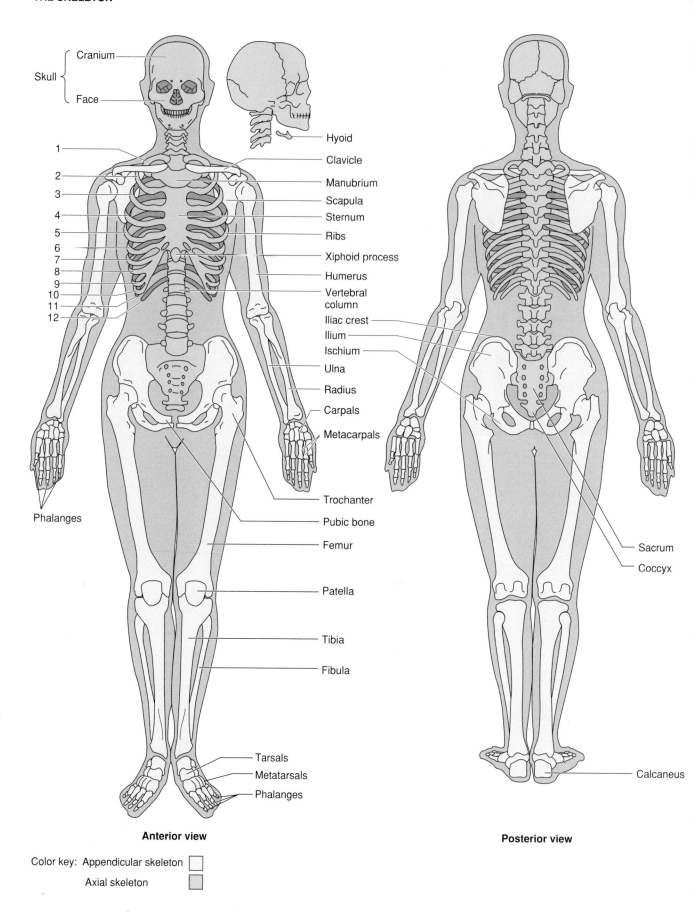

Skull { Cranium
        Face

Hyoid

1
2
3
4
5
6
7
8
9
10
11
12

Clavicle
Manubrium
Scapula
Sternum
Ribs
Xiphoid process
Humerus
Vertebral column
Iliac crest
Ilium
Ischium
Ulna
Radius
Carpals
Metacarpals

Phalanges

Trochanter
Pubic bone
Femur

Patella

Tibia

Fibula

Sacrum
Coccyx

Calcaneus

Tarsals
Metatarsals
Phalanges

Anterior view

Posterior view

Color key: Appendicular skeleton ☐
            Axial skeleton ▨

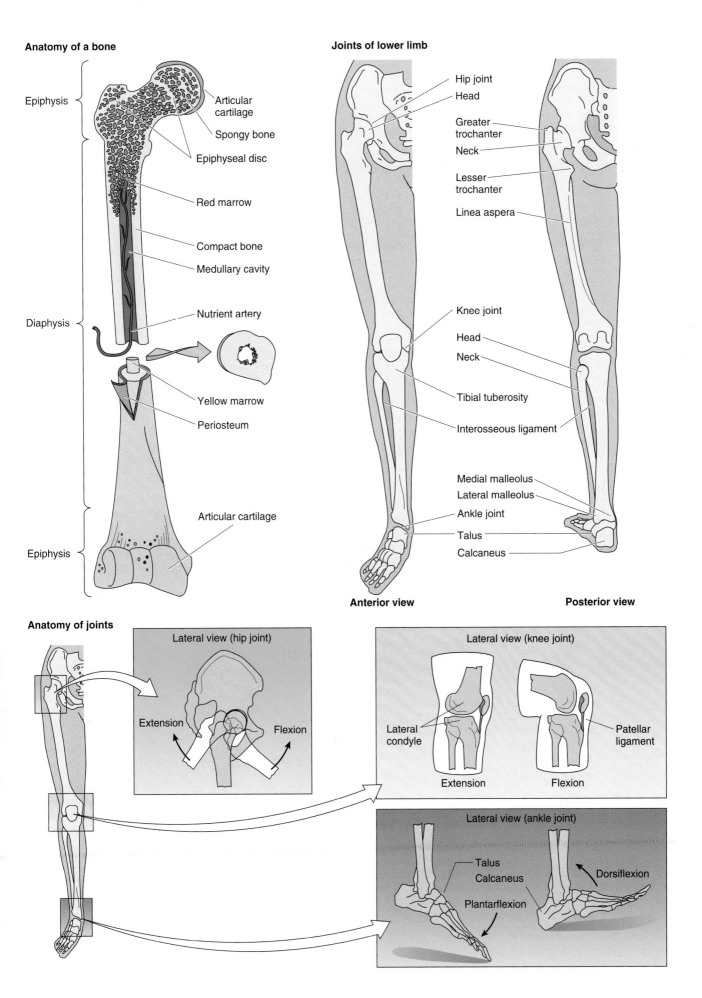

Plate 6

Anatomy of a bone

Epiphysis

Articular cartilage
Spongy bone
Epiphyseal disc

Red marrow

Compact bone
Medullary cavity

Diaphysis

Nutrient artery

Yellow marrow
Periosteum

Articular cartilage

Epiphysis

Joints of lower limb

Hip joint
Head
Greater trochanter
Neck
Lesser trochanter
Linea aspera

Knee joint
Head
Neck
Tibial tuberosity
Interosseous ligament

Medial malleolus
Lateral malleolus
Ankle joint
Talus
Calcaneus

Anterior view

Posterior view

Anatomy of joints

Lateral view (hip joint)
Extension
Flexion

Lateral view (knee joint)
Lateral condyle
Patellar ligament
Extension
Flexion

Lateral view (ankle joint)
Talus
Calcaneus
Dorsiflexion
Plantarflexion

Plate 7

THE SKULL: Anterior view

Frontal bone

Parietal bone

Greater wing of sphenoid bone

Temporal bone

Zygomatic bone

Maxilla bone

Mandible

Supraorbital foramen

Lacrimal bone

Ethmoid bone

Nasal bones

Infraorbital foramen

Median nasal septum

Inferior nasal concha

Mental foramen

THE SKULL: Lateral view

Coronal suture

Frontal bone

Sphenoid bone

Lacrimal bone

Nasal bone

Maxilla

Zygomatic bone

Mandible

Parietal bone

Occipital bone

Temporal bone

External auditory meatus

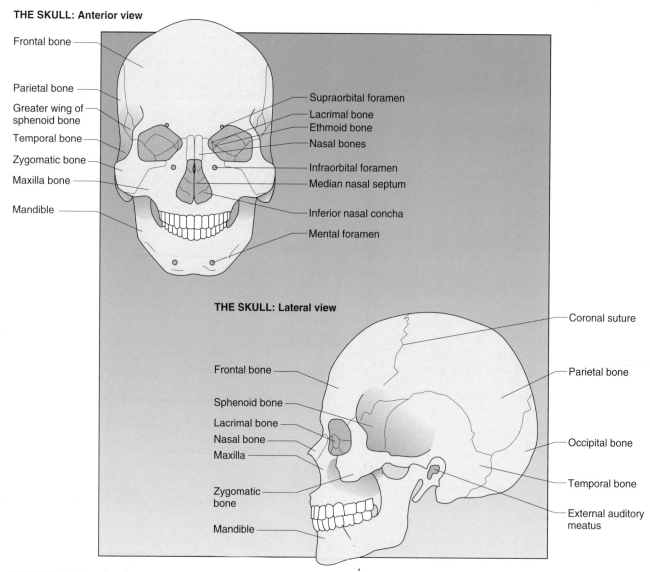

THE SKULL: Superior view

Lambdoidal suture

Sagittal suture

Coronal suture

Occipital bone

Parietal bone

Frontal bone

Nasal bone

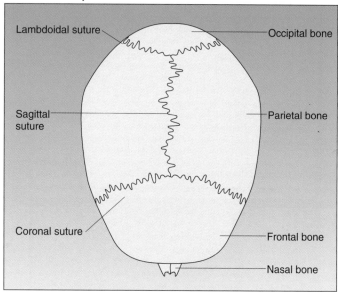

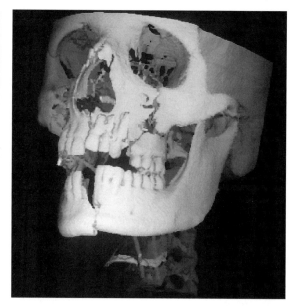

Three-dimensional CT reconstruction of a skull showing traumatic injury to facial bones suffered as the result of a motor vehicle accident.

Plate 8

THE VERTEBRAE: Lateral view

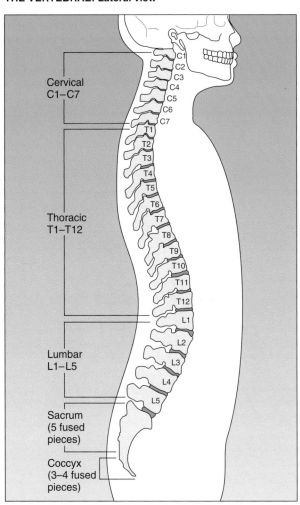

Cervical
C1–C7

Thoracic
T1–T12

Lumbar
L1–L5

Sacrum
(5 fused
pieces)

Coccyx
(3–4 fused
pieces)

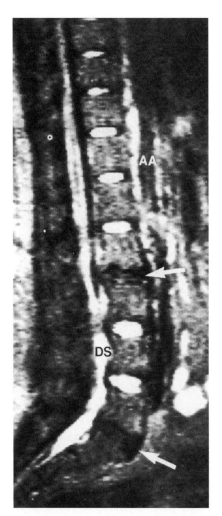

Lateral magnetic resonance image demonstrating degenerative disc disease at the L2 and L5 level (*arrows*). Dural sac (DS) and abdominal aorta (AA) are also visible.

Superior view (L2)

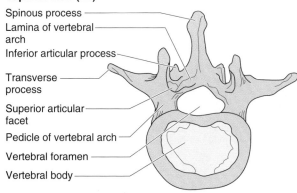

Spinous process
Lamina of vertebral arch
Inferior articular process
Transverse process
Superior articular facet
Pedicle of vertebral arch
Vertebral foramen
Vertebral body

Lateral view (L2)

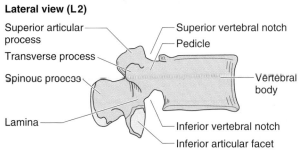

Superior articular process
Superior vertebral notch
Pedicle
Transverse process
Spinous process
Vertebral body
Lamina
Inferior vertebral notch
Inferior articular facet

Lateral view

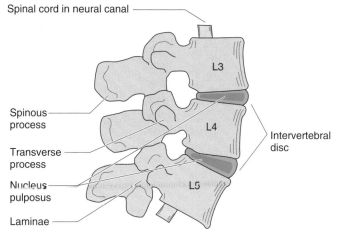

Spinal cord in neural canal
L3
L4
Intervertebral disc
Spinous process
Transverse process
Nucleus pulposus
L5
Laminae

Plate 9

MUSCLES OF THE BODY

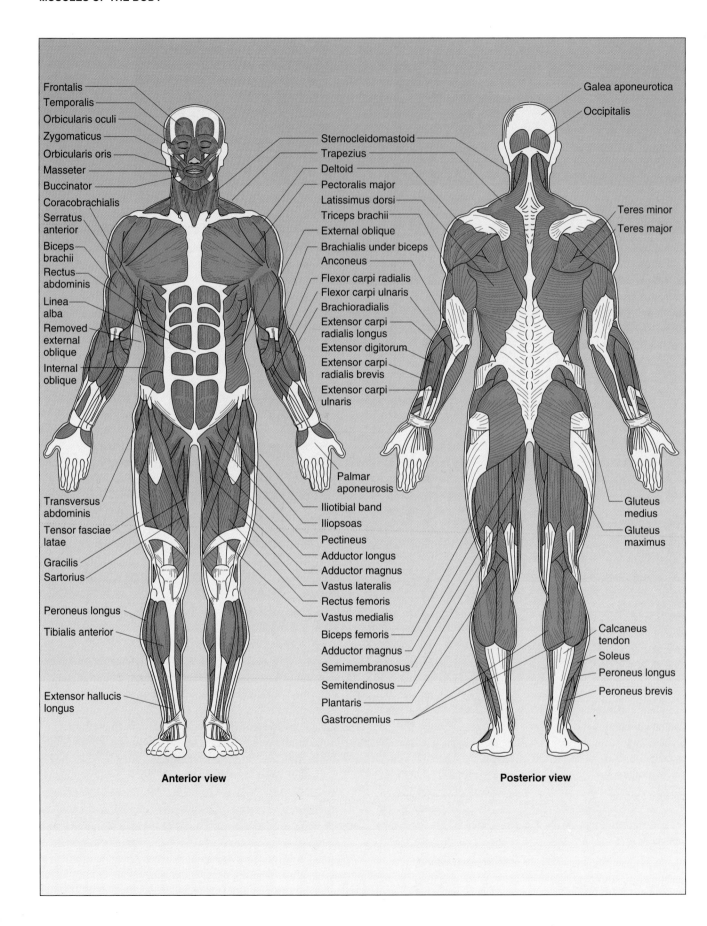

Frontalis
Temporalis
Orbicularis oculi
Zygomaticus
Orbicularis oris
Masseter
Buccinator
Coracobrachialis
Serratus anterior
Biceps brachii
Rectus abdominis
Linea alba
Removed external oblique
Internal oblique

Sternocleidomastoid
Trapezius
Deltoid
Pectoralis major
Latissimus dorsi
Triceps brachii
External oblique
Brachialis under biceps
Anconeus
Flexor carpi radialis
Flexor carpi ulnaris
Brachioradialis
Extensor carpi radialis longus
Extensor digitorum
Extensor carpi radialis brevis
Extensor carpi ulnaris

Palmar aponeurosis

Iliotibial band
Iliopsoas
Pectineus
Adductor longus
Adductor magnus
Vastus lateralis
Rectus femoris
Vastus medialis

Biceps femoris
Adductor magnus
Semimembranosus
Semitendinosus
Plantaris
Gastrocnemius

Transversus abdominis
Tensor fasciae latae
Gracilis
Sartorius
Peroneus longus
Tibialis anterior
Extensor hallucis longus

Galea aponeurotica
Occipitalis

Teres minor
Teres major

Gluteus medius
Gluteus maximus

Calcaneus tendon
Soleus
Peroneus longus
Peroneus brevis

Anterior view

Posterior view

Plate 10

THE ARCHITECTURE OF THE THREE TYPES OF MUSCLE

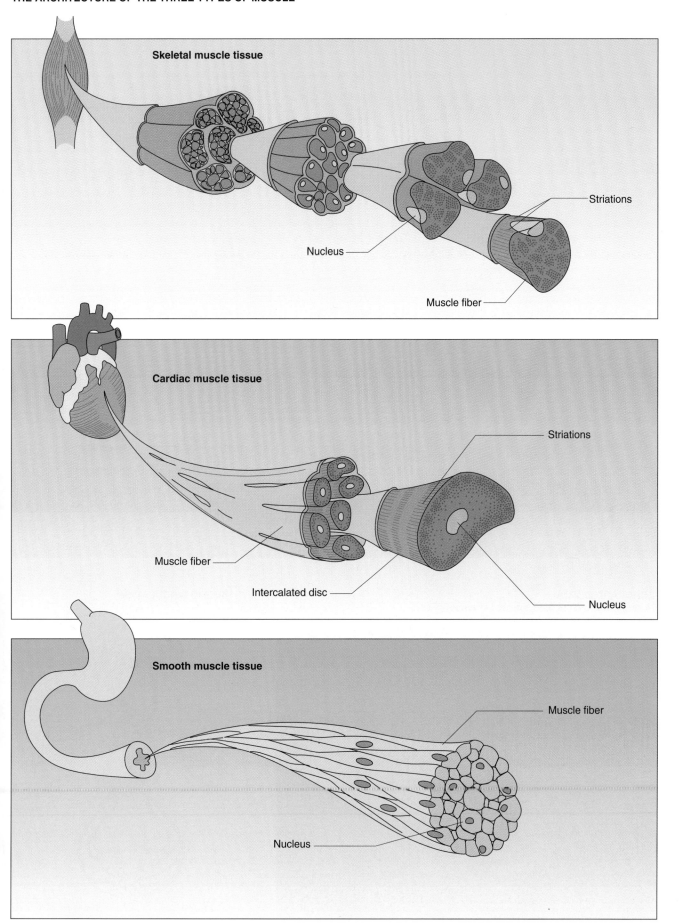

Skeletal muscle tissue

Striations

Nucleus

Muscle fiber

Cardiac muscle tissue

Striations

Muscle fiber

Intercalated disc

Nucleus

Smooth muscle tissue

Muscle fiber

Nucleus

Plate 11

THE HEART

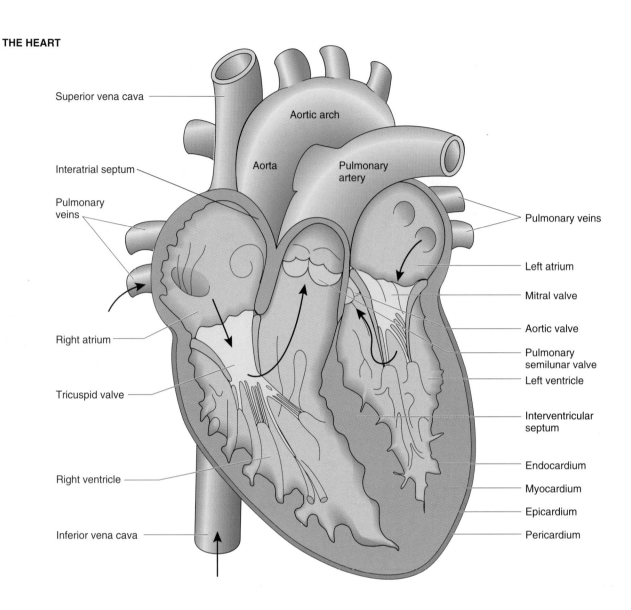

Superior vena cava

Aortic arch

Aorta

Pulmonary artery

Interatrial septum

Pulmonary veins

Pulmonary veins

Left atrium

Mitral valve

Aortic valve

Right atrium

Pulmonary semilunar valve

Left ventricle

Tricuspid valve

Interventricular septum

Endocardium

Myocardium

Right ventricle

Epicardium

Inferior vena cava

Pericardium

ECHOCARDIOGRAM
Normal, two dimensional, apical 4 chamber view
(standard view of American Society)

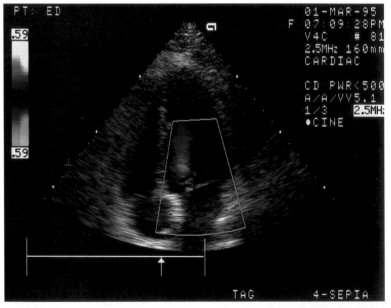

BLOOD CIRCULATION

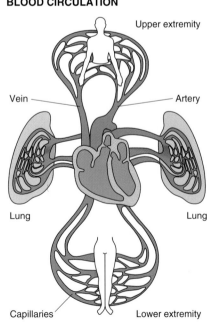

Upper extremity

Vein

Artery

Lung

Lung

Capillaries

Lower extremity

Plate 12

**ANTERIOR VIEW OF
CORONARY ARTERIES**

**POSTERIOR VIEW OF
CORONARY ARTERIES**

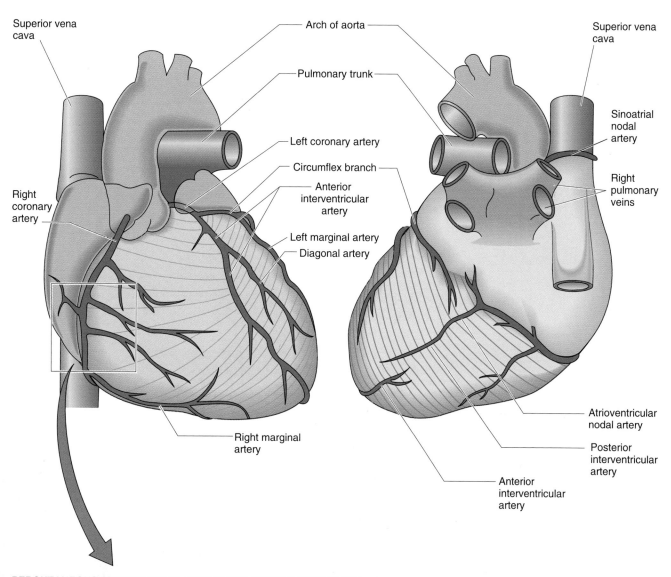

Superior vena
cava

Arch of aorta

Pulmonary trunk

Left coronary artery

Circumflex branch

Anterior
interventricular
artery

Left marginal artery

Diagonal artery

Right
coronary
artery

Right marginal
artery

Superior vena
cava

Sinoatrial
nodal
artery

Right
pulmonary
veins

Atrioventricular
nodal artery

Posterior
interventricular
artery

Anterior
interventricular
artery

PERCUTANEOUS TRANSLUMINAL CORONARY ANGIOPLASTY (PTCA)

Pre-dilation angiogram revealing 99%
stenosis of the right coronary artery (RCA).

PTCA procedure showing catheter
placement and straddling of the balloon
at the occluded site.

Post PTCA angiogram showing
successful dilation.

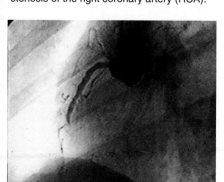

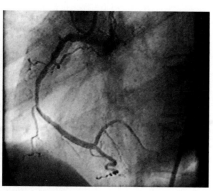

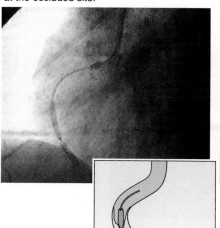

Catheter and wire placement
with balloon inflation.

ARTERIAL BLOOD CIRCULATION

Plate 13

Arteries (carry blood from the heart)

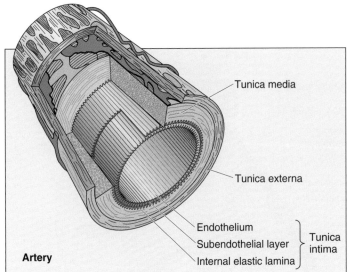

Tunica media

Tunica externa

Endothelium
Subendothelial layer } Tunica intima
Internal elastic lamina

Artery

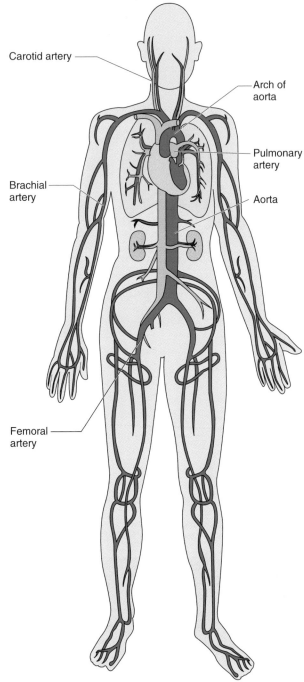

Carotid artery

Arch of aorta

Pulmonary artery

Brachial artery

Aorta

Femoral artery

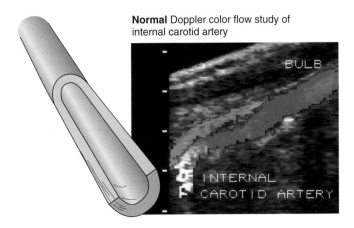

Normal Doppler color flow study of internal carotid artery

BULB

INTERNAL CAROTID ARTERY

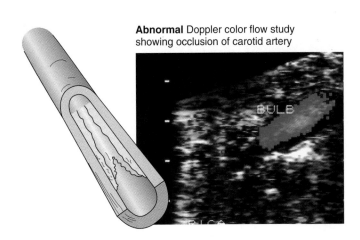

Abnormal Doppler color flow study showing occlusion of carotid artery

BULB

Plate 14

VENOUS CIRCULATION

Veins (carry blood to the heart)

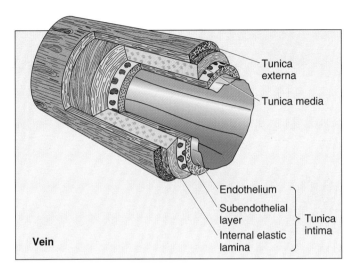

Tunica externa

Tunica media

Endothelium

Subendothelial layer

Internal elastic lamina

Tunica intima

Vein

FEMORAL THROMBUS

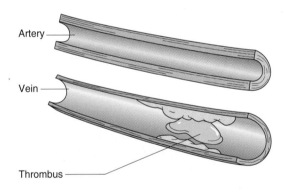

Artery

Vein

Thrombus

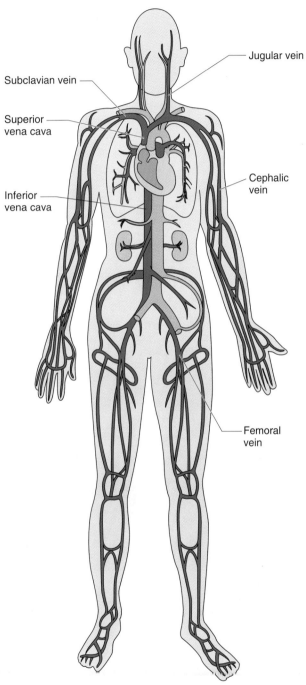

Subclavian vein

Superior vena cava

Inferior vena cava

Jugular vein

Cephalic vein

Femoral vein

Color flow Doppler showing femoral vein thrombus

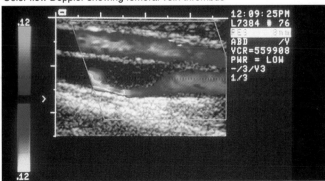

Plate 15

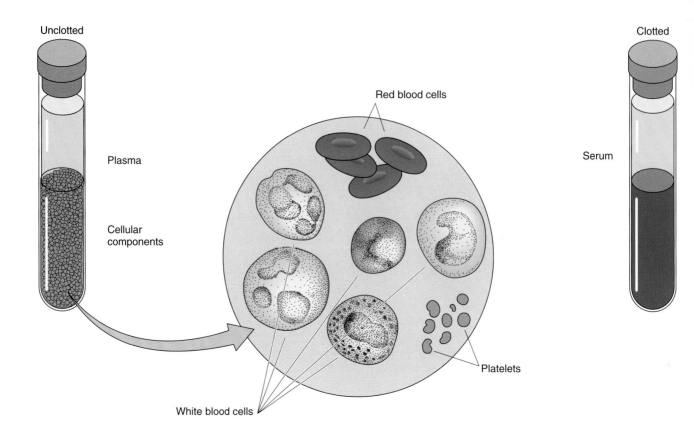

Unclotted

Plasma

Cellular components

Red blood cells

Platelets

White blood cells

Clotted

Serum

CELLULAR COMPONENTS OF THE BLOOD

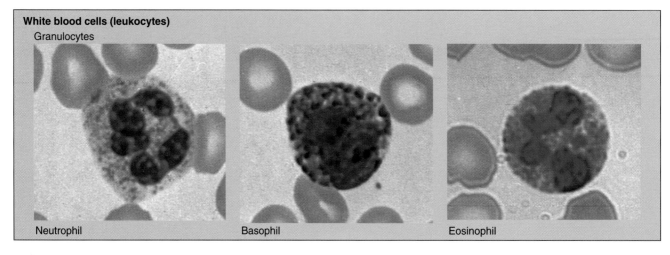

White blood cells (leukocytes)
Granulocytes

Neutrophil

Basophil

Eosinophil

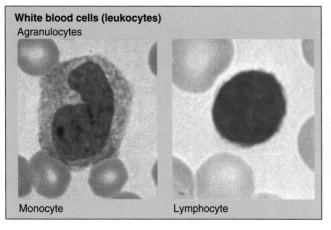

White blood cells (leukocytes)
Agranulocytes

Monocyte

Lymphocyte

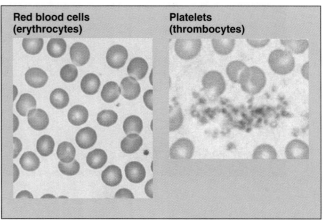

Red blood cells (erythrocytes)

Platelets (thrombocytes)

Plate 16

THE LYMPHATIC SYSTEM

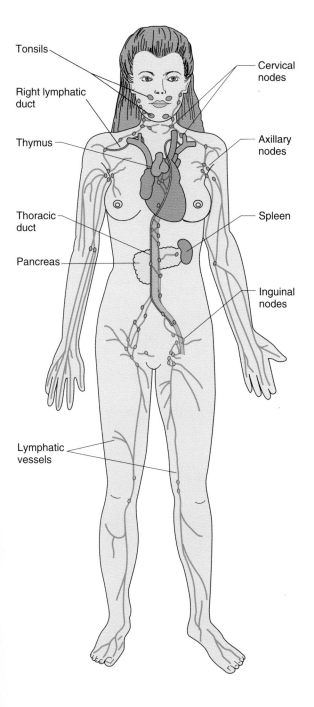

Tonsils

Right lymphatic duct

Thymus

Thoracic duct

Pancreas

Lymphatic vessels

Cervical nodes

Axillary nodes

Spleen

Inguinal nodes

LYMPHATIC DRAINAGE

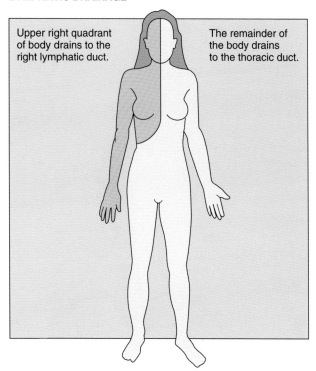

Upper right quadrant of body drains to the right lymphatic duct.

The remainder of the body drains to the thoracic duct.

BLOOD AND LYMPH CIRCULATION

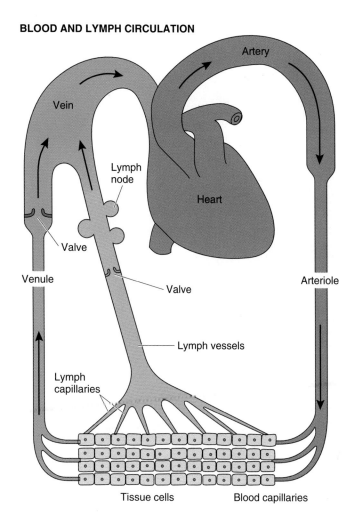

Vein

Artery

Lymph node

Heart

Valve

Venule

Valve

Arteriole

Lymph vessels

Lymph capillaries

Tissue cells

Blood capillaries

Plate 17

THE RESPIRATORY SYSTEM

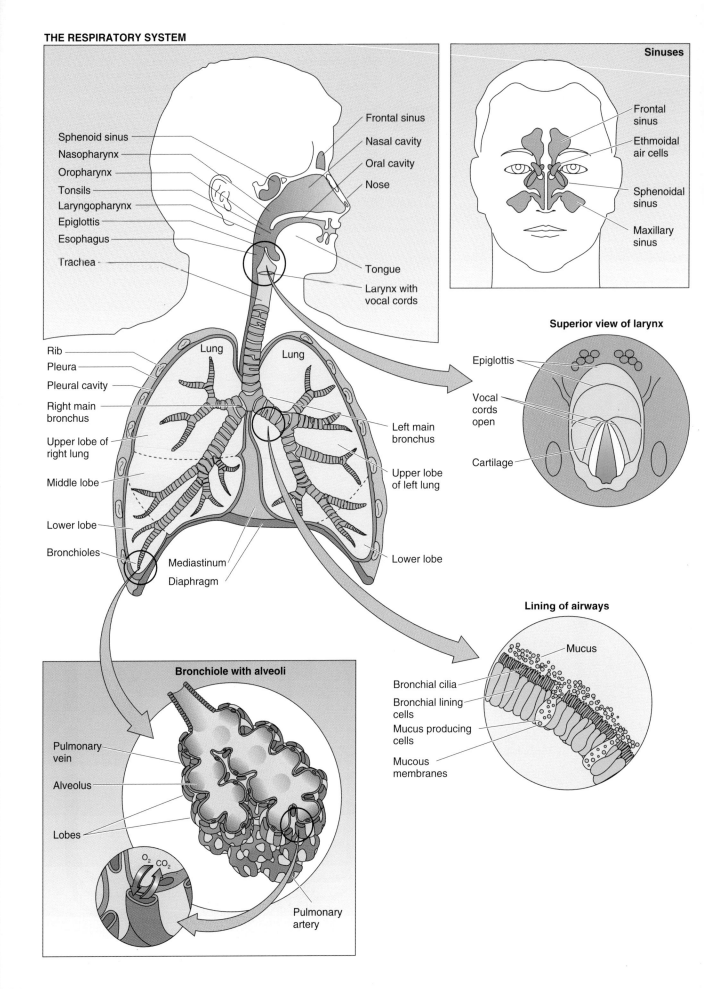

Sinuses

Sphenoid sinus
Nasopharynx
Oropharynx
Tonsils
Laryngopharynx
Epiglottis
Esophagus
Trachea

Frontal sinus
Nasal cavity
Oral cavity
Nose

Tongue
Larynx with vocal cords

Frontal sinus
Ethmoidal air cells
Sphenoidal sinus
Maxillary sinus

Rib
Pleura
Pleural cavity
Right main bronchus
Upper lobe of right lung
Middle lobe
Lower lobe
Bronchioles

Lung   Lung

Left main bronchus
Upper lobe of left lung
Lower lobe

Mediastinum
Diaphragm

Superior view of larynx

Epiglottis
Vocal cords open
Cartilage

Lining of airways

Mucus
Bronchial cilia
Bronchial lining cells
Mucus producing cells
Mucous membranes

Bronchiole with alveoli

Pulmonary vein
Alveolus
Lobes

O_2 CO_2

Pulmonary artery

BRONCHOSCOPY

Plate 18

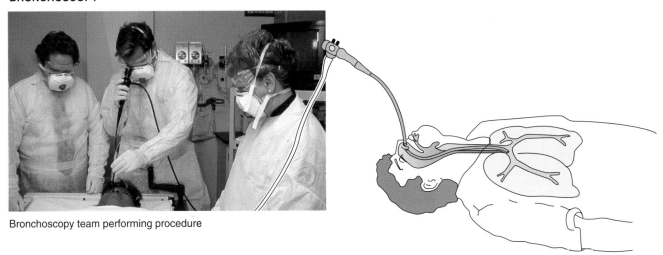

Bronchoscopy team performing procedure

Area of carina

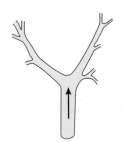

Bronchoscopic views

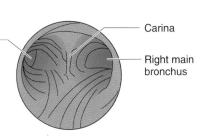

Left main bronchus

Carina

Right main bronchus

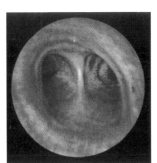

Blood clot

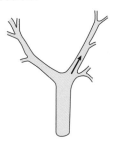

Blood clot occluding right main bronchus

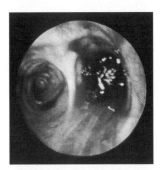

Mucus plug

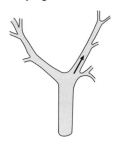

Mucus plug occluding right main bronchus

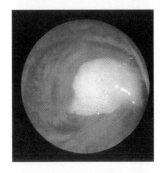

Foreign body

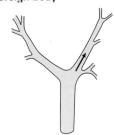

Embedded foreign body

Right upper orifice

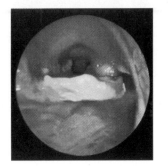

Plate 19

THE BRAIN

Corpus callosum

Meninges

Thalamus

Pineal body

Frontal sinus

Hypothalamus

Pituitary gland

Sphenoid sinus

Pons

Medulla oblongata

Cerebellum

Spinal cord

Midsagittal view of brain

Cranium

Venous sinus

Meninges { Dura mater
Arachnoid
Pia mater

Subdural space

Subarachnoid space

Cerebrum

Magnetic resonance imaging (MRI) of normal brain, midsagittal view

Plate 20

LOBES OF THE BRAIN

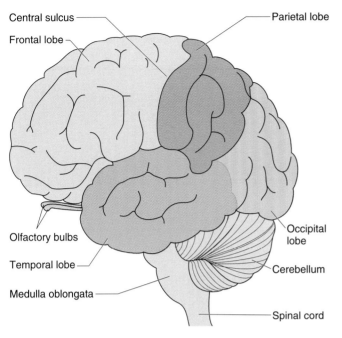

Central sulcus
Frontal lobe
Parietal lobe
Olfactory bulbs
Temporal lobe
Medulla oblongata
Occipital lobe
Cerebellum
Spinal cord

LOCALIZED FUNCTIONS OF THE CEREBRUM

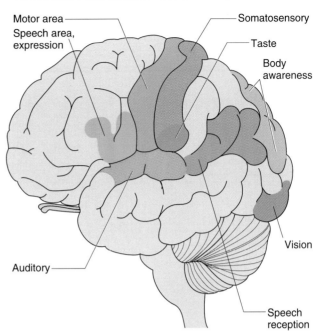

Motor area
Speech area, expression
Somatosensory
Taste
Body awareness
Auditory
Vision
Speech reception

VENTRICLES OF THE BRAIN

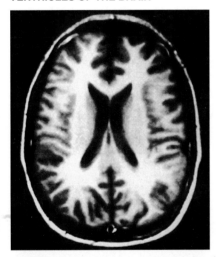

Magnetic resonance image, horizontal view A

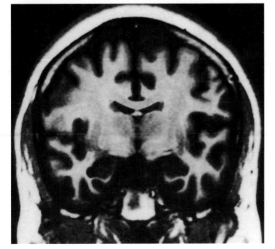

Magnetic resonance image, coronal view B

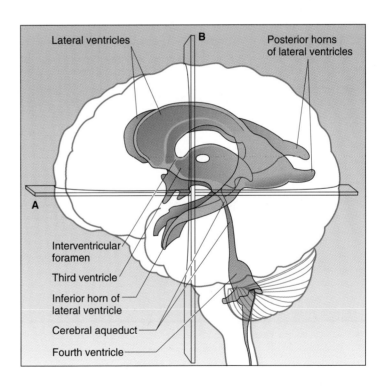

Lateral ventricles
B
Posterior horns of lateral ventricles
A
Interventricular foramen
Third ventricle
Inferior horn of lateral ventricle
Cerebral aqueduct
Fourth ventricle

Plate 21

THE PERIPHERAL NERVOUS SYSTEM

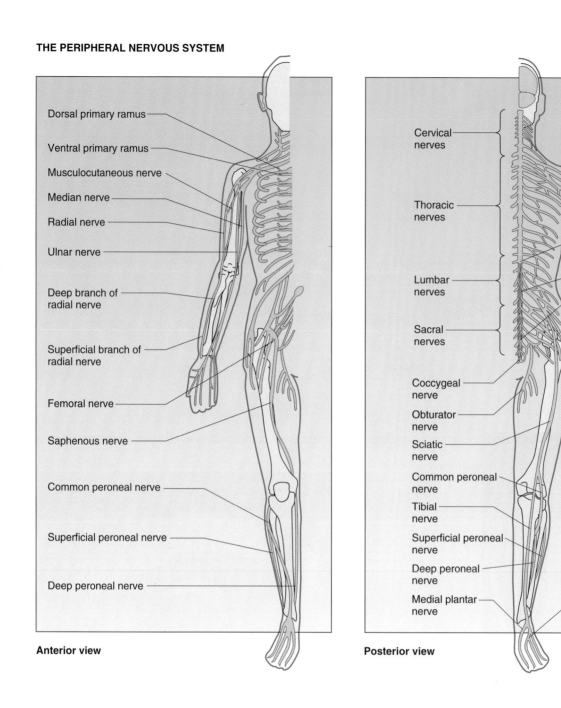

Dorsal primary ramus

Ventral primary ramus

Musculocutaneous nerve

Median nerve

Radial nerve

Ulnar nerve

Deep branch of
radial nerve

Superficial branch of
radial nerve

Femoral nerve

Saphenous nerve

Common peroneal nerve

Superficial peroneal nerve

Deep peroneal nerve

Anterior view

Cervical
nerves

Thoracic
nerves

Lumbar
nerves

Sacral
nerves

Coccygeal
nerve

Obturator
nerve

Sciatic
nerve

Common peroneal
nerve

Tibial
nerve

Superficial peroneal
nerve

Deep peroneal
nerve

Medial plantar
nerve

Filum
terminale

Cauda
equina

Lateral plantar
nerve

Posterior view

A NEURON

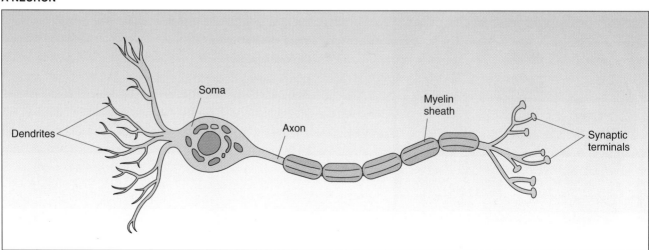

Dendrites

Soma

Axon

Myelin
sheath

Synaptic
terminals

Plate 22

BRAIN DIAGNOSTIC AND IMAGING TECHNIQUES

Electroencephalography (EEG)

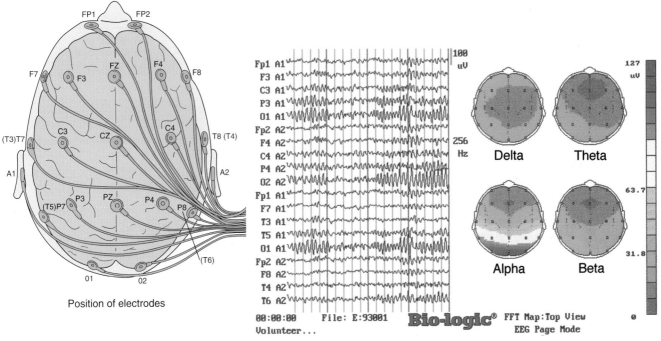

Position of electrodes

Normal EEG wave forms shown on left and computer compilation of frequency bands (delta, theta, alpha, and beta) mapped on right

Positron emission tomography (PET) scans

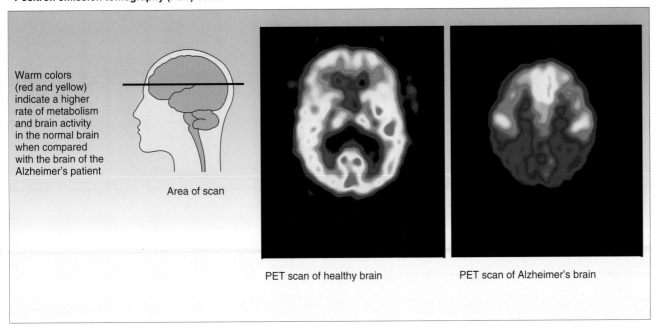

Warm colors (red and yellow) indicate a higher rate of metabolism and brain activity in the normal brain when compared with the brain of the Alzheimer's patient

Area of scan

PET scan of healthy brain

PET scan of Alzheimer's brain

Plate 23

THE ENDOCRINE SYSTEM

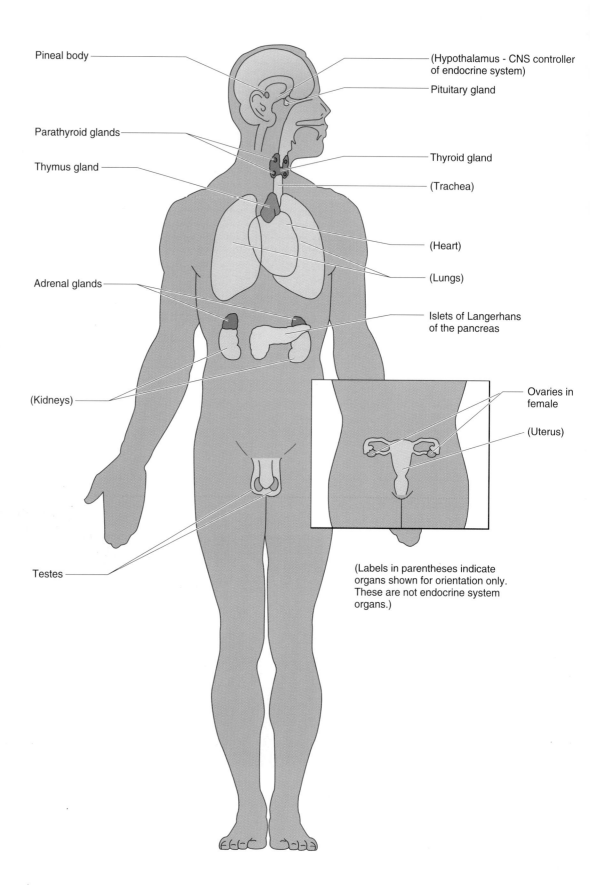

Pineal body

(Hypothalamus - CNS controller of endocrine system)

Pituitary gland

Parathyroid glands

Thyroid gland

Thymus gland

(Trachea)

(Heart)

(Lungs)

Adrenal glands

Islets of Langerhans of the pancreas

(Kidneys)

Ovaries in female

(Uterus)

Testes

(Labels in parentheses indicate organs shown for orientation only. These are not endocrine system organs.)

Plate 24

Endocrine gland	Secretions	Function
* Anterior pituitary (adenohypophysis)	Thyroid-stimulating hormone (TSH)	Stimulates secretion from thyroid gland
	Adrenocorticotrophic hormone (ACTH)	Stimulates secretion from adrenal cortex
	Follicle-stimulating hormone (FSH)	Initiates growth of ovarian follicle; stimulates secretion of estrogen in females and sperm production in males
	Luteinizing hormone (LH)	Causes ovulation; stimulates secretion of progesterone by corpus luteum; causes secretion of testosterone in testes
	Melanocyte-stimulating hormone (MSH)	Affects skin pigmentation
	Growth hormone (GH)	Influences growth
	Prolactin (lactogenic hormone)	Stimulates breast development and milk production during pregnancy
* Posterior pituitary (neurohypophysis)	Antidiuretic hormone (ADH)	Influences the absorption of water by kidney tubules
	Oxytocin	Influences uterine contraction
Pineal body	Melatonin	Exact function unknown, affects onset of puberty
	Serotonin	Serves as a precursor to melatonin
Thyroid gland	Triiodothyronine (T_3), thyroxine (T_4)	Regulate metabolism
	Calcitonin	Regulates calcium and phosphorus metabolism
Parathyroid glands	Parathyroid hormone (PTH)	Regulates calcium and phosphorus metabolism
Pancreas (islets of Langerhans)	Insulin, glucagon	Regulates carbohydrate/sugar metabolism
Thymus gland	Thymosin	Regulates immune response
Adrenal glands (suprarenal glands)	Steroid hormones: glucocorticoids, mineral corticosteroids, androgens	Regulate carbohydrate metabolism and salt and water balence; some effect on sexual characteristics.
	Epinephrine, norepinephrine	Affect sympathetic nervous system in stress response
Ovaries	Estrogen, progesterone	Responsible for the development of female secondary sex characteristics, and regulation of reproduction
Testes	Testosterone	Affects masculinization and reproduction

* Release of hormones in pituitary is controlled by hypothalamus

Plate 25

THE EYE

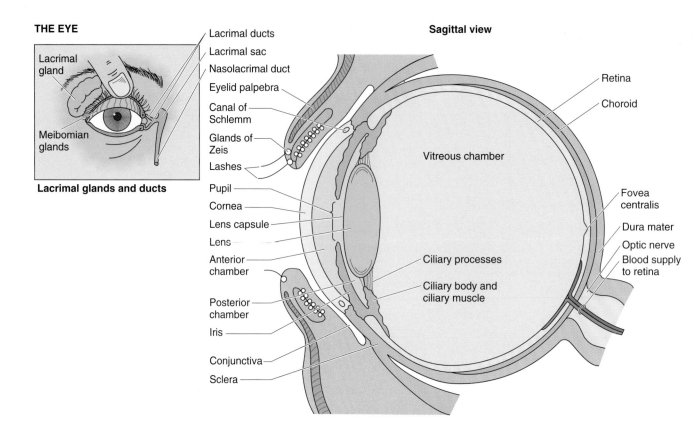

Lacrimal gland

Meibomian glands

Lacrimal glands and ducts

Lacrimal ducts
Lacrimal sac
Nasolacrimal duct
Eyelid palpebra
Canal of Schlemm
Glands of Zeis
Lashes
Pupil
Cornea
Lens capsule
Lens
Anterior chamber
Posterior chamber
Iris
Conjunctiva
Sclera

Sagittal view

Vitreous chamber

Ciliary processes

Ciliary body and ciliary muscle

Retina
Choroid
Fovea centralis
Dura mater
Optic nerve
Blood supply to retina

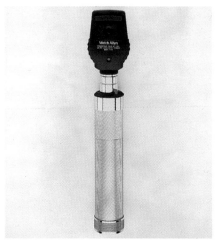

Ophthalmoscope

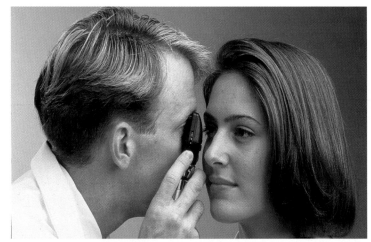

Doctor examining patient using ophthalmoscope

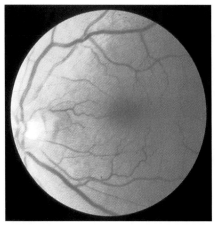

Normal retina

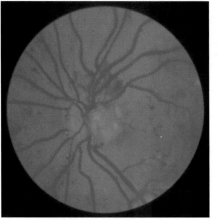

Aneurysms seen in proliferative diabetic retinopathy

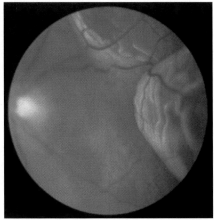

Retinal detachment

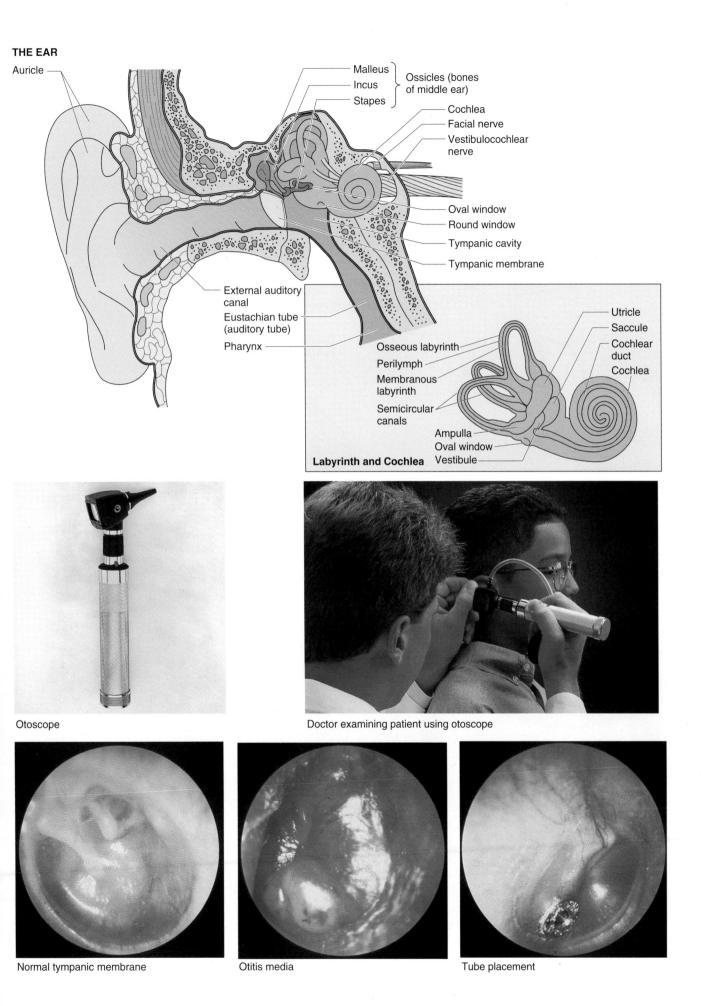

Auricle

Malleus
Incus
Stapes
Ossicles (bones of middle ear)

Cochlea
Facial nerve
Vestibulocochlear nerve

Oval window
Round window
Tympanic cavity
Tympanic membrane

External auditory canal
Eustachian tube (auditory tube)
Pharynx

Osseous labyrinth
Perilymph
Membranous labyrinth
Semicircular canals

Utricle
Saccule
Cochlear duct
Cochlea

Ampulla
Oval window
Vestibule

Labyrinth and Cochlea

Otoscope

Doctor examining patient using otoscope

Normal tympanic membrane

Otitis media

Tube placement

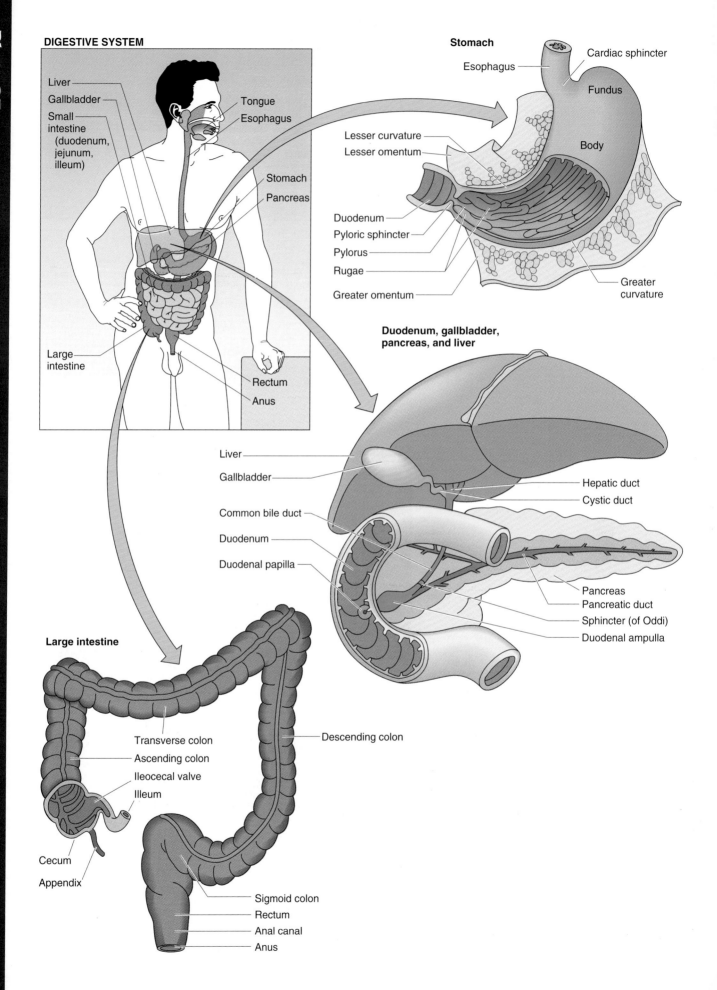

Plate 27

DIGESTIVE SYSTEM

Liver
Gallbladder
Small intestine (duodenum, jejunum, illeum)
Tongue
Esophagus
Stomach
Pancreas
Large intestine
Rectum
Anus

Stomach

Esophagus
Cardiac sphincter
Fundus
Body
Lesser curvature
Lesser omentum
Duodenum
Pyloric sphincter
Pylorus
Rugae
Greater omentum
Greater curvature

Duodenum, gallbladder, pancreas, and liver

Liver
Gallbladder
Common bile duct
Duodenum
Duodenal papilla
Hepatic duct
Cystic duct
Pancreas
Pancreatic duct
Sphincter (of Oddi)
Duodenal ampulla

Large intestine

Transverse colon
Ascending colon
Ileocecal valve
Illeum
Cecum
Appendix
Descending colon
Sigmoid colon
Rectum
Anal canal
Anus

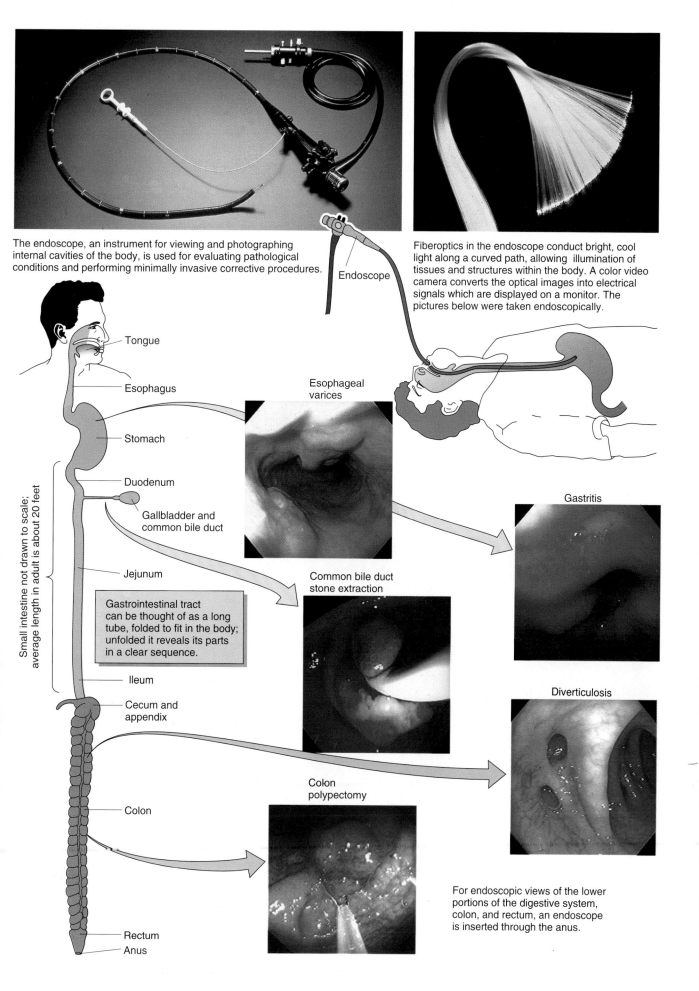

Plate 28

The endoscope, an instrument for viewing and photographing internal cavities of the body, is used for evaluating pathological conditions and performing minimally invasive corrective procedures.

Endoscope

Fiberoptics in the endoscope conduct bright, cool light along a curved path, allowing illumination of tissues and structures within the body. A color video camera converts the optical images into electrical signals which are displayed on a monitor. The pictures below were taken endoscopically.

Tongue

Esophagus

Esophageal varices

Stomach

Duodenum

Gallbladder and common bile duct

Gastritis

Jejunum

Small intestine not drawn to scale; average length in adult is about 20 feet

Common bile duct stone extraction

Gastrointestinal tract can be thought of as a long tube, folded to fit in the body; unfolded it reveals its parts in a clear sequence.

Ileum

Cecum and appendix

Diverticulosis

Colon polypectomy

Colon

For endoscopic views of the lower portions of the digestive system, colon, and rectum, an endoscope is inserted through the anus.

Rectum

Anus

Plate 29

THE URINARY SYSTEM

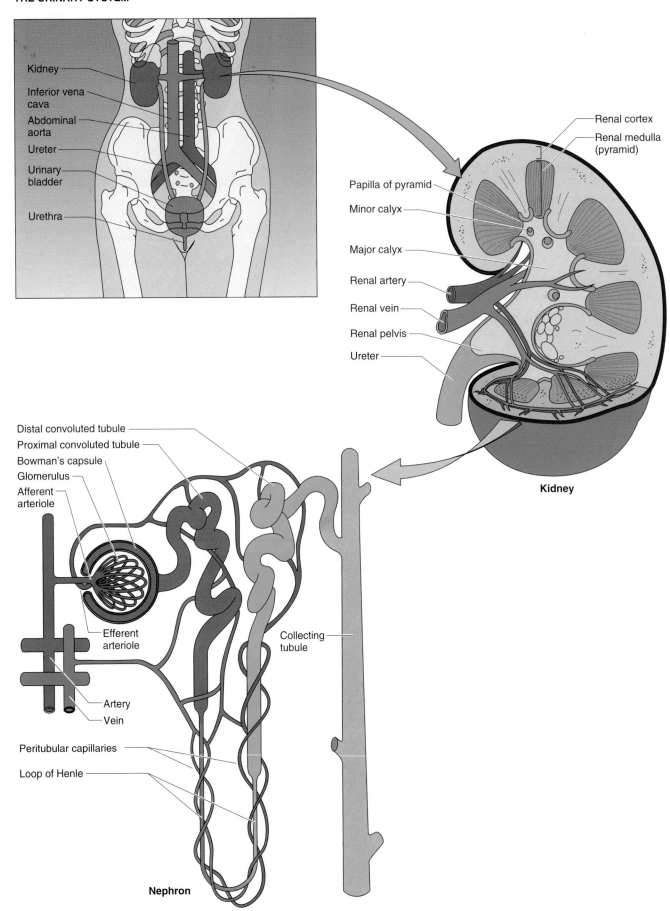

Kidney
Inferior vena cava
Abdominal aorta
Ureter
Urinary bladder
Urethra

Renal cortex
Renal medulla (pyramid)
Papilla of pyramid
Minor calyx
Major calyx
Renal artery
Renal vein
Renal pelvis
Ureter

Kidney

Distal convoluted tubule
Proximal convoluted tubule
Bowman's capsule
Glomerulus
Afferent arteriole
Efferent arteriole
Artery
Vein
Peritubular capillaries
Loop of Henle
Collecting tubule

Nephron

THE MALE REPRODUCTIVE SYSTEM

Plate 30

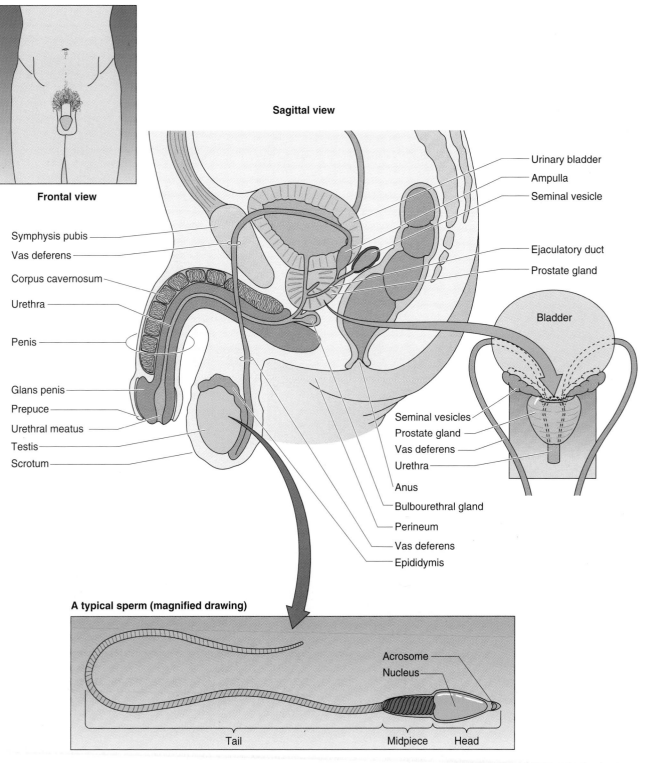

Frontal view

Sagittal view

Symphysis pubis

Vas deferens

Corpus cavernosum

Urethra

Penis

Glans penis

Prepuce

Urethral meatus

Testis

Scrotum

Urinary bladder

Ampulla

Seminal vesicle

Ejaculatory duct

Prostate gland

Bladder

Seminal vesicles

Prostate gland

Vas deferens

Urethra

Anus

Bulbourethral gland

Perineum

Vas deferens

Epididymis

A typical sperm (magnified drawing)

Acrosome

Nucleus

Tail

Midpiece

Head

Abnormal sperm

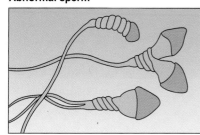

Plate 31

THE FEMALE REPRODUCTIVE SYSTEM

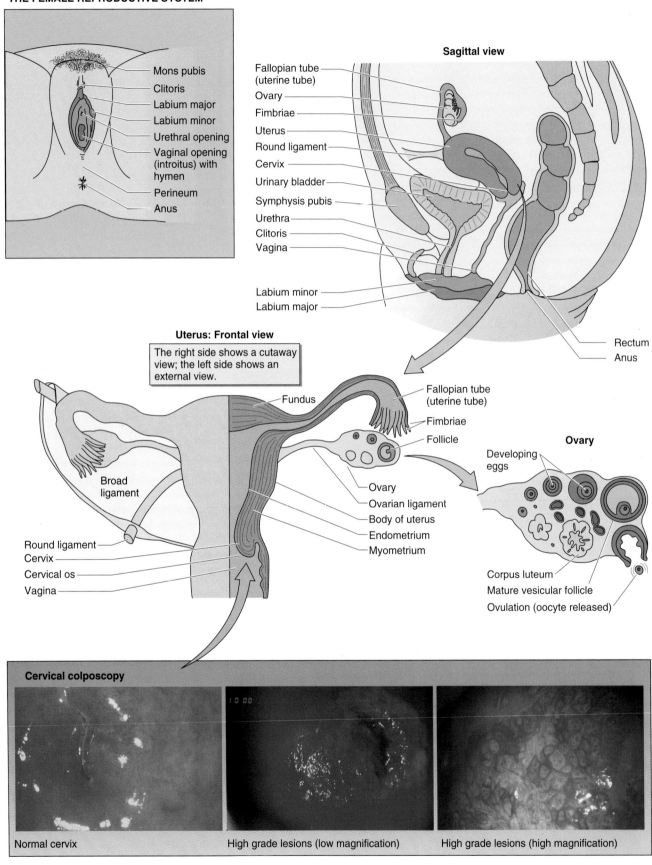

Mons pubis
Clitoris
Labium major
Labium minor
Urethral opening
Vaginal opening (introitus) with hymen
Perineum
Anus

Sagittal view

Fallopian tube (uterine tube)
Ovary
Fimbriae
Uterus
Round ligament
Cervix
Urinary bladder
Symphysis pubis
Urethra
Clitoris
Vagina
Labium minor
Labium major
Rectum
Anus

Uterus: Frontal view

The right side shows a cutaway view; the left side shows an external view.

Fundus
Fallopian tube (uterine tube)
Fimbriae
Follicle
Broad ligament
Ovary
Ovarian ligament
Body of uterus
Endometrium
Myometrium
Round ligament
Cervix
Cervical os
Vagina

Ovary

Developing eggs
Corpus luteum
Mature vesicular follicle
Ovulation (oocyte released)

Cervical colposcopy

Normal cervix
High grade lesions (low magnification)
High grade lesions (high magnification)

Plate 32

Sperm and ovum

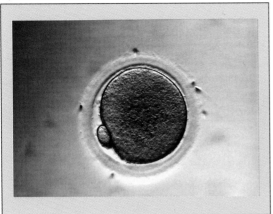

Obstetrical sonograms

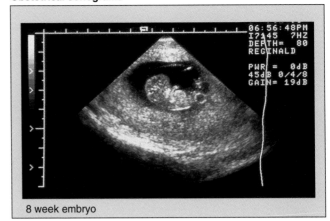

8 week embryo

Fetus in utero

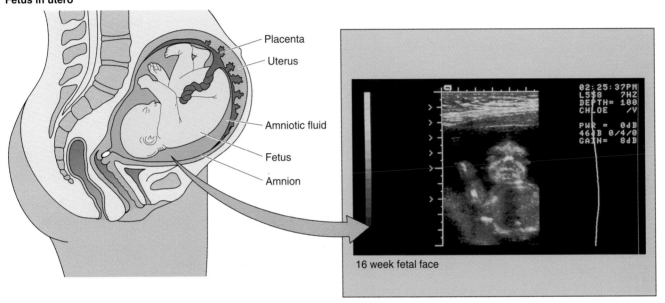

Placenta

Uterus

Amniotic fluid

Fetus

Amnion

16 week fetal face

Breast

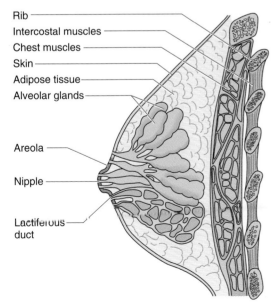

Rib

Intercostal muscles

Chest muscles

Skin

Adipose tissue

Alveolar glands

Areola

Nipple

Lactiferous
duct

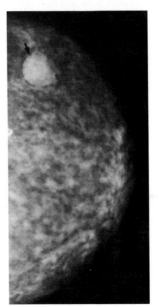

Mammogram showing breast lump

A33

5 Integumentary System

OBJECTIVES

After completion of this chapter you will be able to

1. **Define common combining forms used in relation to the integumentary system**

2. **Define basic anatomical terms related to the integumentary system**

3. **Identify common symptomatic, diagnostic, operative, and therapeutic terms referring to the integumentary system**

4. **List common diagnostic tests and procedures related to the integumentary system**

5. **Explain the terms and abbreviations used in documenting medical records involving the integumentary system**

Combining Forms

Combining Form	Meaning	Example
adip/o	fat	**adiposis** ad-i-pō′sis
lip/o		**lipoma** li-pō′ma
steat/o		**steatoma** stē-ă-tō′mă
derm/o	skin	**hypodermic** hī′pō-der′mik
dermat/o		**dermatology** der-mă-tol′ō-jē
cutane/o		**subcutaneous** sŭb-kyū-tā′nē-ŭs
diaphor/o	profuse sweating	**diaphoretic** dī-ă-fō-ret′ik
erythr/o	red	**erythrodermatitis** ĕ-rith-rō-der′mă-tī′tis
hidr/o	sweat	**anhidrosis** an-hī-drō′sis
hist/o	tissue	**histology** his-tol′ō-jē
histi/o		**histiogenic** his′tē-ō-jen′ik
kerat/o	hard	**keratosis** ker-ă-tō′sis
leuk/o	white	**leukonychia** lū-kō-nik′ē′ă
melan/o	black	**melanocyte** mel′ă-nō-sīt
myc/o	fungus	**mycosis** mī-kō′sis
onych/o	nail	**onychodystrophy** on′i-kō-dis′trō-fē
plas/o	formation	**dysplastic** dis-plas′tik
purpur/o	purple	**purpuric** pŭr′pū′rik

continued

Combining Form	Meaning	Example
seb/o	sebum (oil)	**seborrhea** seb-ō-rē′ă
squam/o	scale	**squamous** skwā′mŭs
trich/o	hair	**trichorrhexis** trik-ō-rek′sis
xer/o	dry	**xerosis** zē-rō′sis
xanth/o	yellow	**xanthoma** zan-thō′mă

Integumentary System Overview

The integumentary system is composed of the skin (also called the *integument*) and its appendages, including hair, nails, sweat glands, and sebaceous glands. It protects the body from injury or intrusion of microorganisms, helps microorganisms, helps regulate body temperature, and houses the receptors for the sense of touch, including pain and sensation (Fig. 5.1).

The skin is the largest organ in the body. Skin layers are divided into an outer layer called the epidermis and an inner layer called the dermis.

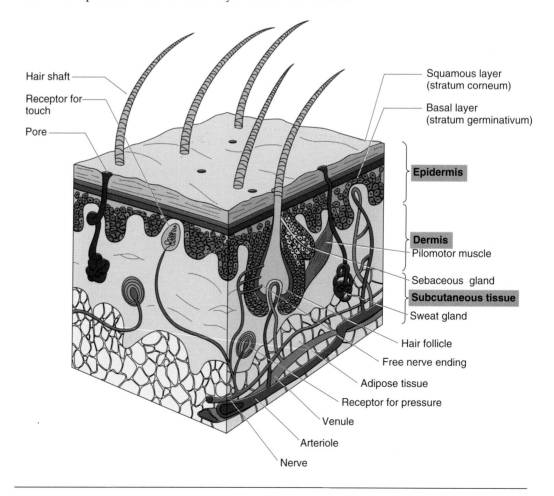

Figure 5.1. The skin.

Epidermis

The epidermis consists of several layers of stratified squamous (scale-like) epithelium. The two significant layers are the innermost layer, known as the *basal layer* (stratum germinativum), and the outermost layer, called the *squamous layer* (stratum corneum). The cells of the basal layer are constantly being produced, moving the older cells up toward the surface. As these cells are being pushed up, they flatten, become filled with a hard protein substance called *keratin*, and soon die. As a result, many layers of tightly packed dead cells accumulate in the outermost squamous layer where they are sloughed off from the surface of the skin.

Melanocytes, which produce the pigment called *melanin* that gives color to the skin, are found in the basal layer.

Dermis

The dermis, also called the *corium*, is the connective tissue layer; it contains blood and lymphatic vessels, nerves and nerve endings, glands, and hair follicles within a network of elastic and collagen fibers. Collagen is a fibrous protein material that is tough and resistant. These fibers give the skin its qualities of toughness and elasticity.

Subcutaneous Layer

The subcutaneous layer is below the dermis and is composed of loose connective tissue and adipose (fatty) tissue.

Anatomical Terms

Term	Meaning
epithelium ep-i-thē′lē-ŭm	cells covering external and internal surfaces of the body
epidermis ep-i-derm′is	thin, cellular outer layer of the skin
squamous cell layer skwā′mŭs	flat scale-like epithelial cells comprising outermost layers of epidermis
basal layer bā′săl	deepest region of epidermis
melanocyte mel′ă-nō-sīt	a cell found in the basal layer that gives color to the skin
melanin mel′ă-nin	dark brown to black pigment contained in melanocytes
dermis	dense, fibrous connective tissue layer of the skin (also known as corium)
sebaceous glands sē-bā′shŭs	oil glands in the skin

continued

Term	Meaning
sebum se′bŭm	oily substance secreted by the sebaceous glands
sudoriferous glands sū-dō-rif′er-ŭs	sweat glands (sudor = sweat; ferre = to bear)
subcutaneous layer sŭb-kyū-ta′ne-ŭs	connective and adipose tissue layer just under the dermis
collagen kol′lă-jen	protein substance found in skin and connective tissue (koila = glue; gen = producing)
hair	outgrowth of the skin composed of keratin
nail	outgrowth of the skin attached to the distal end of each finger and toe, composed of keratin
keratin ker′ă-tin	hard protein material found in the epidermis, hair, and nails

Symptomatic Terms

Term	Meaning
lesion le′zhŭn	an area of pathologically altered tissue (two types: primary and secondary) (Fig. 5.2) (see Color Atlas, plate 4)
primary lesions	lesions arising from previously normal skin

Flat, Nonpalpable Changes in Skin Color

macule mak′yūl	a flat discolored spot on the skin up to 1 cm across (e.g., a freckle)
patch	a flat discolored area on the skin larger than 1 cm (e.g., vitiligo)

Elevated, Palpable, Solid Masses

papule pap′yūl	a solid mass on the skin up to 0.5 cm in diameter [e.g., a nevus (mole)]
plaque plāk	a solid mass greater than 1 cm in diameter, limited to the surface of the skin
nodule nod′yūl	a solid mass greater than 1 cm, which extends deeper into the epidermis
tumor tu′mŏr	solid mass larger than 1–2 cm
wheal hwēl	an area of localized skin edema (swelling) (e.g., a hive)

Elevation Formed by Fluid within a Cavity

vesicle ves′ĭ-kl	little bladder; an elevated fluid-filled sac (blister) within or under the epidermis up to 0.5 cm diameter (e.g., a fever blister)
bulla bul′ă	a blister larger than 0.5 cm (e.g., a second degree burn) (bulla = bubble)

continued

PRIMARY LESIONS

Flat discolored, nonpalpable changes in skin color

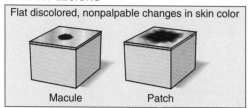

Elevated, palpable solid masses

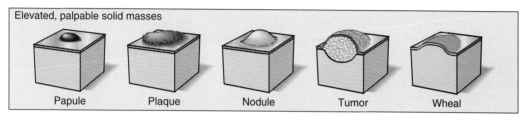

Elevation formed by fluid in a cavity

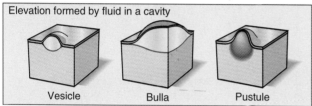

SECONDARY LESIONS

Loss of skin surface

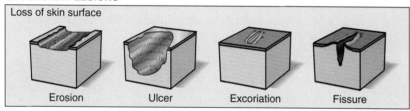

Material on skin surface

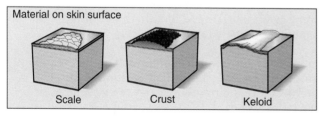

VASCULAR LESIONS

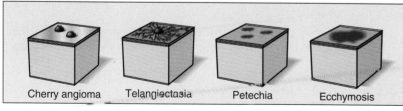

Figure 5.2. Types of primary, secondary, and vascular lesions.

Term	Meaning
pustule pŭs′chūl	a pus filled sac (e.g., a pimple)
secondary lesions	lesions that result in changes in primary lesions
Loss of Skin Surface	
erosion ē-rō′zhŭn	to gnaw away; loss of superficial epidermis leaving an area of moisture but no bleeding (e.g., area of moisture after rupture of a vesicle)
ulcer	an open sore on the skin or mucous membrane that can bleed and scar and is sometimes accompanied by infection (e.g., decubitus ulcer)
excoriation eks-kō′rē-ā′shŭn	a scratch mark
fissure fish′ŭr	a linear crack in the skin
Material on Skin Surface	
scale	a thin flake of exfoliated epidermis (e.g., dandruff)
crust	dried residue of serum (body liquid), pus, or blood on the skin (e.g., in impetigo)
Other Secondary Lesions	
cicatrix of the skin sik′ă-triks	mark left by the healing of a sore or wound showing the replacement of destroyed tissue by fibrous tissue (cicatrix = scar)
keloid kē′loyd	an abnormal overgrowth of scar tissue that is thick and irregular (kele = tumor)
vascular lesions	lesions of a blood vessel
cherry angioma chār′ē an-jē-ō′mă	a small, round, bright red blood vessel tumor on the skin, often on the trunk of the elderly
telangiectasia tel-an′jē-ek-tā′zē-ă **spider angioma** spī′der an-jē-ō′mă	a tiny, red blood vessel lesion formed by the dilation of a group of blood vessels radiating from a central arteriole, most commonly seen on the face, neck, or chest (telos = end)
purpuric lesions pŭr′pū-rik	purpura; lesions as a result of hemorrhages into the skin
petechia pe-tē′ke-ă	spot; reddish-brown, minute hemorrhagic spots on the skin that indicate a bleeding tendency—small purpura
ecchymosis ek-i-mō′sis	bruise; a black and blue mark—large purpura (chymo = juice)
epidermal tumors	skin tumors arising from the epidermis
nevus nē′vŭs	birthmark; a congenital malformation on the skin that can be epidermal or vascular—also called a mole (see Color Atlas, plate 4)

continued

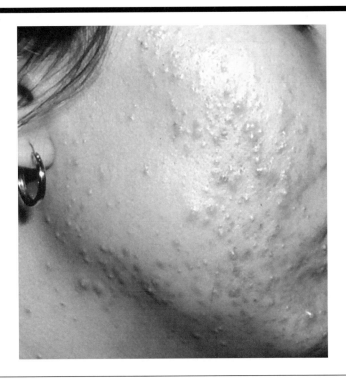

Figure 5.5. Acne.

Term	Meaning
rubeola rū-bē′ō-lă	reddish; 14-day measles
varicella var-ĭ-sel′ă	a tiny spot; chicken pox
eczema ek′zĕ-mă	to boil out; skin condition characterized by the appearance of inflamed, swollen papules and vesicles that crust and scale, often with sensations of itching and burning
furuncle fyū′rŭng-kl	boil; a painful nodule formed in the skin by inflammation originating in a hair follicle—caused by staphylococcosis
carbuncle kar′bŭng-kl	skin infection consisting of clusters of furuncles (carbo = small glowing embers)
abscess ab′ses	localized collection of pus in a cavity formed by the inflammation of surrounding tissues that heals when drained or excised (abscessus = a going away)
gangrene gang′grēn	an eating sore; death of tissue associated with a loss of blood supply
herpes simplex virus Type 1 (HSV-1) her′pēz	transient viral vesicles (e.g., cold sores or fever blisters) that infect the facial area, especially the mouth and nose (herpes = creeping skin disease)
herpes simplex virus Type 2 (HSV-2)	sexually transmitted ulcer-like lesions of the genital and anorectal skin and mucosa; after initial infection the virus lies dormant in the nerve cell root and may recur at times of stress (see Color Atlas, plate 4)

continued

Term	Meaning
herpes zoster her′pēz zos′ter	a viral disease affecting the peripheral nerves characterized by painful blisters that spread over the skin following the affected nerves, usually unilateral—also known as shingles (zoster = girdle)
impetigo im-pe-tī′gō	highly contagious, bacterial skin inflammation marked by pustules that rupture and become crusted—most often occurs around mouth and nostrils
keratoses ker-ă-tō′sez	thickened areas of epidermis
actinic keratoses ak-tin′ik	
solar keratoses	localized thickening of the skin caused by excessive exposure to sunlight—known precursor to cancer (actinic = ray; solar = sun)
seborrheic keratoses seb-ō-rē′ik	benign wart-like tumors (seen especially on elderly skin) (Fig. 5.6)
lupus lū′pŭs	a chronic autoimmune disease characterized by inflammation of various parts of the body (lupus = wolf)
cutaneous lupus kyū-tā′nē-ŭs	limited to the skin; evidenced by a characteristic rash especially on the face, neck and scalp
systemic lupus erythematosus (SLE) sis-tem′ik lū′pŭs er-i-them′ă-tō-sis	a more severe form of lupus involving the skin, joints, and often vital organs (e.g., lungs or kidneys)
malignant cutaneous neoplasm mă-lig′nănt kyū-tā′nē-ŭs nē′ō-plazm	skin cancer
squamous cell carcinoma skwā′mŭs sel kar-si-nō′mă	malignant tumor of squamous epithelium (see Color Atlas, plate 3)
basal cell carcinoma bā′săl sel kar-si-nō′mă	malignant tumor of the basal layer of the epidermis [most common type of skin cancer (see Color Atlas, plate 3)]
malignant melanoma mă-lig′nănt mel′ă-nō′mă	a malignant tumor composed of melanocytes—most develop from a pigmented nevus over time (see Color Atlas, plate 3)
Kaposi's sarcoma kăp′ō-sēz sar-kō′mă	a malignant tumor of the walls of blood vessels appearing as painless dark bluish-purple plaques on the skin, often spreads to lymph nodes and internal organs
onychia ō-nik′ē-ă	inflammation of fingernail or toenail
paronychia par-ō-nik′ē-ă	inflammation of nail fold (Fig. 5.7)
pediculosis pĕ-dik′yū-lō′sis	infestation with lice that causes itching and dermatitis (pediculo = louse) (Fig. 5.8)
pediculosis capitis pĕ-dik′yū-lō′sis kap′i-tis	head lice (capitis = head)

continued

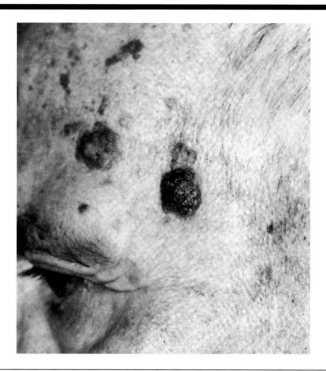

Figure 5.6. Multiple raised, brown lesions of the skin typical of seborrheic keratosis.

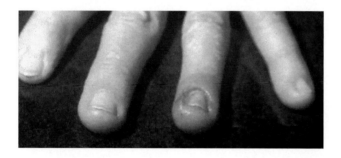

Figure 5.7. Chronic paronychia.

Term	Meaning
pediculosis pubis pĕ-dik′yū-lō′sis pyū′bis	lice that generally infect the pubic region, but hair of the axilla, eyebrows, lashes, beard, or other hairy body surfaces may also be involved—also called crabs (pubis = groin)
psoriasis sō-rī′ă-sis	an itching; a chronic, recurrent skin disease marked by silver-gray scales covering red patches on the skin that result from overproduction and thickening of skin cells—elbows, knees, genitals, arms, legs, scalp, and nails are common sites of involvement
scabies skā′bēz	a contagious disease caused by a parasite (mite) that invades the skin, causing an intense itch—most often found at articulations between the fingers or toes, elbow, etc. (scabo = to scratch)

continued

TINEA. Tinea is Latin for a grub, a gnawing worm; it is used to describe the gnawed or moth-eaten appearance of the skin in this condition.

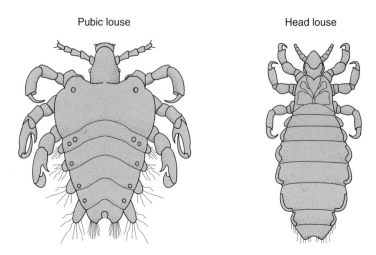

Pubic louse   Head louse

Figure 5.8. Pediculosis.

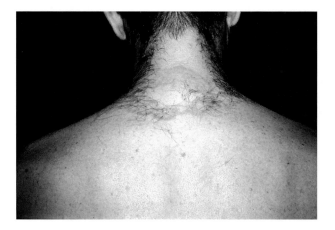

Figure 5.9. Tinea corporis.

Term	Meaning
seborrhea seb-ō-rē'ă	a skin condition marked by the hypersecretion of sebum from the sebaceous glands
tinea tin'ē-ă	a group of fungal skin diseases identified by the body part that is affected, including tinea corporis (body), commonly called ringworm, and tinea pedis (foot), also called athlete's foot (Fig. 5.9)

Diagnostic Tests and Procedures

Term	Meaning
biopsy (Bx) bī′op-sē	removal of a small piece of tissue for microscopic pathological examination (Fig. 5.10)
excisional Bx	removal of an entire lesion
incisional Bx	removal of a selected portion of a lesion
shave Bx	a technique using a surgical blade to "shave" tissue from epidermis and upper dermis
culture and sensitivity (C&S)	technique of isolating and growing colonies of microorganisms to identify a pathogen and to determine which drugs might be effective in combating the infection it has caused
frozen section (FS)	a surgical method involving cutting a thin piece of tissue from a frozen specimen for immediate pathological examination
skin tests	methods for determining the reaction of the body to a given substance by applying it to, or injecting it into, the skin—commonly seen in treating allergy
scratch test	substance is applied to the skin through a scratch
patch test	substance is applied topically to the skin on a small piece of blotting paper or wet cloth

SUTURE. Suture is derived from the Latin sutura, meaning a seam, a sewing together. In surgery, a suture is a thread or other material used for sewing. Also, to suture is to sew up or stitch together. Numbers indicate thickness of the thread (i.e., lower numbers denote thicker thread; higher numbers denote thinner thread).

Operative Terms (Fig. 5.11)

Term	Meaning
chemosurgery kem′ō-ser-jer-ē **chemical peel**	a technique for restoring wrinkled, scarred, or blemished skin by application of an acid solution to "peel" away the top layers of the skin

continued

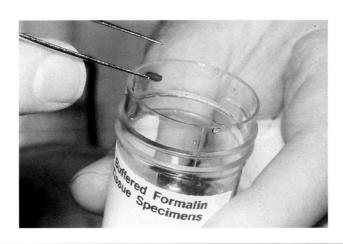

Figure 5.10. Collection of a biopsy specimen.

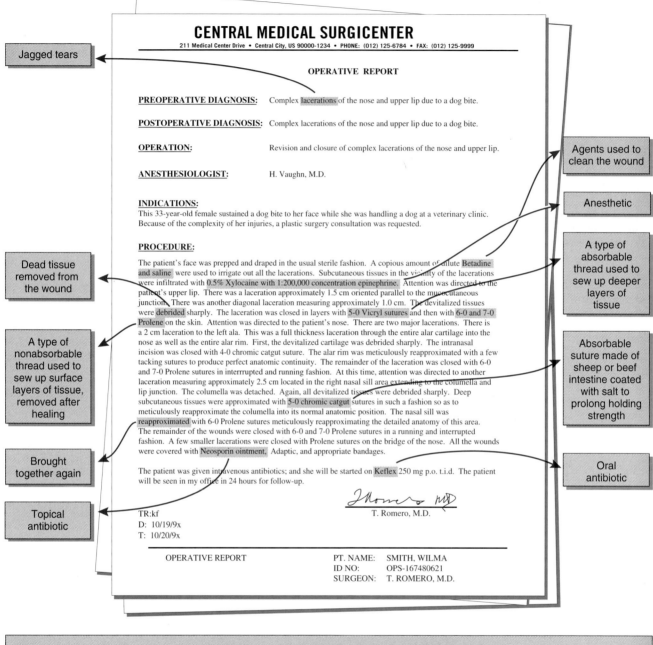

Jagged tears

Agents used to clean the wound

Anesthetic

A type of absorbable thread used to sew up deeper layers of tissue

Dead tissue removed from the wound

A type of nonabsorbable thread used to sew up surface layers of tissue, removed after healing

Absorbable suture made of sheep or beef intestine coated with salt to prolong holding strength

Brought together again

Oral antibiotic

Topical antibiotic

CENTRAL MEDICAL SURGICENTER
211 Medical Center Drive • Central City, US 90000-1234 • PHONE: (012) 125-6784 • FAX: (012) 125-9999

OPERATIVE REPORT

PREOPERATIVE DIAGNOSIS: Complex lacerations of the nose and upper lip due to a dog bite.

POSTOPERATIVE DIAGNOSIS: Complex lacerations of the nose and upper lip due to a dog bite.

OPERATION: Revision and closure of complex lacerations of the nose and upper lip.

ANESTHESIOLOGIST: H. Vaughn, M.D.

INDICATIONS:
This 33-year-old female sustained a dog bite to her face while she was handling a dog at a veterinary clinic. Because of the complexity of her injuries, a plastic surgery consultation was requested.

PROCEDURE:
The patient's face was prepped and draped in the usual sterile fashion. A copious amount of dilute Betadine and saline were used to irrigate out all the lacerations. Subcutaneous tissues in the vicinity of the lacerations were infiltrated with 0.5% Xylocaine with 1:200,000 concentration epinephrine. Attention was directed to the patient's upper lip. There was a laceration approximately 1.5 cm oriented parallel to the mucocutaneous junction. There was another diagonal laceration measuring approximately 1.0 cm. The devitalized tissues were debrided sharply. The laceration was closed in layers with 5-0 Vicryl sutures and then with 6-0 and 7-0 Prolene on the skin. Attention was directed to the patient's nose. There are two major lacerations. There is a 2 cm laceration to the left ala. This was a full thickness laceration through the entire alar cartilage into the nose as well as the entire alar rim. First, the devitalized cartilage was debrided sharply. The intranasal incision was closed with 4-0 chromic catgut suture. The alar rim was meticulously reapproximated with a few tacking sutures to produce perfect anatomic continuity. The remainder of the laceration was closed with 6-0 and 7-0 Prolene sutures in interrupted and running fashion. At this time, attention was directed to another laceration measuring approximately 2.5 cm located in the right nasal sill area extending to the columella and lip junction. The columella was detached. Again, all devitalized tissues were debrided sharply. Deep subcutaneous tissues were approximated with 5-0 chromic catgut sutures in such a fashion so as to meticulously reapproximate the columella into its normal anatomic position. The nasal sill was reapproximated with 6-0 Prolene sutures meticulously reapproximating the detailed anatomy of this area. The remainder of the wounds were closed with 6-0 and 7-0 Prolene sutures in a running and interrupted fashion. A few smaller lacerations were closed with Prolene sutures on the bridge of the nose. All the wounds were covered with Neosporin ointment, Adaptic, and appropriate bandages.

The patient was given intravenous antibiotics; and she will be started on Keflex 250 mg p.o. t.i.d. The patient will be seen in my office in 24 hours for follow-up.

T. Romero MD
T. Romero, M.D.

TR:kf
D: 10/19/9x
T: 10/20/9x

OPERATIVE REPORT   PT. NAME: SMITH, WILMA
                          ID NO: OPS-167480621
                          SURGEON: T. ROMERO, M.D.

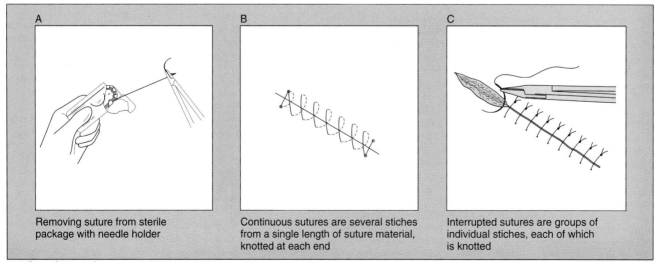

A

Removing suture from sterile package with needle holder

B

Continuous sutures are several stiches from a single length of suture material, knotted at each end

C

Interrupted sutures are groups of individual stiches, each of which is knotted

Term	Meaning
cryosurgery krī-ō-ser′jer-ē	destruction of tissue by freezing—involves application of an extremely cold chemical (e.g., liquid nitrogen)
dermabrasion der-mă-brā′zhŭn	surgical removal of frozen epidermis using wire brushes and emery papers to remove scars, tattoos, and/or wrinkles; aerosol spray is used to freeze the skin
debridement dā-brēd-mon′	removal of dead tissue from a wound or burn site to promote healing and prevent infection
curettage kyū-rĕ-tahzh′	to clean; scraping of a wound using a spoon-like cutting instrument called a curette; this technique is used in debridement
electrosurgical procedures	use of electric currents to destroy tissue—type and strength of the current and method of application varies (Fig. 5.12)
electrocautery ē-lek′trō-caw′ter-ē	use of an instrument heated by electric current (cautery) to coagulate bleeding areas by burning the tissue (e.g., to sear a blood vessel)
electrodesiccation ē-lek′trō-des-i-kā′shŭn	use of short, high-frequency, electric currents to destroy tissue by drying—the active electrode makes direct contact with the skin lesion (desicco = to dry up)
fulguration ful-gŭ-rā′shŭn	to lighten; use of long, high-frequency, electric sparks to destroy tissue; the active electrode does *not* touch the skin
incision and drainage (I&D)	incision and drainage of an infected skin lesion (e.g., an abscess)
laser surgery lā′zer	surgery using a laser in various dermatological procedures to remove lesions, scars, tattoos, etc.
laser	an acronym for light amplification by stimulated emission of radiation; an instrument that concentrates high frequencies of light into a small, extremely intense beam that is precise in depth and diameter; it is applied to body tissues to destroy lesions or for dissection (cutting of parts for study)

CAUTERY. A Greek word meaning branding iron refers to the surgical use of flame or heat to destroy tissue, control bleeding of wound sites, etc. The ancients used actual cautery with a metallic instrument heated in a flame and potential cautery with a caustic chemical.

continued

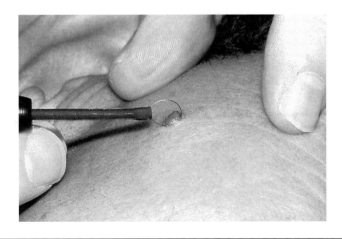

Figure 5.12. Excision of a skin lesion.

Term	Meaning
Mohs' surgery mōz	a technique used to excise tumors of the skin by removing fresh tissue layer by layer until a tumor-free plane is reached
skin grafting	transfer of skin from one body site to another to replace skin lost through burns or injury
autograft aw'tō-graft	transfer to a new position in the body of the same person (auto = self)
heterograft het'er-ō-graft	a graft transfer from one animal species to one of another species (hetero = different)
homograft hō'mō-graft **allograft** al'ō-graft	donor transfer between persons of the same species such as human to human (homo = same)

Therapeutic Terms

Term	Meaning
chemotherapy kēm'ō-ther-ă-pē	treatment of malignancies, infections, and other diseases with chemical agents that destroy selected cells or impair their ability to reproduce
radiation therapy rā'dē-ā'shŭn	treatment of neoplastic disease by using ionizing radiation to deter proliferation of malignant cells
sclerotherapy sklēr-ō-ther'ă-pē	use of sclerosing agents in treating diseases (e.g., injection of a saline solution into a dilated blood vessel tumor in the skin, resulting in hardening of the tissue within and eventual sloughing away of the lesion)
ultraviolet therapy ŭl-tră-vī'ō-let	use of ultraviolet light to promote healing of a skin lesion (e.g., an ulcer)

Common Therapeutic Drug Classifications

anesthetic an-es-thet'ik	a drug that temporarily blocks transmission of nerve conduction to produce a loss of sensations (e.g., pain)
antibiotic an'tē-bī-ot'ik	a drug that kills or inhibits the growth of microorganisms
antifungal an-tē-fŭng'ăl	a drug that kills or prevents the growth of fungi
antihistamine an-tē-his'tă-mēn	a drug that blocks the effects of histamine in the body
histamine his'tă-mēn	a regulating body substance released in excess during allergic reactions causing swelling and inflammation of tissues [e.g., in urticaria (hives), hay fever, etc.]
anti-inflammatory an'tē-in-flam'ă-tor-ē	a drug that reduces inflammation
antipruritic an'tē-prū-rit'ik	a drug that relieves itching
antiseptic an-tă-sep'tik	an agent that inhibits the growth of infectious microorganisms

PRACTICE EXERCISES

For the following terms, draw a line or lines to separate prefixes, combining forms, and suffixes. Then define the term.

1. pachyonychia _____

2. keratomycosis_____

3. dermatologist _____

4. histotrophic _____

5. hyperonychia _____

6. leukotrichia _____

7. keratosis _____

8. pachydermatosis _____

9. epidermis _____

10. lipoma _____

11. subcutaneous _____

12. anhidrosis _____

13. histodialysis _____

14. dysplasia _____

15. xanthoderma _____

16. dysplastic _____

17. pachydermatocele _____

18. erythrodermatitis _____

19. histotoxic _____

20. melanocyte _____

21. xerosis _____

22. purpuric _____

23. squamous _____

24. seborrhea _____

25. steatolysis _____

Write the correct medical term for each of the following:

26. death of tissue associated with loss of blood supply _____

27. transfer of skin to a new position in the body of the same person _____

28. black and blue mark _____

29. itching _____

30. a cluster of furuncles _____

31. fungal skin disease _____

32. hives _____

33. a graft transfer from one animal species to one of another species _____

34. pubic lice _____

35. a boil _____

36. freckle _____

37. flake of exfoliated epidermis _____

38. head lice_____

39. baldness _____

40. virus that causes cold sores _____

41. study of tissue _____

42. redness of skin _____

43. a blackhead _____

44. mark left by healed wound _____

45. a linear crack in the skin _____

46. profuse sweating _____

47. excision of tissue for microscopic study _____

48. appearance of a skin lesion _____

49. abnormal scar formation _____

Complete the medical term by writing the missing part:

50. _____ oma = black tumor

51. sebo _____= discharge of oil

52. _____ derma = thick skin

53. _____ coriation = scratch mark on skin

54. _____ derma = white skin

55. _____ section = type of microscopic study of fresh tissue

56. _____ derma = red skin

57. _____ derma = hard skin

58. _____ keratoses = thickened skin tumors seen in old age

59. _____ oma = fat tumor

60. _____derma = yellow skin

61. _____osis = presence of fungus

62. _____dermic = pertaining to below the skin

63. _____ angioma = bright red, round blood vessel tumor

64. _____derma = dry skin

Give the medical terms for the following viral diseases:

65. German measles _____

66. chickenpox _____

67. 14-day measles _____

Match the following terms with the primary lesions described:

68. vesicle   _____   a. a tiny, flat discolored spot on the skin, up to 1 cm diameter

69. pustule   _____   b. a large, flat discolored area on the skin, larger than 1 cm diameter

70. papule   _____   c. raised spot on skin less than 0.5 cm diameter

71. bulla   _____   d. a solid mass greater than 1 cm that extends into the epidermis

72. nodule   _____   e. a solid mass greater than 1 cm limited to the skin's surface

73. wheal   _____   f. a small blister

74. macule   _____   g. area of localized skin edema, such as a hive

75. tumor   _____   h. a large blister

76. patch   _____   i. a pus-filled sac

77. plaque   _____   j. a solid mass larger than 1–2 cm diameter

Write the full medical term from the following abbreviations:

78. HSV-2 _____

79. Bx _____

80. FS _____

81. I & D _____

Write the plural forms of the following terms:

82. keratosis _____

83. ecchymosis _____

84. bulla _____

85. macula _____

86. nevus _____

Match the following terms with their meanings:

87. scabies   _____   a. chemical peel

88. cryosurgery   _____   b. crabs

89. telangiectasia   _____   c. mites

90. nevus   _____   d. freezing treatment

91. cicatrix   _____   e. intense light

92. actinic keratoses   _____   f. desiccation

93. radiation therapy   _____   g. spider angioma

94. petechia   _____   h. mole

95. liposis   _____   i. scar

96. verruca   _____   j. cancer treatment

97. chemosurgery   _____   k. wart

98. electrosurgery   _____   l. solar keratoses

99. pediculosis   _____   m. purpuric lesion

100. laser   _____   n. adipose

Medical Record Analyses

MEDICAL RECORD 5.1

After ignoring various skin problems for months, Robert Fuller consulted his doctor in October when he became alarmed by what he saw happening on his right hand. His doctor referred him to Dr. Luong, a dermatologist, who then diagnosed and treated Mr. Fuller.

Directions

Read Medical Record 5.1 for Robert Fuller (page 111) and answer the following questions. This record is a progress note in a POMR dictated by Dr. Luong immediately after the treatment of Mr. Fuller and transcribed the next day by his assistant.

Questions about Medical Record 5.1

Write your answers in the spaces provided.

1. Below are medical terms used in this record that you have not yet encountered in this text. Underline each where it appears in the record and define below.

   vulgaris _____

   verruciform _____

2. In your own words, not using medical terminology, briefly describe Mr. Fuller's complaint.

   _____

   _____

   _____

3. In your own words, not using medical terminology, briefly describe Dr. Luong's three objective findings:

   a. _____

   b. _____

   c. _____

4. Define the three diagnoses for those three objective findings:

   a. _____

   b. _____

   c. _____

5. Briefly describe the treatments for those three diagnoses:

   a. _____

   b. _____

   c. _____

6. What did Dr. Luong tell Mr. Fuller might occur in the future? Check *all* that apply:

   _____ scarring where the lesions were

   _____ nausea and possible vomiting from the nitrogen

   _____ red freckle-like spots appearing on right hand

   _____ possible regrowth of lesions

   _____ self-desiccating tissue destruction

MEDICAL RECORD 5.2

About five months ago Patricia Brown saw Dr. Luong, the dermatologist, and was treated for a skin problem. Since she was told then that there was a chance of recurrence, she has watched that area of her skin carefully. When what looked to her like a small dot appeared in the same area, she called Dr. Luong for another appointment.

Directions

Read Medical Record 5.2 for Patricia Brown (page 113) and answer the following questions. This record is the progress note dictated by Dr. Luong after treating her and transcribed the next day by his assistant.

Questions about Medical Record 5.2

Write your answers in the spaces provided.

1. Below are medical terms used in this record you have not yet encountered in this text. Underline each where it appears in the record and define below.

   pigmented _____

   margin _____

   defect _____

2. In your own words, not using medical terminology, briefly describe what Dr. Luong found in the first visit five months ago and the treatment he then gave.

   _____

   _____

   _____

CENTRAL MEDICAL GROUP, INC.

Department of Dermatology

201 Medical Center Drive • Central City, US 90000-1234 • PHONE: (012) 125-8888 • FAX: (012) 125-3434

CHART NOTE

PATIENT: FULLER, ROBERT K.

DATE: October 19, 199x

SUBJECTIVE: The patient presents with a growth on the right hand, multiple lesions, and other growths.

OBJECTIVE: Ulcerated growth on the right hand, marked A; one verruciform tumor on the left hand; erythematous keratotic patches on the arms.

ASSESSMENT: Basal cell carcinoma, verruca vulgaris, and actinic keratoses.

PLAN: Following full counseling on healing with scarring, keloids, and possible recurrence, the growth from the right hand was excised. The site was anesthetized with Xylocaine 2% without epinephrine, 2 cc. Following excision, the bases of the growths were treated with fulguration and electrodesiccation. Desiccation was also performed on 0.3 cm of normal surrounding skin. The wart was treated with liquid nitrogen, two cycles. Freezing time: 8-10 seconds. Ten erythematous keratotic patches were also treated with liquid nitrogen, two cycles. Freezing time: 10-14 seconds.

D. Luong, M.D.

DL:ti

D: 10/19/9x
T: 10/20/9x

Medical Record 5.1.

3. Dr. Malloy analyzed a tissue sample for Dr. Luong five months ago and diagnosed the lesion marked C. Translate into lay language her diagnosis:

_____

_____

_____

4. Before initiating treatment of the recurrent lesion in this visit, Dr. Luong fully explained to Ms. Brown the likely and possible results. What three specific things (in nonmedical language) did she agree to accept as possible risks?

   a. _____

   b. _____

   c. _____

5. Treatment of the recurrent lesion involved several steps. Put the following actions in correct order by numbering them 1 to 5:

   _____ sample sent to lab

   _____ suture removal

   _____ excision of tumor and surrounding area

   _____ patient's permission given

   _____ suturing the wound

6. What, briefly, is Dr. Malloy's role *this* time? Is this the same as or different from her role in Ms. Brown's first treatment?

   _____

   _____

   _____

MEDICAL RECORD 5.3

Mary Chen's physician, Dr. Ogawa, treated her for a skin lesion more than two months ago and more recently did a biopsy after that carcinoma apparently recurred. Dr. Ogawa then referred Mary to Dr. Volkman, a dermatologic surgeon.

Directions

Read Medical Record 5.3 (pages 114–115) for Mary Chen and answer the following questions. This record is the operative report dictated by Dr. Volkman after performing the surgery.

CENTRAL MEDICAL GROUP, INC.

Department of Dermatology

201 Medical Center Drive • Central City, US 90000-1234 • PHONE: (012) 125-8888 • FAX: (012) 125-3434

CHART NOTE

PATIENT: BROWN, PATRICIA D.

DATE: May 11, 199x

SUBJECTIVE:	Recurrence of growth on the patient's left leg. The patient was in my office on December 12, 199x. At that time, three changing moles were excised: one on the left leg, marked C; one on the back; and one on the right of the chest. The one marked C was read by Dr. Malloy, the pathologist, as a pigmented compound nevus with mild atypical melanocytic hyperplasia, margins free and adequate.
OBJECTIVE:	Very small pigmented lesion, approximately 2-3 mm in diameter, in the same area.
ASSESSMENT:	Atypical and dysplastic nevus, possible recurrence.
PLAN:	Fully counseled patient regarding healing with scarring and keloid; however, due to the nature of the nevus and the recurrence, we will need to remove a minimum of 4-5 mm of normal surrounding skin. With the patient's full acceptance of scarring, a keloid, and the possibility of recurrence, the tumor was re-excised with a large area surrounding the brown pigment, approximately 3-4 mm. The defect was then closed using 4-0 Vicryl x 3 and 4-0 Prolene x 4 interrupted. The specimen was marked C-1 and was sent to DermLab again to Dr. Malloy who read the patient's slide on December 12, 199x. The patient is to return in two weeks for suture removal. An aftercare handout was given and discussed.

_____
D. Luong, M.D.

DL:ti

D: 5/11/9x
T: 5/12/9x

Medical Record 5.2.

CENTRAL MEDICAL SURGICENTER

211 Medical Center Drive • Central City, US 90000-1234 • PHONE: (012) 125-6784 • FAX: (012) 125-9999

OPERATIVE REPORT

DATE OF OPERATION:	May 6, 199x
LOCATION:	Mohs' surgery suite.
PREOPERATIVE DIAGNOSIS:	Recurrent basal cell carcinoma, left nasal tip.
POSTOPERATIVE DIAGNOSIS:	Recurrent basal cell carcinoma, left nasal tip, with extension and full-thickness loss.
OPERATION PERFORMED:	Mohs' histographic surgery, fresh tissue technique.
SURGEON:	E. Volkman, M.D.
ASSISTANT:	K. Ball, M.D.
ANESTHESIA:	Local.

INDICATIONS:
The patient is a 64-year-old white female with a history of a lesion over the left nasal tip which was biopsied on March 27, 199x, slide number K-476-9x. Findings revealed recurrent basal cell carcinoma. Examination revealed a 12 x 10 mm ill-defined area of the left tip with waxiness and indistinct margins. The patient was referred by Dr. Ogawa who performed the above biopsy and additionally had treated the patient in February 199x for a basal cell carcinoma with a shave curettage and desiccation, slide number K-159-9x. In light of this, it was thought that Mohs' surgery would be appropriate. I discussed it with the patient. The patient fully understands the aims, risks, alternatives, and possible complications and elects to proceed. There are no medical or surgical contraindications to the procedure.

PROCEDURE:
The patient was placed in the supine position on the operating table in the Mohs' surgery suite. The area was prepared and draped in a standard manner. Gentian violet was used to outline the clinical margins of the tumor, and thereafter, local anesthesia with 1% Lidocaine with 1:100,000 epinephrine mixed with 0.5% Marcaine was administered; a total amount of 7.2 cc was used throughout the entire procedure. All of the grossly visible tumor was removed, and an underlying

(continued)

OPERATIVE REPORT Page 1	PT. NAME: CHEN, MARY S. ID NO: OP-078919 SURGEON: EARL VOLKMAN, M.D.

Medical Record 5.3.

CENTRAL MEDICAL SURGICENTER

211 Medical Center Drive • Central City, US 90000-1234 • PHONE: (012) 125-6784 • FAX: (012) 125-9999

OPERATIVE REPORT

layer was taken and was processed by the Mohs' technique. Hemostasis was obtained with electrocautery. The tumor was found to be present on the gross vertical and extended deep between cartilages and throughout the left alar tip. The first Mohs' layer consisted of seven sections with seven slides being evaluated. The second Mohs' layer consisted of seven sections with seven slides being evaluated. The third Mohs' layer consisted of three sections with three slides being evaluated. A total of the vertical and 17 slides were examined under the microscope via the Mohs' technique. A cancer-free plane was reached after the third layer. The final size of the defect was 25 x 23 mm. The wound was covered with an antibiotic ointment and a nonadherent dressing between stages.

Estimated blood loss for the total procedure was 4 cc.

Total operative time, including tissue processing in the Mohs' laboratory and microscopic Mohs' frozen section slide review per Dr. O'Connor, was four hours. The patient tolerated the procedure well and left the operating room in good condition. There was full-thickness loss of the left ala (wing-like flap of the nostril composed of cartilage). The patient was placed on Keflex 250 mg 1 p.o. q.i.d. and was referred to Dr. Jensen in plastic surgery who will see the patient later today for consideration of reconstructive repair which may indeed require a forehead flap. She is to take Tylenol with Codeine 1 q 4 h p.r.n. pain and will also be followed by Dr. Ogawa.

Earl Volkman MD

Earl Volkman, M.D.

EV:ti

D: 5/6/9x
T: 5/7/9x

OPERATIVE REPORT	PT. NAME:	CHEN, MARY S.
Page 2	ID NO:	OP-078919
	SURGEON:	EARL VOLKMAN, M.D.

Medical Record 5.3. *Continued.*

Questions about Medical Record 5.3

Write your answers in the spaces provided.

1. Below are medical terms used in this record you have not yet encountered in this text. Underline each where it appears in the record and define below.

   supine _____

   gentian (crystal) violet _____

   hemostat _____

   flap (full thickness) _____

2. In your own words, not using medical terminology, briefly describe Ms. Chen's preoperative diagnosis:

   _____

   Now describe the meaning of the addition to that diagnosis in the postoperative diagnosis:

   _____

3. In your own words, describe Dr. Ogawa's earlier treatment of Ms. Chen's lesion:

   _____

   _____

4. The surgery was performed with Ms. Chen in what position?

   a. lying flat face down

   b. lying flat face up

   c. lying on side

   d. sitting

5. Put the following surgical actions in correct order to describe the surgery by numbering them 1 to 8:

   _____ removing the gross tumor

   _____ stopping the bleeding

   _____ applying antibiotics

   _____ outlining clinical margins of the tumor

   _____ removing first underlying layer

_____ evaluating tissues microscopically

_____ administering local anesthetic

_____ removing second and third layers

6. Translate the surgeon's phrase "Hemostasis was obtained with electrocautery":

_____

_____

7. Describe a "frozen section": _____

_____

How many frozen sections were analyzed in this surgery? _____

8. For the other two physicians mentioned, give their specializations and their roles in treating Ms. Chen now and in the future:

Dr. O'Connor specialization _____

role in treatment _____

Dr. Jensen specialization _____

role in treatment _____

9. Translate the instructions for the two medications Ms. Chen will be taking post-operatively:

Drug Name	Route of Administration	Dose	Frequency of Dose
_____	_____	_____	_____
_____	_____	_____	_____

10. In your own words, not using medical terminology, briefly describe the additional treatment to be considered for Ms. Chen:

_____

_____

_____

CHAPTER

6 Musculoskeletal System

OBJECTIVES

After completion of this chapter you will be able to

1. Define common combining forms used in relation to the musculoskeletal system

2. Describe the anatomical position

3. List the planes of the body

4. Describe the anatomical position and body planes using positional and directional terms

5. Define the terms related to body movements

6. Define the basic anatomical terms referring to the musculoskeletal system

7. Define common symptomatic, diagnostic, operative, and therapeutic terms related to the musculoskeletal system

8. List common diagnostic tests and procedures related to the musculoskeletal system

9. Explain the terms and abbreviations used in documenting medical records involving the musculoskeletal system

Combining Forms

Combining Form	Meaning	Example
ankyl/o	crooked or stiff	ankylotic ang-ki-lot′ik
arthr/o	joint	arthritis ar-thrı′tis
articul/o		articular ar-tik′yu-lăr
brachi/o	arm	brachium bra′ke-ŭm
cervic/o	neck	cervical ser′vĭ-kal
chondr/o	cartilage (gristle)	chondral kon′drăl
cost/o	rib	intercostal in-ter-kos′tăl
crani/o	skull	cranial kra′ne-ăl
dactyl/o	digit (finger or toe)	dactylomegaly dak′til-o-meg′ă-le
fasci/o	fascia (a band)	fasciodesis fas-e-od′ĕ-sis
femor/o	femur	femoral fem′ŏ-răl
fibr/o	fiber	fibrous fı′brŭs
kyph/o	humped	kyphosis kı-fo′sis
lei/o	smooth	leiomyoma lı′o-mı-o′mă
lord/o	bent	lordosis lŏr-do′sis
lumb/o	loin (lower back)	lumbar lŭm′bar
myel/o	bone marrow or spinal cord	myelitis mı-ĕ-lı′tis
my/o	muscle	myalgia mı-al′je-ă
myos/o		myositis mı-ō-sī′tis
muscul/o		muscular mŭs′kyu-lăr
oste/o	bone	osteomyelitis os′te-o-mı-ĕ-lı′tis
patell/o	knee cap	patellar pa-tel′ăr

continued

SKELETON. Skeleton is derived from a Greek word meaning "dried up." The Greeks used the term in reference to a mummy or dried up body. The word was never used by them in the modern meaning of the bony framework of the body. The first recorded use of the modern term in English is in 1578.

Combining Form	Meaning	Example
pelv/i	hip bone or pelvic cavity	pelvimeter pel-vim′ĕ-ter
pelv/o		pelvic pel′vik
radi/o	radius	radial ra′de-ăl
rhabd/o	rod shaped or striated (skeletal)	rhabdomyoma rab′do-mı-o′mă
sarc/o	flesh	sarcoma sar-ko′mă
scoli/o	twisted	scoliosis sko-le-o′sis
spondyl/o	vertebra	spondylitis spon-di-lı′tis
vertebr/o		vertebral ver′tĕ-brăl
stern/o	sternum (breastbone)	sternocostal ster′no-kos′tăl
ten/o	tendon (to stretch)	tenodesis tĕ-nod′e-sis
tend/o		tendolysis ten-dol′i-sis
tendin/o		tendinitis ten-di-nı′tis
thorac/o	chest	thoracic tho-ras′ik
ton/o	tone or tension	myotonia mı-o-to′ne-ă
uln/o	ulna	ulnar ŭl′năr

Musculoskeletal System Overview

The musculoskeletal system provides support and gives shape to the body (Fig. 6.1) (see Color Atlas, plates 5–10).

The skeleton gives structure to the body by providing a framework of bones and cartilage. Also, the bones store calcium and other minerals and produce certain blood cells within the bone marrow.

The muscles cover the bones where they hinge (articulate) and supply the forces that make movement possible. They also provide a protective covering for internal organs and produce body heat.

Anatomical Terms Related to Bones (see Color Atlas, plates 5–8)

Term	Meaning
appendicular skeleton ap′en-dik′yu-lăr	bones of shoulder, pelvis, and upper and lower extremities
axial skeleton ak′se-ăl	bones of skull, vertebral column, chest, and hyoid bone (U-shaped bone lying at the base of the tongue); refer to Color Atlas, plate 8 for abbreviated identification and numbering of cervical, thoracic, and lumbar vertebrae

continued

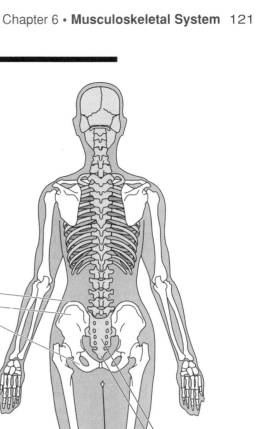

Skull { Cranium
Face

Hyoid
Clavicle
Manubrium
Scapula
Sternum
Ribs
Xiphoid process
Humerus
Vertebral column
Iliac crest
Ilium
Ischium
Ulna
Radius
Carpals
Metacarpals

1
2
3
4
5
6
7
8
9
10
11
12

Phalanges

Trochanter
Pubic bone
Femur

Patella

Tibia

Fibula

Sacrum
Coccyx

Calcaneus

Tarsals
Metatarsals
Phalanges

Anterior view

Posterior view

Color key: Appendicular skeleton ☐
Axial skeleton ▨

Figure 6.1. The skeleton.

Term	Meaning
bone	specialized connective tissue composed of osteocytes (bone cells) forming the skeleton

Types of Bone Tissue

compact bone	tightly solid, strong bone tissue resistant to bending
spongy (cancellous) bone spŭn′je kan′sĕ-lŭs	mesh-like bone tissue containing marrow and fine branching canals through which blood vessels run

continued

BURSA. A Latin word for a purse was given to the small synovial pouch associated with a joint. The meaning stems from the use of a purse by the bursar, the man who holds the purse in order to pay out of it. Most anatomical terms come from the names of familiar objects [e.g., patella (dish), acetabulum (bowl), etc.].

Term	Meaning
Classification of Bones	
long bones	bones of arms and legs
short bones	bones of wrist and ankles
flat bones	bones of ribs, shoulder blades, pelvis, and skull
irregular bones	bones of vertebrae and face
sesamoid bones ses'ă-moyd	round bones that are found near joints (e.g., patella)
Parts of a Long Bone (Fig. 6.2)	
epiphysis e-pif'i-sis	wide ends of a long bone (physis = growth)
diaphysis dī-af'i-sis	shaft of a long bone
metaphysis mĕ-taf'i-sis	growth zone between epiphysis and diaphysis during development of a long bone
endosteum en-dos'tē-ŭm	membrane lining the medullary cavity of a bone
medullary cavity med'ŭ-lār-ē	cavity within the shaft of the long bones filled with bone marrow
bone marrow mar'ō	soft connective tissue within the medullary cavities of bones
red bone marrow	found in cavities of most bones in infants; functions in formation of red blood cells, some white blood cells, and platelets; in adults, red bone marrow is found most often in the flat bones
yellow bone marrow	gradually replaces red bone marrow in adult bones, functions as storage for fat tissue, and is inactive in formation of blood cells
periosteum per-ē-os'tē-ŭm	a fibrous, vascular membrane that covers the bone
articular cartilage ar-tik'yū-lăr kar'ti-lij	a gristle-like substance found on bones where they articulate

Anatomical Terms Related to Joints and Muscles

Term	Meaning
articulation ar'tik-yū-lā'shŭn	a joint; the point where two bones come together (Fig. 6.3)
bursa ber'să	a fibrous sac between certain tendons and bones that is lined with a synovial membrane that secretes synovial fluid
disc*	a flat plate-like structure composed of fibrocartilaginous tissue found between the vertebrae to reduce friction (see Color Atlas, plate 8)

continued

* Disc can also be spelled disk.

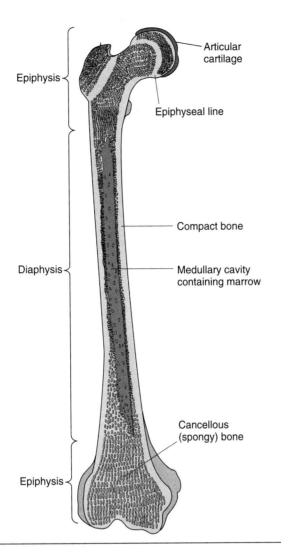

Figure 6.2. Parts of a long bone.

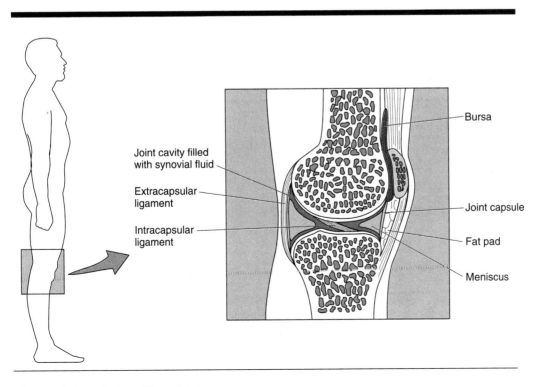

Figure 6.3. Lateral view of knee joint.

FASCIA. Fascia is derived from a Latin word for a band or bandage derived from fascis, a bundle (the bandage that ties up a bundle, especially a band around a bundle of sticks). Fasces were bundles of sticks from which an ax projected; they were carried by Roman officials. In the 20th century, fasces were adopted in Italy as a party badge, hence the term "fascist." In anatomy, the sheets of connective tissue that wrap the muscles or other parts are called fascia. Many are named for those who first described them, e.g., Camper, Scarpa, Colles, etc.

Term	Meaning
nucleus pulposus nu'klē-ŭs pŭl-pō'sŭs	soft, fibrocartilaginous, central portion of intervertebral disc
ligament lig'ă-ment	a flexible band of fibrous tissue that connects bone to bone
synovial membrane si-nō've-ăl mem'brăn	membrane lining the capsule of a joint
synovial fluid si-nō've-ăl flū'id	lubricating fluid secreted by the synovial membrane
muscle mŭs'ĕl	tissue composed of fibers that can contract, causing movement of an organ or part of the body (see Color Atlas, plate 10)
striated (skeletal) muscle strı'ā-ted (skel'e-tăl)	voluntary striated muscle attached to the skeleton
smooth muscle	involuntary muscle found in internal organs
cardiac muscle	muscle of the heart
origin of a muscle	end attached to the bone that does not move when the muscle contracts
insertion of a muscle	end attached to the bone that moves when the muscle contracts
tendon ten'dŏn	a band of fibrous tissue that connects muscle to bone
fascia fash'e-ă	a band; a sheet of fibrous connective tissue that covers, supports, and separates muscle

Anatomical Position and Terms of Reference

To communicate effectively about the body, health professionals use terms with specific meanings to refer to body positions, directions, and planes. These terms of reference are based on the body being in anatomical position, in which the person is assumed to be standing upright (erect), facing forward, feet pointed forward and slightly apart, arms at the sides with palms facing forward. The patient is visualized in this pose before applying any other term of reference.

With the body in an anatomical position, three different imaginary lines divide the body in half, forming body *planes* (Fig. 6.4). In addition to the three body planes, *positional and directional terms* are used to indicate the location or direction of body parts in respect to each other.

Term	Meaning
Body Planes	
coronal or frontal plane kōr'ŏ-năl frŭn'tăl	vertical division of body into front (anterior) and back (posterior) portions
sagittal plane saj'i-tăl	vertical division of body into right and left portions
transverse plane trans-vers'	horizontal division of body into upper and lower portions

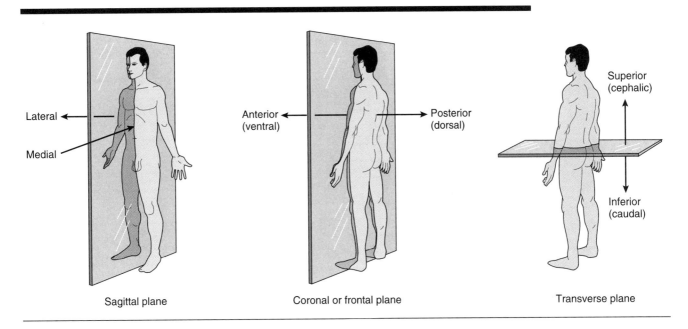

Figure 6.4. Body planes.

Term	Meaning
Directional Terms	
anterior (A) (ventral) an-tēr′ē-ōr ven′trăl	front of the body
posterior (P) (dorsal) pos-tēr′ē-ōr dor′săl	back of the body
anterior-posterior (AP)	from front to back; commonly associated with the direction of an x-ray beam
posterior-anterior (PA)	from back to front; commonly associated with the direction of an x-ray beam
superior (cephalic) su-pēr′ē-ōr se-fal′ik	situated above another structure, toward the head
inferior (caudal) in-fē′rē-ōr kaw′dăl	situated below another structure, away from the head
proximal prok′si-măl	toward the beginning or origin of a structure
distal dis′tăl	away from the beginning or origin of a structure
medial mē′dē-ăl	toward the middle (midline)
lateral lat′er-ăl	toward the side
axis ak′sis	line that runs through the center of the body or a body part
Body Positions	
erect ĕ-rĕkt′	normal standing position

continued

Term	Meaning
lateral decubitus dē-kyū′bi-tŭs	to lie down; lying on the side
prone prōn	lying face down and flat
recumbent rē-kŭm′bent	lying down
supine sū-pīn′	horizontal recumbent; lying flat on the back—"on the spine"

Body Movements (Fig. 6.5)

Term	Meaning
flexion flek′shŭn	bending at the joint so that the angle between the bones is decreased
extension eks-ten′shŭn	straightening at the joint so that the angle between the bones is increased
abduction ab-dŭk′shŭn	movement away from the body
adduction ă-duk′shŭn	movement toward the body
rotation rō-tā′shŭn	circular movement around an axis
eversion ē-ver′zhŭn	turning outward
inversion in-ver′zhŭn	turning inward
supination sū′pi-nā′shŭn	turning upward or forward of the palmar surface (palm of the hand) or plantar surface (sole of the foot)
pronation prō-nā′shŭn	turning downward or backward of the palmar surface (palm of the hand) or plantar surface (sole of the foot)
dorsiflexion dōr-si-flek′shŭn	bending of the foot or the toes upward
plantar flexion plan′tăr	bending of the sole of the foot by curling the toes toward the ground
range of motion (ROM)	total amount of motion in a joint, described by the terms related to body movements (e.g., the elbow extends to 80 degrees)
goniometer gō-nē-om′ĕ-ter	instrument used to measure joint angles (gonio = angle) (Fig. 6.6)

Symptomatic and Diagnostic Terms

Term	Meaning
Symptomatic	
arthralgia ar-thral′jē-ă	joint pain

continued

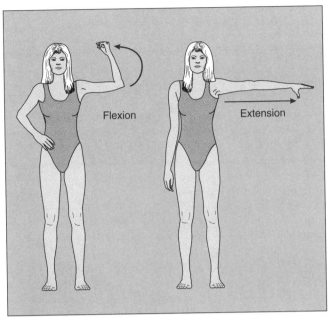
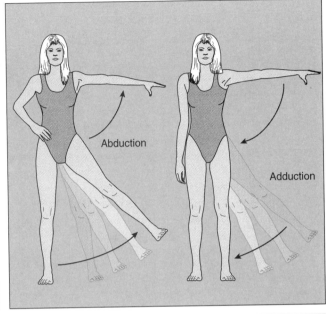
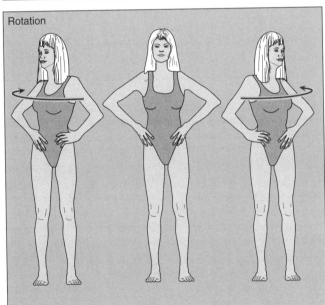
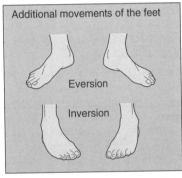
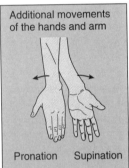
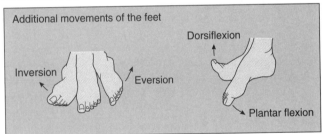

Figure 6.5. Body movements.

Term	Meaning
atrophy at'rō-fē	shrinking of muscle size
crepitation krep-i-tā'shŭn **crepitus** krep-i-tŭs	grating sound made by movement of some joints or broken bones
exostosis eks-os-tō'sis	a projection arising from a bone that develops from cartilage

continued

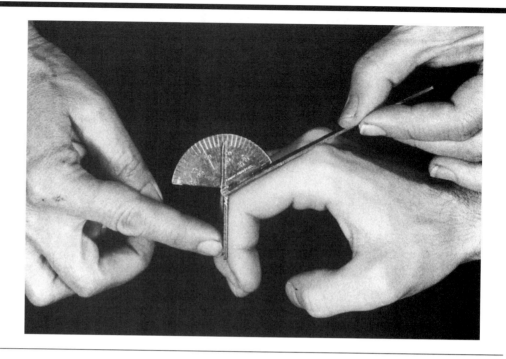

Figure 6.6. Dorsal placement of goniometer used when measuring digital motion.

Term	Meaning
flaccid flas′id	flabby, relaxed, or having defective or absent muscle tone
hypertrophy hī-per′trō-fē	increase in the size of a muscle
hypotonia hī′pō-tō′ne-ă	reduced muscle tension
myalgia mī-al′jē-ă **myodynia** mī′ō-din′e-ă	muscle pain
ostealgia os-tē-al′jē-ă **osteodynia** os-tē-o-din′e-ă	bone pain
rigor or rigidity rig′er ri-jid′i-tē	stiffness; stiff muscle
spasm spazm	drawing in; involuntary contraction of muscle
spastic spas′tik	uncontrolled contractions of skeletal muscles causing stiff and awkward movements (resembles spasm)
tetany tet′ă-nē	tension; prolonged, continuous muscle contraction
tremor trem′er	shaking; rhythmic muscular movement

continued

Term	Meaning
Diagnostic	
ankylosis ang'ki-lō'sis	stiff joint condition
arthritis ar-thrī'tis	inflammation of the joints characterized by pain, swelling, redness, warmth, and limitation of motion—there are more than 100 different types of arthritis
osteoarthritis os'tē-ō-ar-thrī'tis **degenerative arthritis** dē-jen'er-ă-tiv ar-thrī'tis **degenerative joint disease** (DJD) dē-jen'er-ă-tiv joynt di-zēz'	most common form of arthritis that especially affects weight bearing joints (e.g., knee or hip) characterized by the erosion of articular cartilage (Fig. 6.7)
rheumatoid arthritis rū'mă-toyd ar-thrī'tis	most crippling form of arthritis characterized by a chronic, systemic inflammation most often affecting joints and synovial membranes (especially in the hands and feet) causing ankylosis and deformity (Fig. 6.8)

continued

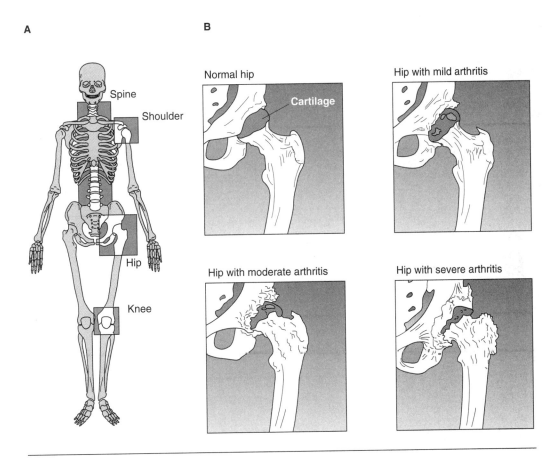

Figure 6.7. Osteoarthritis. **A.** Common sites of osteoarthritis. **B.** How osteoarthritis affects the hip.

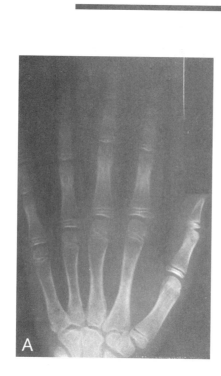

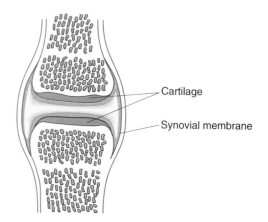

Cartilage

Synovial membrane

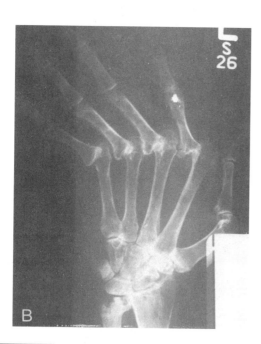

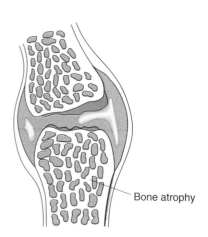

Bone atrophy

Figure 6.8. Joints of the hand affected by rheumatoid arthritis. **A.** X-ray of normal hand. **B.** X-ray of hand with rheumatoid arthritis.

Term	Meaning
gouty arthritis gow'tē ar-thrī'tis	acute attacks of arthritis usually in a single joint (especially the great toe) caused by hyperuricemia (an excessive level of uric acid in the blood)
bony necrosis nĕ-krō'sis **sequestrum** sē-kwes'trŭm	something laid aside; dead bone tissue from loss of blood supply (e.g., after a fracture)
bunion bŭn'yŭn	swelling of the joint at the base of the great toe caused by inflammation of the bursa
bursitis ber-sī'tis	inflammation of a bursa
chondromalacia kon'dro-mă-lā'shē-ă	softening of cartilage
epiphysitis e-pif-i-sī'tis	inflammation of epiphyseal regions of the long bone
fracture (Fx) frak'chŭr	broken or cracked bone (Fig. 6.9)
closed fracture	broken bone with no open wound
open fracture	compound fracture; broken bone with an open wound
simple fracture	a nondisplaced fracture involving one fracture line that does not require extensive treatment to repair (e.g., hairline Fx, stress Fx, or a crack)
complex fracture	a displaced fracture that requires manipulation or surgery to repair
fracture line	line made by broken bone (e.g., oblique, spiral, or transverse)
comminuted fracture kom'i-nū-ted	broken in many little pieces
greenstick fracture	bending and incomplete break of a bone—most often seen in children
herniated disc or disk her'nē-ā-ted	protrusion of a degenerated or fragmented intervertebral disk so that the nucleus pulposus protrudes, causing compression on the nerve root (Fig. 6.10)
myeloma mī-ĕ-lō'mă	bone marrow tumor
myositis mī-ō-sī'tis	inflammation of muscle
myoma mī-ō'mă	muscle tumor
leiomyoma lī'ō-mī-ō'mă	smooth muscle tumor
leiomyosarcoma lī'ō-mī'ō-sar-kō'mă	malignant smooth muscle tumor

GOUT. The Latin word gutta means a drop. Known to the ancients, the condition was thought to be caused by a liquid secretion that was distilled drop by drop on the diseased part.

continued

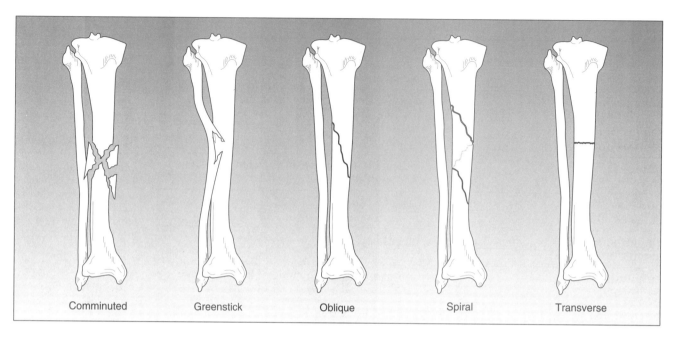

Comminuted   Greenstick   Oblique   Spiral   Transverse

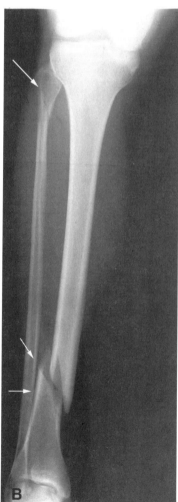

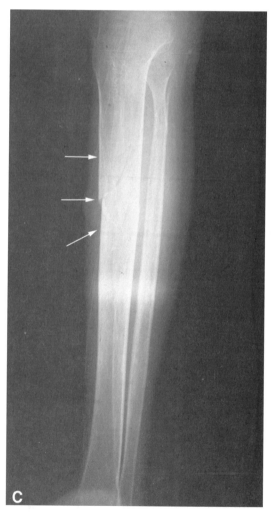

Figure 6.9. A. Types of common fracture. **B.** AP radiograph of lower leg demonstrating open fractures of tibia and fibia (*arrows*).
C. Lateral view radiograph demonstrating a closed spiral fracture of tibia (*arrows*).

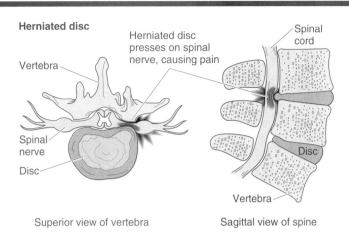

Herniated disc

Vertebra

Herniated disc presses on spinal nerve, causing pain

Spinal cord

Spinal nerve

Disc

Superior view of vertebra

Disc

Vertebra

Sagittal view of spine

Figure 6.10. Herniated disc (disk).

Term	Meaning
rhabdomyoma rab′dō-mī-o′mă	skeletal muscle tumor
rhabdomyosarcoma rab′dō-mī-ō-sar-kō′mă	malignant skeletal muscle tumor
muscular dystrophy mŭs′kyū-lăr dis′trō-fē	a category of genetically transmitted diseases characterized by progressive atrophy of skeletal muscles (Duchenne's type is most common)
osteoma os-tē-ō′mă	bone tumor
osteosarcoma os′tē-ō-sar-kō′mă	malignant bone tumor
osteomalacia os′tē-ō-mă-lā′shē-ă	disease marked by softening of the bone caused by calcium and vitamin D deficiency
rickets rik′ets	osteomalacia in children (causes bone deformity)
osteomyelitis os′tē-ō-mī-ĕ-lī′tis	infection of bone and bone marrow causing inflammation
osteoporosis os′tē-ō-pō-rō′sis	condition of decreased bone density and increase in porosity, causing bones to become brittle and liable to fracture (porosis = passage) (Fig. 6.11)
spinal curvatures (Fig. 6.12) spī′năl	
kyphosis kī-fō′sis	abnormal posterior curvature
lordosis lōr-dō′sis	abnormal anterior curvature

continued

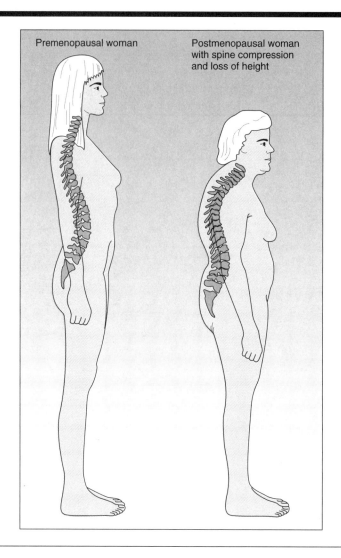

Premenopausal woman

Postmenopausal woman with spine compression and loss of height

Figure 6.11. Osteoporosis.

Term	Meaning
scoliosis skō-lē-ō'sis	abnormal lateral curvature (Fig. 6.13)
spondylolisthesis spon'di-lō-lis-thē'sis	forward slipping of a lumbar vertebra (listhesis = slipping)
spondylosis spon-di-lō'sis	stiff, immobile condition of vertebrae
sprain sprān	injury to a ligament caused by joint trauma but without joint dislocation or fracture
subluxation sŭb-lŭk-sā'shŭn	a partial dislocation (Fig. 6.14)
tendinitis ten-di-nī'tis **tendonitis** ten-dō-nī'tis	inflammation of a tendon

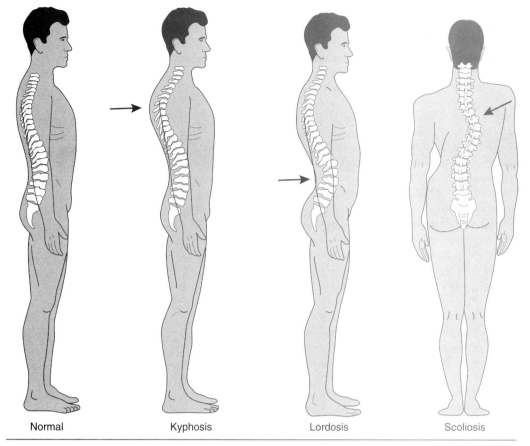

Figure 6.12. Spinal curvatures.

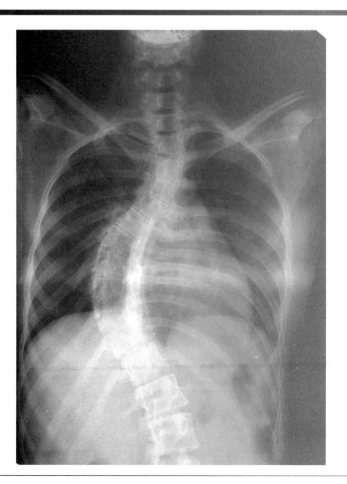

Figure 6.13. AP thoracic spine radiograph demonstrating scoliosis.

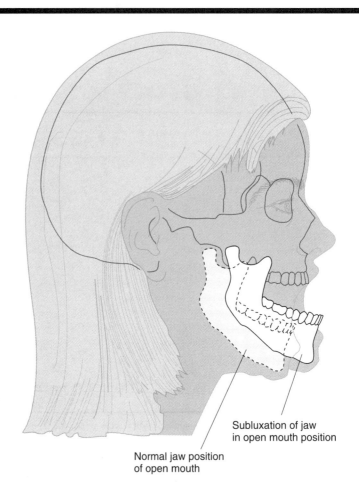

Subluxation of jaw
in open mouth position

Normal jaw position
of open mouth

Figure 6.14. Subluxation.

Diagnostic Tests and Procedures

Test or Procedure	Explanation
electromyogram (EMG) ē-lek-trō-mī′ō-gram	a neurodiagnostic graphic record of the electrical activity of muscle at rest and during contraction to diagnose neuromusculoskeletal disorders [e.g., muscular dystrophy (usually performed by a neurologist)]
magnetic resonance imaging (MRI) măg-nĕt′ik rez′ō-nans im′ă-jing	a nonionizing (no x-ray) imaging technique using magnetic fields and radio frequency waves to visualize anatomical structures—useful in detecting joint, tendon, and vertebral disc disorders (Fig. 6.15)
nuclear medicine imaging nū′klē-er **radionuclide organ imaging** rā′dē-ō-nū′klīd	a diagnostic imaging technique using injected or ingested radioactive isotopes and a gamma-camera for determining size, shape, location, and function of various body parts
bone scan	a nuclear scan of bone tissue to detect tumor, malignancy, etc. (Fig. 6.16)

continued

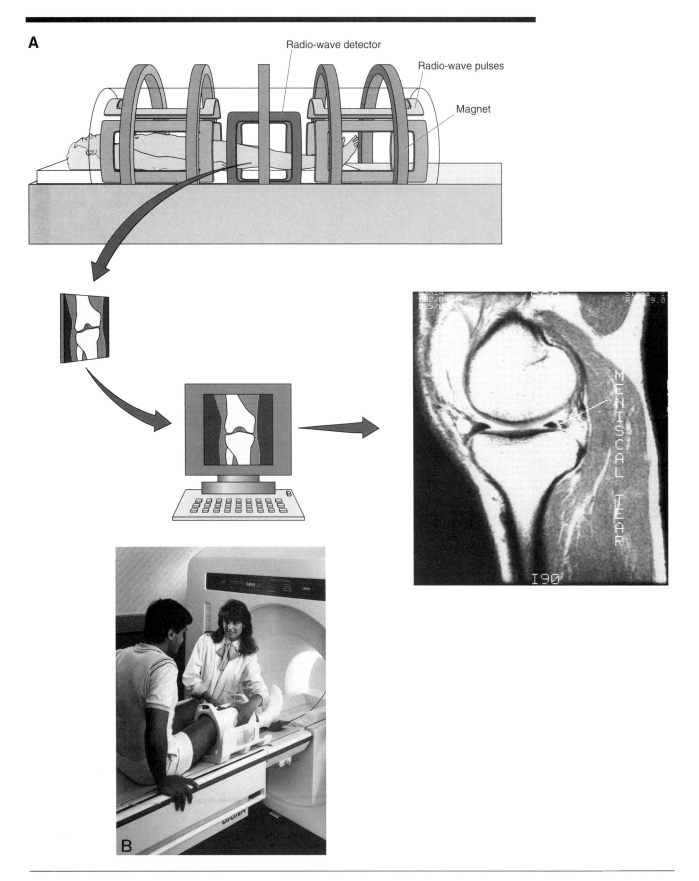

Figure 6.15. A. Principles of magnetic resonance imaging (MRI). Patient is positioned within a magnetic field as radiowave signals are conducted through selected body part. Energy is absorbed by tissues and then released. Computer processes the released energy and formulates image. *Inset,* magnetic resonance image of knee (lateral view) identifying a torn meniscus. **B.** MRI unit.

X-RAYS. Wilhelm Roentgen discovered x-rays in 1895. He used the expression rays for the sake of brevity and named them x-rays to distinguish them from others of the same name. The first x-ray image was made of Roentgen's wife's hand.

Test or Procedure	Meaning
radiography (x-ray) rā′dē-og′ră-fē	an imaging modality using x-rays (ionizing radiation) to diagnose a condition or impairment somewhere in the body (e.g., extremities, ribs, back, shoulders, joint) (Fig. 6.17)
arthrogram ar′thrō-gram	an x-ray of a joint taken after injection of a contrast medium
computed tomography (CT) tō-mog′ră-fē	a radiologic procedure using a machine called a scanner to examine a body site by taking a series of cross-sectional images one slice at a time in a full circle rotation; a computer then calculates and converts the rates of absorption and density of the x-rays into a picture on a screen (Fig. 6.18)
computed axial tomography (CAT)	
sonography sŏ-nog′ră-fē	use of high frequency sound waves (ultrasound) to visualize tissues or structures (e.g., muscles, ligaments, displacements or dislocations, arthroscopic visualizations, etc.)

continued

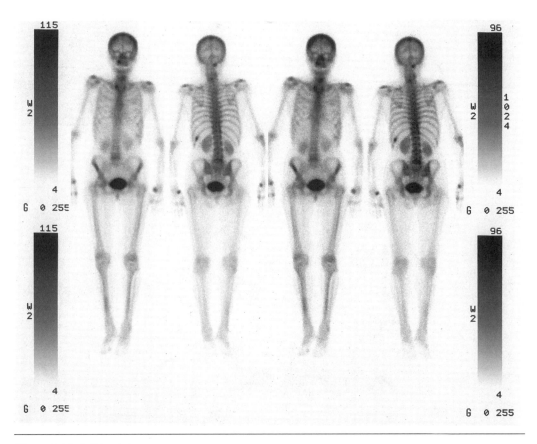

Figure 6.16. Full body bone scan.

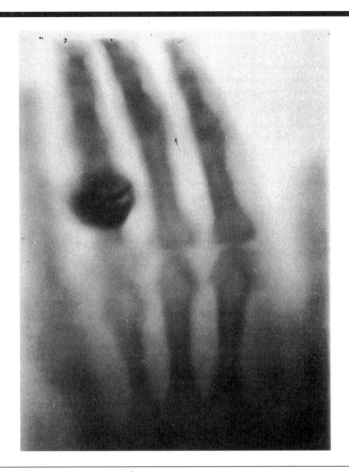

Figure 6.17. First published x-ray image of the hand and signet ring of Professor Roentgen's wife was produced December 22, 1895.

Operative Terms

Term	Meaning
amputation am-pyū-tā′shŭn	to cut around; partial or complete removal of a limb; AKA, above knee amputation; BKA, below knee amputation
arthrocentesis ar′thrō-sen-tē′sis	puncture for aspiration of a joint
arthrodesis ăr-thrō-dē′sĭs	binding or fusing of joint surfaces
arthroplasty ar′thrō-plas-tē	repair or reconstruction of a joint (Fig. 6.19)
arthroscopy ar-thros′kă-pē	procedure with an arthroscope to examine, diagnose, and repair a joint from within (Fig. 6.20)
bone grafting	transplantation of a piece of bone from one site to another to repair a skeletal defect
bursectomy ber-sek′tō-mē	excision of a bursa

continued

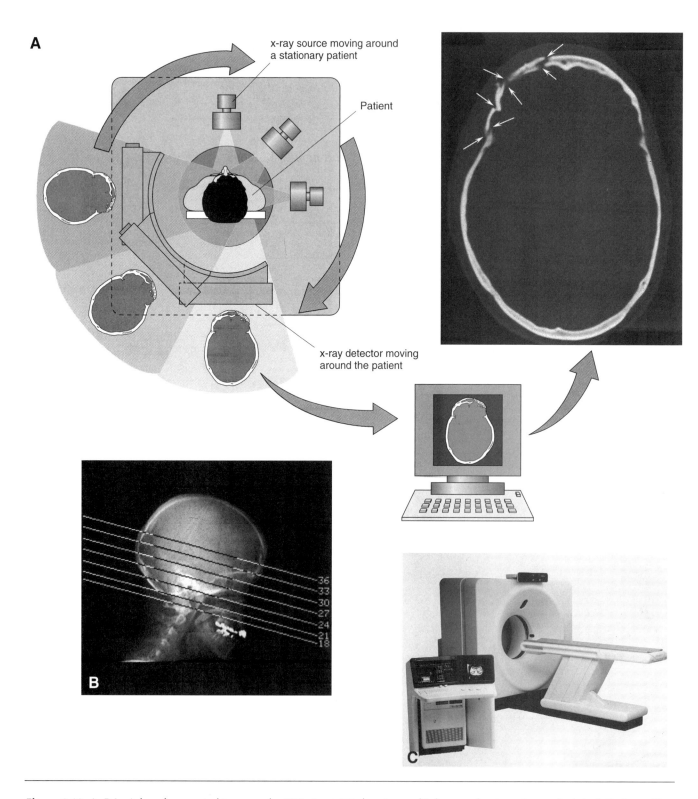

Figure 6.18. A. Principles of computed tomography (CT). *Inset,* CT showing multiple open fractures (*arrows*) of skull. **B.** Scout film of skull identifying CT slices. **C.** CT unit.

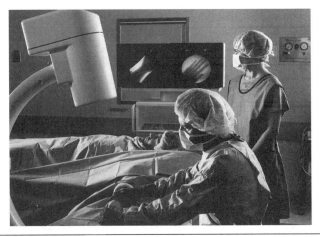

Figure 6.19. X-ray of hand performed during arthroplasty.

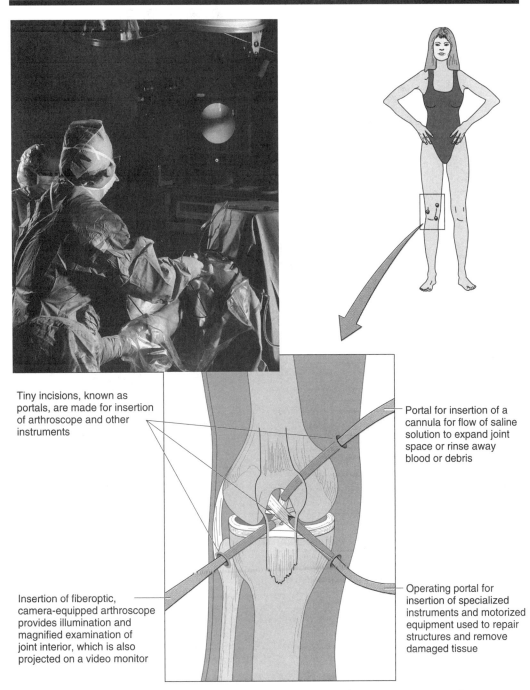

Tiny incisions, known as portals, are made for insertion of arthroscope and other instruments

Portal for insertion of a cannula for flow of saline solution to expand joint space or rinse away blood or debris

Insertion of fiberoptic, camera-equipped arthroscope provides illumination and magnified examination of joint interior, which is also projected on a video monitor

Operating portal for insertion of specialized instruments and motorized equipment used to repair structures and remove damaged tissue

Figure 6.20. Scene of arthroscopic knee surgery with projection of surgeon's view on video monitor.

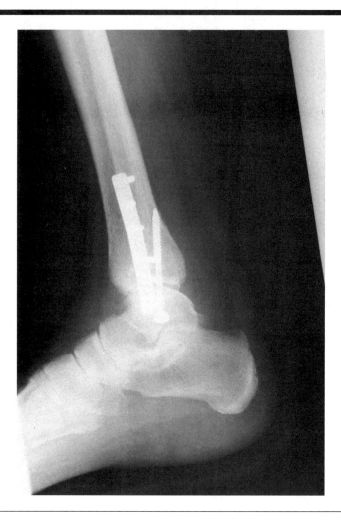

Figure 6.21. An x-ray image taken after open reduction, internal fixation (ORIF) of right ankle (see Medical Record 6.1).

Term	Meaning
myoplasty mī′ō-plas-tē	repair of muscle
open reduction, internal fixation (ORIF)	internal surgical repair of a fracture by bringing bones back into alignment and fixing them into place, often utilizing plates, screws, pins, etc. (Fig. 6.21)
osteotomy os-tē-ot′ō-mē	an incision into bone
osteoplasty os′tē-ō-plas-tē	repair of bone
spondylosyndesis spon′di-lō-sin-dē′sis	spinal fusion
tenotomy te-not′ō-mē	division by incision of a tendon to repair a deformity caused by shortening of a muscle

Therapeutic Terms

Term	Meaning
closed reduction, external fixation of a fracture	manipulation of a fracture to regain alignment from the outside along with application of an external device to protect and hold the fracture while healing
casting	use of a stiff, solid dressing around a limb or other body part to immobilize it during healing (Fig. 6.22)
splinting	use of a rigid device to immobilize or restrain a broken bone or injured body part (Fig. 6.23)
traction (Tx) trak'shŭn	application of a pulling force to a fractured bone or dislocated joint to maintain proper position during healing (Fig. 6.24)
closed reduction, percutaneous fixation of a fracture	manipulation of a fracture from the outside to regain alignment followed by insertion of a pin to maintain position (Fig. 6.25)
orthosis or-thō'sis	use of an orthopedic appliance to maintain bony position or provide limb support (e.g., back, knee, or wrist brace) (Fig. 6.26)

continued

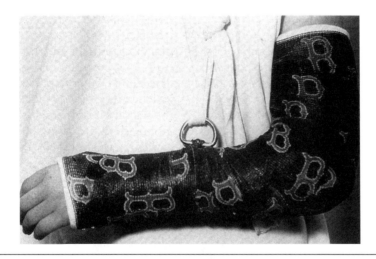

Figure 6.22. Patient in long arm cast.

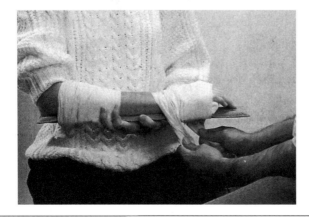

Figure 6.23. Arm splint.

144

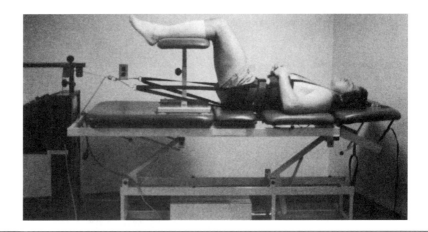

Figure 6.24. Mechanical lumbar traction.

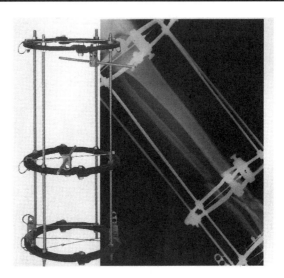

Figure 6.25. Closed reduction, percutaneous fixation of a fracture is indicated for 37-year-old with gunshot wound to right lower extremity (open comminuted distal tib/fib fracture).

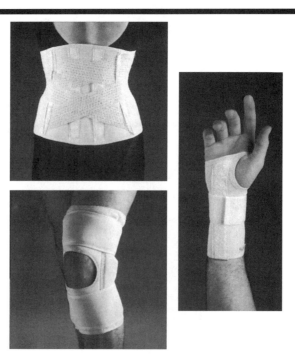

Figure 6.26. Examples of orthoses: back, knee, and wrist.

Term	Meaning
physical therapy (PT) fĭz′ĭ-kăl thĕr′ă-pē	treatment to rehabilitate patients disabled by illness or injury, involving many different modalities (methods) such as exercise, hydrotherapy, diathermy, ultrasound, etc. (Fig. 6.27)
prosthesis pros′thĕ-sis	an artificial replacement for a missing body part or a device used to improve a body function such as an artificial limb, hip, joint, etc. (Fig. 6.28)

continued

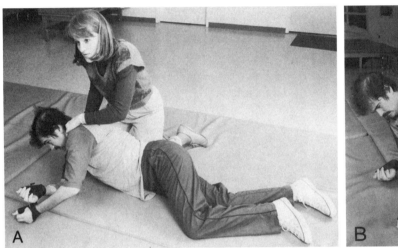
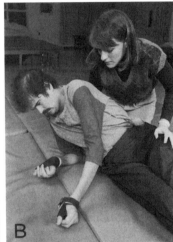

Figure 6.27. Physical therapist assists patients regaining neuromuscular function.

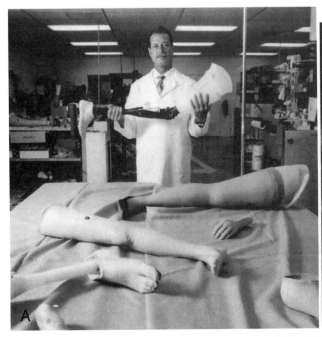
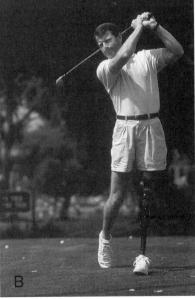

Figure 6.28. A. Prosthetist holding an above-the-knee prosthesis with an array of prostheses on table in foreground. **B.** Prosthetic leg makes it possible for above-the-knee amputee to lead active life.

Term	Meaning

Common Therapeutic Drug Classifications

Term	Meaning
analgesic an-ăl-jē'zik	a drug that relieves pain
narcotic nar-kot'ik	a potent analgesic that has addictive properties
anti-inflammatory an'tē-in-flam'ă-tō-rē	a drug that reduces inflammation
antipyretic an'tē-pī-ret'ik	a drug that relieves fever
nonsteroidal anti-inflammatory drug (NSAID) non-stēr'oy-dăl	a group of drugs with analgesic, anti-inflammatory, and antipyretic properties (e.g., ibuprofen, aspirin) commonly used to treat arthritis

PRACTICE EXERCISES

For the following terms, draw a line or lines to separate prefixes, combining forms, and suffixes. Then define the term.

1. hemipelvectomy _____

2. arthritis _____

3. myofascial _____

4. arthropathy _____

5. spondylolysis _____

6. osteogenic _____

7. chondrectomy _____

8. myonecrosis _____

9. spondylosyndesis _____

10. periosteitis _____

11. leiomyosarcoma _____

12. myelocyte _____

13. costotomy _____

14. spondylomalacia _____

15. osteoarthritis _____

16. intercostal _____

17. orthosis _____

18. craniotomy _____

19. myotonia _____

20. kyphosis _____

21. craniectomy _____

22. arthrodesis _____

23. osteoplasty _____

24. fibromyalgia _____

25. rhabdomyoma _____

26. arthrogram _____

27. intraarticular _____

28. lordosis _____

29. syndactylism _____

30. tenomyotomy _____

31. cervicobrachial _____

32. hypotonia _____

33. arthroscopy _____

34. lumbodynia _____

35. thoracic _____

36. ostealgia _____

37. costovertebral _____

Write the correct medical term for each of the following:

38. lateral curvature of the spine _____

39. joint pain _____

40. bone tumor _____

41. muscle tumor _____

42. grating sound made by movement of broken bones _____

43. bone pain _____

44. x-ray of a joint _____

45. line that divides the body into right and left halves _____

46. surgical reconstruction of bone _____

47. plane that divides the body into front and back portions _____

48. opposite of hypertrophy _____

49. striated (skeletal) muscle tumor _____

50. test to record muscle response to electrical stimulation _____

51. smooth muscle tumor _____

52. application of a pulling force to a fractured or dislocated joint to maintain proper position during healing

    _____

53. flabby (relaxed muscle) _____

54. lying flat on the back _____

55. bone marrow tumor _____

56. arthritis caused by hyperuricemia _____

57. horizontal plane that divides the body into superior and inferior portions

    _____

58. turning downward or backward of the palm of the hand or sole of the foot

    _____

59. stiff joint _____

60. a partial dislocation _____

61. toward the beginning of a structure _____

62. lying face down and flat _____

63. an artificial replacement for a missing body part _____

64. diagnostic test that uses nuclear imaging techniques to visualize bone tissue

65. above another structure or toward the head _____

66. bending of the foot or toes upward _____

67. internal surgical repair of a fracture by bringing bones into alignment _____

68. osteomalacia in children _____

69. diagnostic imaging technique using high-frequency sound waves to visualize body tissues and structures

    _____

70. physician specializing in x-ray technology _____

71. stiff muscle _____

Complete the medical term by writing the missing part:

72. inter_____ al = pertaining to between the *ribs*

73. _____ myosarcoma = malignant *striated or skeletal* muscle tumor

74. hyper _____ = excessive *nourishment or development* (increase in the size of a muscle)

75. myo_____ = *suture* of a muscle

76. spondylosyn_____ = *binding* together of vertebrae

77. _____ myoma = *smooth* muscle tumor

78. osteo_____ = *softening* of bone

79. _____ listhesis = slipping of *vertebra*

80. arthro_____ = *x-ray* of a joint

81. _____ tomy = incision into *bone*

82. epiphys_____ = *inflammation* of the ends of the long bones

83. _____ al = pertaining to the *neck*

84. bone _____ osis = *dead* bone tissue

85. _____ oma = tumor of *cartilage*

86. arthro_____ = *puncture for aspiration* of a joint

Match the following terms with the appropriate body movements:

87. flexion   _____   a. movement toward the body

88. inversion   _____   b. straightening

89. adduction   _____   c. bending

90. extension   _____   d. to turn inward

91. abduction   _____   e. to turn outward

92. eversion   _____   f. movement away from the body

Define the following abbreviations:

93. CT _____

94. PT _____

95. Tx _____

96. ROM _____

97. Fx _____

Medical Record Analyses

MEDICAL RECORD 6.1

As Alice Toohey was playing with her young granddaughter, she stepped on a toy dump truck and fell down her porch steps, wrenching her ankle violently. Because of the sharp pain and immediate swelling, Ms. Toohey was taken immediately to the hospital. After being seen by the emergency room physician, she was admitted and scheduled for surgery.

Directions

Read Medical Record 6.1 for Alice Toohey (page 154) and answer the following questions. This record is the operative report dictated by the surgeon, Dr. Ricardo Rodriguez, immediately after the operation and processed by a medical transcriptionist.

Questions about Medical Record 6.1

Write your answers in the spaces provided.

1. Below are medical terms used in this record you have not yet encountered in this text. Underline each where it appears in the record and define below.

   malleolus _____

   oblique _____

   sterile _____

2. In your own words, not using medical terminology, briefly describe the preoperative diagnosis for Ms. Toohey.

   _____

   _____

   _____

3. Put the following operative steps in correct order by numbering them 1 to 10.

   _____ x-ray of the screws that were too long

   _____ incision on the outer side of the ankle

   _____ plate placed onto fibula

   _____ sewing the incisions

   _____ x-ray of satisfactory screw position

   _____ towel clip positioned

   _____ removal of medial hematoma

_____ removal of lateral hematoma

_____ placement of screw into lower tibia

_____ incision on the inner side of the right ankle

4. In this operation the surgeon redid one step after using a diagnostic procedure to check whether that step was as effective as possible. In your own words, explain what Dr. Rodriguez changed and why.

_____

_____

_____

5. Describe the fracture line: _____

6. When Dr. Rodriguez examined the ankle after making the first incision, he found a problem he could not and did not repair. In your own words, what had been destroyed in Ms. Toohey's injury? _____

_____

7. Which of the following actions did *not* occur in this operation?

   a. washing the wound with antibiotic

   b. taping the fracture line

   c. drilling holes in the bone

   d. stapling the skin closed

8. Describe Ms. Toohey's condition when transferred to PAR after the operation:

_____

_____

_____

CENTRAL MEDICAL CENTER

211 Medical Center Drive • Central City, US 90000-1234 • PHONE: (012) 125-6784 • FAX: (012) 125-9999

OPERATIVE REPORT

PREOPERATIVE DIAGNOSIS: Trimalleolar fracture, right ankle/fracture dislocation.

POSTOPERATIVE DIAGNOSIS: Trimalleolar fracture, right ankle/fracture dislocation.

OPERATION PERFORMED: Open reduction and internal fixation of medial malleolus and lateral malleolus, right ankle.

ANESTHESIOLOGIST: K. Teglam, M.D.

ANESTHESIA: General.

DESCRIPTION OF OPERATION: After successful general anesthesia, the right lower extremity was prepped and draped in a sterile fashion. A pneumatic tourniquet was used in the case at 300 mm Hg (mercury) for 51 minutes. The medial side was opened first; the skin was incised, and this was carried down through the subcutaneous tissue down to the periosteum which was incised enough at the fracture site for visualization of a large transverse medial malleolar fracture. A hematoma was evacuated by curettage and irrigation. Unfortunately, there was some debris within the joint which was articular cartilage destruction and damage on the talus.

Attention was then directed laterally where an incision was made and carried through the skin and subcutaneous tissue. The fracture was brought into full view very easily. The fracture was long and oblique. This was curetted of hematoma and irrigated, and using a bone clamp, it was clamped in a reduced position. A 6-hole semitubular fibular-type plate was then bent to position and placed onto the fibula; and after predrilling, premeasuring, and pretapping, six cortical 3.5 mm diameter screws were used to hold the plate to the fractured fibula.

Attention was then directed medially. The fracture was reduced and held in place with a towel clip, and a 60 mm long malleolar screw was then inserted into the fragment into the distal tibia. X-rays revealed that three of the screws laterally were too long, and these were changed. The medial malleolus screw was also tightened down further. Repeat film revealed very satisfactory position of all the screws. The posterior malleolar fragment was felt to be adequately positioned. All the wounds were then irrigated with goodly amounts of antibiotic solution. Vicryl sutures, 0 and 2-0, were used to close the subcutaneous tissue on both sides; and staples were used for the skin. A bulky Jones dressing was applied with splints anteriorly and posteriorly.

The patient tolerated the procedure well and was transferred to the recovery room with stable vital signs.

R. Rodriguez, M.D.

RR:mb

D: 10/19/9x
T: 10/20/9x

OPERATIVE REPORT	PT. NAME:	TOOHEY, ALICE M.
	ID NO:	IP-236701
	ROOM NO:	729
	ATT. PHYS:	R. RODRIGUEZ, M.D.

Medical Record 6.1.

MEDICAL RECORD 6.2

Jay Dorn, a retired construction worker, has had intermittent back pain for the last two months. When he began also having shooting pains in his legs, he went to his doctor at Central Medical Center. After a physical examination, Mr. Dorn underwent a series of back x-rays.

Directions

Read Medical Record 6.2 for Jay Dorn (page 156) and answer the following questions. This record is the radiographic report dictated by Dr. Mary Volz, the radiographer, after studying Mr. Dorn's x-rays and later transcribed for the record.

Questions about Medical Record 6.2

Write your answers in the spaces provided.

1. Below are medical terms used in this record you have not yet encountered in this text. Underline each where it appears in the record and define below.

    eburnation _____

    lipping _____

    discogenic _____

2. What phrase in the report indicates more than one x-ray was taken?

    _____

    Does the report state how many x-rays were taken?

    _____ no _____ yes   If yes, how many? _____

3. In your own words, not using medical terminology, describe the three diagnoses Dr. Volz makes:

    a. _____

    b. _____

    c. _____

4. Not using any abbreviations, explain what test Dr. Volz says may be useful for Mr. Dorn to have next.

    _____

5. Which of the following is *not* mentioned in the report as a finding?

    a. lateral curvature of spine

    b. forward slipping of vertebra

    c. immobile condition of spine

    d. inflammation of bone marrow

    e. inflammation of both hips

CENTRAL MEDICAL CENTER

211 Medical Center Drive • Central City, US 90000-1234 • PHONE: (012) 125-6784 • FAX: (012) 125-9999

X-RAY REPORT

LUMBOSACRAL SPINE:

Multiple views reveal no evidence of fracture. There is slight lumbar spondylosis with slight lipping and minimal bridging. The disc spaces appear maintained except for slight narrowing at L4-L5 and L5-S1. There is also a Grade I spondylolisthesis of L5 on S1 and evidence of spondylolysis at L5 on the left. There is also slight dextroscoliosis in the lumbar region and slight increased lordosis in the lumbosacral region. The bony architecture is unremarkable except for eburnation between the articulating facets at L5-S1. The SI joints appear unremarkable. Incidentally noted are slight osteoarthritic changes involving both hips.

CONCLUSION:

1. Slight lumbar spondylosis with hypertrophic lipping and slight narrowing of the L4-L5 and L5-S1 disc spaces, 'rule out discogenic disease. If clinically indicated, CT of the lumbosacral spine may prove helpful in further evaluation.

2. Grade I spondylolisthesis of L5 on S1 with evidence of spondylolysis at L5 on the left.

3. Slight dextroscoliosis in the lumbar region and slight increased lordosis in the lumbosacral region.

M. Volz M.D.
M. Volz, M.D.

MV:ti

D: 10/19/9x
T: 10/20/9x

X-RAY REPORT	PT. NAME:	DORN, JAY F.
	ID NO:	RL-483091
	ATT. PHYS:	T. LIGHT, M.D.

Medical Record 6.2.

Cardiovascular System

OBJECTIVES

After completion of this chapter you will be able to

1. Define common combining forms used in relation to the cardio-vascular system

2. Identify basic anatomical terms referring to the heart and blood vessels

3. Trace the flow of blood through the heart

4. Define blood pressure

5. Describe the pathway of electrical conduction in the heart

6. Define common symptomatic, diagnostic, operative, and therapeutic terms referring to the cardiovascular system

7. List common diagnostic tests and procedures related to the cardiovascular system

8. Explain terms and abbreviations used in documenting medical records involving the cardiovascular system

Combining Forms

Combining Form	Meaning	Example
angi/o	vessel	**angiogram** an'jē-ō-gram
vas/o		**vasospasm** vā'sō-spazm
vascul/o		**vascular** vas'ku-lar
aort/o	aorta	**aortic** ā-ōr'tik
arteri/o	artery	**arteriostenosis** ar-tēr'ē-ō-stĕ-nō'sis
ather/o	fat	**atheroma** ath-er-ō'mă
atri/o	atrium	**atrioventricular** a'trē-ō-ven-trik'yū-lăr
cardi/o	heart	**cardiology** kar-dē-ol'ō-jē
coron/o	circle or crown	**coronary** kōr'o-nār-ē
pector/o	chest	**pectoral** pek'tŏ-ral
steth/o		**stethoscope** steth'ō-skōp
sphygm/o	pulse	**sphygmomanometer** sfig'mō-mă-nom'ĕ-ter
thrombo	clot	**thrombocyte** throm'bō-sīt
ven/o	vein	**venous** vē'nŭs
phleb/o		**phlebitis** flĕ-bī'tis
varic/o	swollen, twisted vein	**varicosis** vār-i-kō'sis
ventricul/o	ventricle (belly or pouch)	**ventricular** ven-trik'yū-lăr

Cardiovascular System Overview

The cardiovascular system consists of the heart and blood vessels that transport blood throughout the body (see Color Atlas, plates 11–14).

The heart is the muscular organ that pumps blood throughout the body (Fig. 7.1). Its hollow interior has four chambers: the *right atrium* and *left atrium* (upper chambers) and the *right ventricle* and *left ventricle* (lower chambers). A partition, called the *septum*, divides the heart into right and left portions. The atria are separated by the *interatrial septum*, and the ventricles are separated by the *interventricular septum*. The valves of the heart open and close with the heartbeat to maintain the one-way flow of blood through the heart. They include the *tricuspid valve*, the *mitral (bicuspid) valve*, the *pulmonary semilunar valve*, and the *aortic valve*.

There are three layers of the heart: endocardium, myocardium, and epicardium. The *endocardium* is the membrane that lines the interior cavities of the heart. The *myocardium* is the thick, muscular layer, and the *epicardium* is the outer membrane. Surrounding and enclosing the heart is a loose, protective sac called the *pericardium*.

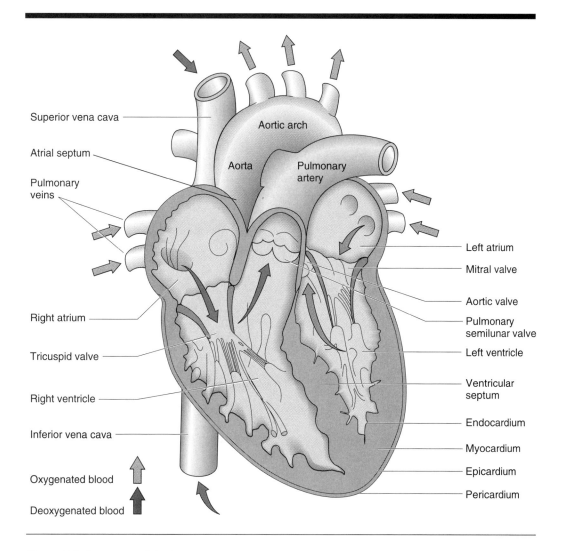

Figure 7.1. Structures of the heart.

Blood transports essential elements within the body. It is circulated throughout the body via *arteries, arterioles, capillaries, venules,* and *veins.* (Blood is discussed separately in Chapter 8.) Blood flow through the heart is as follows.

Deoxygenated (depleted of oxygen) blood returning from circulation in the body enters the heart through the *superior vena cava* and *inferior vena cava* into the right atrium. During atrial contraction, the tricuspid valve opens to allow blood to flow into the right ventricle. Contraction of the ventricle causes blood to be pushed through the pulmonary semilunar valve into the pulmonary artery. The *pulmonary artery* carries the blood through two branches going to the lungs and on through the *pulmonary circulation* (a network of arteries, capillaries, air sacs, and veins in the lung) where it is oxygenated (supplied with oxygen) and gives off carbon dioxide waste. The oxygenated blood returns to the heart via the *pulmonary veins* into the left atrium. With atrial contraction, the mitral valve (also called bicuspid valve) opens to allow blood flow into the left ventricle. Contraction of the left ventricle causes blood to be pushed through the aortic valve into the aorta. Blood is then carried to all parts of the body through the *systemic circulation* (arteries, arterioles, capillaries, and veins) to provide transport for oxygen and nutrients. Notice that the right side of the heart, right heart, handles deoxygenated blood and the left side of the heart, left heart, handles oxygenated blood.

The heart is the first organ to receive oxygenated blood via the coronary circulation. Branching from the aorta, the right and left coronary arteries divide to distribute blood throughout the entire heart (Fig. 7.2).

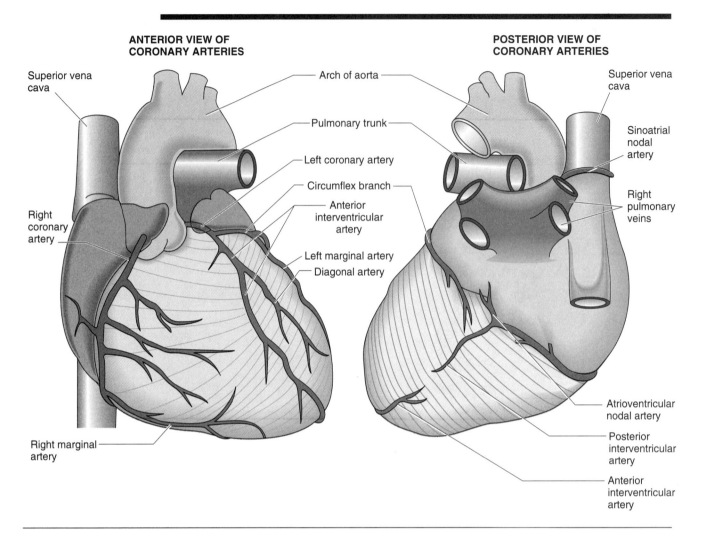

Figure 7.2. Coronary arteries.

Anatomical Terms

Term	Meaning
Septa and Layers of Heart	
atrium ā′trē-ŭm	upper right or left chamber of heart
endocardium en-dō-kar′dē-ŭm	membrane lining the cavities of the heart
epicardium ep-i-kar′dē-ŭm	membrane forming the outer layer of the heart
interatrial septum in-ter-ā′trē-ăl sep′tŭm	partition between right and left atrium
interventricular septum in-ter-ven-trik′yū-lăr sep′tŭm	partition between right and left ventricle
myocardium mī-ō-kar′dē-ŭm	heart muscle

continued

Term	Meaning
pericardium per-i-kar'dē-ŭm	protective sac enclosing the heart composed of two layers with fluid between
visceral pericardium vis'er-ăl	layer closest to the heart (visceral = pertaining to organ)
parietal pericardium pă-rī'ĕ-tăl	outer layer (parietal = pertaining to wall)
pericardial cavity pĕr-ĭ-kar'dē-ăl	fluid-filled cavity between the pericardial layers
ventricle ven'tri-kăl	lower right and left chamber of the heart

Valves of Heart and Veins

Term	Meaning
heart valves	structures within the heart that open and close with the heartbeat to regulate the one-way flow of blood
aortic valve ā-ōr'tik	heart valve between the left ventricle and the aorta
mitral or bicuspid valve mī'trăl bī-kŭs'pid	heart valve between the left atrium and left ventricle (cuspis = point)
pulmonary semilunar valve pŭl'mō-nār-ē sem-ē-lū'năr	heart valve opening from the right ventricle to the pulmonary artery (luna = moon)
tricuspid valve trī-kŭs'pid	valve between the right atrium and the right ventricle
valves of the veins	valves located at intervals within the lining of veins, especially in the legs, which constrict with muscle action to move the blood returning to the heart

Blood Vessels (Fig. 7.3)

Term	Meaning
arteries ăr'tĕr-ēz	vessels that carry blood *from* the heart to arterioles (see Color Atlas, plate 13)
aorta ā-ōr'tă	large artery that is the main trunk of the arterial system branching from the left ventricle
arterioles ăr-tēr'ē-ōlz	small vessels that receive blood from the arteries
capillaries kap'i-lār-ēz	tiny vessels that join arterioles and venules
venules ven'yūlz	small vessels that gather blood from the capillaries into the veins
veins vānz	vessels that carry blood to the heart from the venules (see Color Atlas, plate 14)

Circulation

Term	Meaning
systemic circulation sis-tĕm'ik	circulation of blood throughout the body through arteries, arterioles, capillaries, and veins to deliver oxygen and nutrients to body tissues

continued

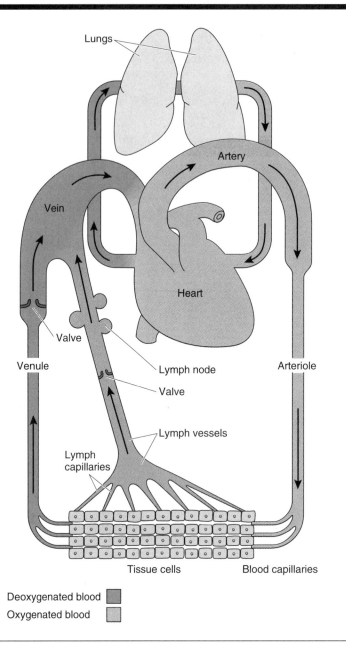

Figure 7.3. Blood and lymph circulation.

Term	Meaning
coronary circulation kōr'o-nār-ē	circulation of blood through the coronary blood vessels to deliver oxygen and nutrients to the heart muscle tissue
pulmonary circulation pŭl'mō-nār-ē	circulation of blood from the pulmonary artery through the vessels in the lungs and back to the heart via the pulmonary vein, providing for the exchange of gases

Blood Pressure

Blood pressure is the force exerted by circulating blood on the walls of the arteries, veins, and heart chambers. This pressure is determined by the volume of blood, the space within the arteries and arterioles, and the force of heart contractions (Fig. 7.4).

Blood pressure (BP) technique involves measuring pressure within the walls of an artery during the period of contraction of the heart, or *systole,* and during the period of relaxation of the heart, or *diastole.* When blood pressure is written, the systolic measurement is recorded first, followed by a slash, then the diastolic measurement (e.g., BP 120/80 means that the systolic reading is 120 and the diastolic reading is 80).

Blood Pressure Terms

Term	Meaning
diastole dī-as′tō-lē	to expand; period in the cardiac cycle when blood enters the relaxed ventricles from the atria
systole sis′tō-lē	to contract; period in the cardiac cycle when the heart is in contraction and blood is ejected through the aorta and pulmonary artery
normotension nōr-mō-ten′shŭn	normal blood pressure
hypotension hī′pō-ten′shŭn	low blood pressure

continued

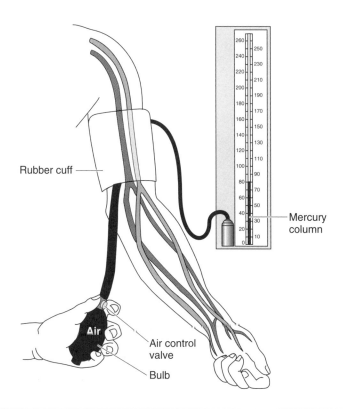

Figure 7.4. Blood pressure determination.

Term	Meaning
hypertension hī′per-ten′shŭn	high blood pressure

Symptomatic Terms (Fig. 7.5)

Term	Meaning
arteriosclerosis ar-tēr′ē′ō′skler-ō′sis	thickening, loss of elasticity, and calcification of arterial walls
atherosclerosis ath′er-ō-skler-ō′sis	buildup of fatty substances within the walls of arteries
atheromatous plaque ath-er-ō′mă-tŭs plak	a swollen area within the lining of an artery caused by the buildup of fat (lipids)
thrombus throm′bŭs	a stationary blood clot
embolus em′bō-lŭs	a clot (air, fat, foreign object, etc.) carried in the bloodstream (embolus = a stopper)
stenosis ste-nō′sis	narrowing of a part
constriction kon-strik′shŭn	compression of a part
occlusion ŏ-klū′zhŭn	plugging; obstruction or a closing off

continued

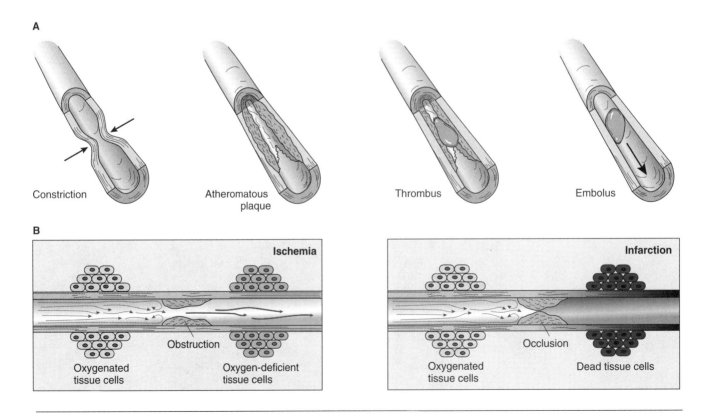

Figure 7.5. A. Examples of conditions causing reduction of blood flow. **B.** Effects of reduction of blood flow.

Term	Meaning
ischemia is-kē′mē-ă	to hold back blood; decreased blood flow to tissue, caused by constriction or occlusion of a blood vessel
perfusion deficit per-fyū′zhŭn def′i-sit	a lack of flow through a blood vessel caused by narrowing, occlusion, etc.
infarct in′farkt	to stuff; a localized area of necrosis caused by ischemia as a result of occlusion of a blood vessel
angina pectoris an′ji-nă pek′tō-ris	chest pain caused by a temporary loss of oxygenated blood to heart muscle often caused by narrowing of coronary arteries (angina = to choke)
aneurysm an′yū-rizm	a widening; bulging of the wall of the heart, aorta, or artery caused by congenital defect or acquired weakness (Fig. 7.6)
saccular săk′ū-lăr	a sac-like bulge on one side
fusiform fū′zĭ-form	a spindle-shaped bulge
dissecting dī-sĕkt′ing	a split or tear of the vessel wall
claudication klaw-di-kā′shŭn	limping; pain in a limb (especially the calf) while walking that subsides after rest; it is caused by inadequate blood supply
heart murmur hart mer′mer	an abnormal sound from the heart produced by defects in the chambers or valves
palpitation pal-pi-tā′shŭn	subjective experience of pounding, skipping, or racing heartbeats
vegetation vej-ĕ-tā′shŭn	to grow; an abnormal growth of tissue around a valve, generally a result of infection (Fig. 7.7)

continued

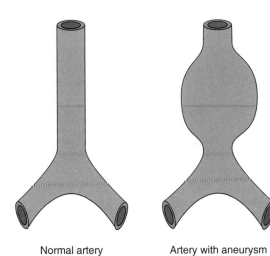

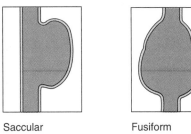
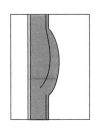

Common types of aneurysms

Normal artery   Artery with aneurysm   Saccular   Fusiform   Dissecting

Figure 7.6. Aneurysm.

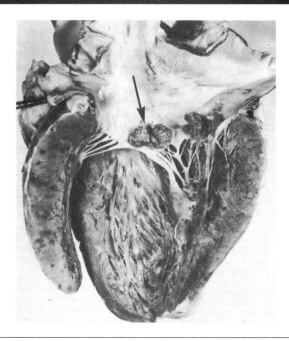

Figure 7.7. *Arrow,* large vegetations attached to mitral valve, present in endocarditis.

Cardiac Conduction

The *cardiac cycle* is the repeated action of the heart during which an electrical impulse is conducted from the sinoatrial (SA) node (the pacemaker of the heart) to the atrioventricular (AV) node, to the bundle of His, to the left and right bundle branches, and to the Purkinje fibers, causing contraction of the heart and circulation of blood (Fig. 7.8).

Initiated by the SA node, each myocardial cell responds to stimulation conducted by electrical impulses, changing from a resting state (polarized) to a state of contraction (depolarized) and then returning to a resting state by recharging (repolarizing); it is then ready again to begin the continuous cycle of contraction and relaxation of the myocardium that pumps blood through the heart.

Cardiac Conduction Terms

Term	Meaning
sinoatrial node (SA node) sī′nō-ā′trē-ăl nōd	the pacemaker; highly specialized neurological tissue impeded in the wall of the right atrium responsible for initiating electrical conduction of the heartbeat, causing the atria to contract and firing conduction of impulses to the AV node
atrioventricular node (AV node) ā′trē-ō-ven-trik′yū-lăr	neurological tissue in the center of the heart that receives and amplifies the conduction of impulses from the SA node to the bundle of His

continued

Term	Meaning
bundle of His bŭn'dl	neurological fibers extending from the AV node to the right and left bundle branches that fire the impulse from the AV node to the Purkinje fibers
Purkinje fibers (network) pŭr-kin'jē fi'berz	fibers in the ventricles that transmit impulses to the right and left ventricles, causing them to contract
polarization pō'lăr-i-zā'shŭn	resting; resting state of a myocardial cell
depolarization dē-pō-lăr-i-zā'shŭn	change of a myocardial cell from a polarized (resting) state to a state of contraction (de = not; polarization = resting)
repolarization rē-pō-lăr-i-zā'shŭn	recharging of the myocardial cell from a contracted state back to a resting state (re = again; polarization = resting)
normal sinus rhythm (NSR)	regular rhythm of the heart cycle stimulated by the SA node

continued

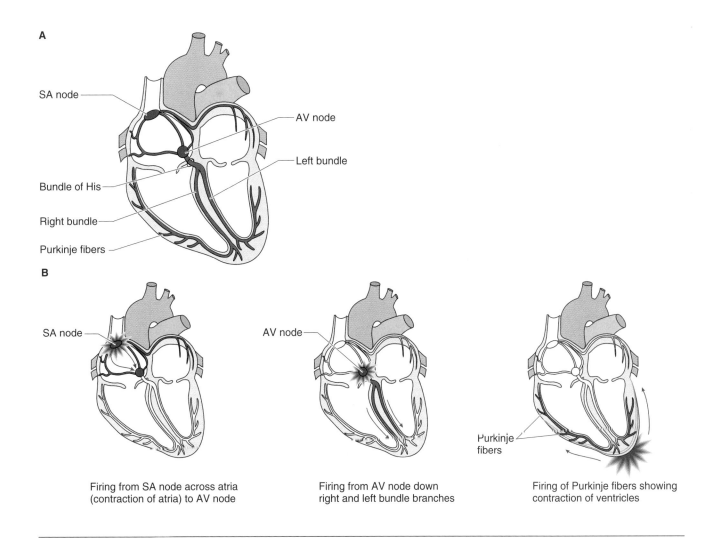

A

SA node

AV node

Left bundle

Bundle of His

Right bundle

Purkinje fibers

B

SA node

AV node

Purkinje fibers

Firing from SA node across atria (contraction of atria) to AV node

Firing from AV node down right and left bundle branches

Firing of Purkinje fibers showing contraction of ventricles

Figure 7.8. Cardiac conduction.

Term	Meaning
Diagnostic Terms (Fig. 7.9)	
arrhythmia ă-rith′mē-ă	any of several kinds of irregularity or loss of rhythm of the heartbeat (Fig. 7.9)
bradycardia brad-ē-kar′dē-ă	slow heart rate (<60 beats/minute)
fibrillation fib-ri-lā′shŭn	chaotic, irregular contractions of the heart as in atrial or ventricular fibrillation
flutter flŭt′er	extremely rapid but regular contractions of heart as in atrial or ventricular flutter
heart block hart blok	an interference with the normal electrical conduction of the heart defined by the location of the block (e.g., AV block)
premature ventricular contraction (PVC) prē-mă-tūr′ ven-trik′yū-lăr kon-trak′shŭn	a ventricular contraction preceding the normal impulse initiated by the SA node (pacemaker)
tachycardia tak′i-kar′dē-ă	fast heart rate (>100 beats/minute)
arteriosclerotic heart disease (ASHD) ar-tēr′ē-ō-skler-ot′ik	a degenerative condition of the arteries characterized by thickening of the inner lining, loss of elasticity, and susceptibility to rupture—seen most often in the aged or smokers
bacterial endocarditis bak-tēr′ē-ăl en′dō-kar-dī′tis	a bacterial inflammation that affects the endocardium or the heart valves
cardiac tamponade kar′dē-ak tam-pŏ-nād′	compression of the heart produced by the accumulation of fluid in the pericardial sac as results from pericarditis or trauma, causing rupture of a blood vessel within the heart (tampon = a plug)
cardiomyopathy kar′dē-ō-mī-op′ă-thē	a general term for disease of the heart muscle [e.g., alcoholic cardiomyopathy (damage to the heart muscle caused by excessive consumption of alcohol)]
congenital anomaly of the heart kon-jen′i-tăl ă-nom′ă-lē	malformations of the heart present at birth (anomaly = irregularity)
atrial septal defect (ASD) ā′trē-ăl sep′tăl dē′fekt	an opening in the septum separating the atria
coarctation of the aorta kō-ark-tā′shŭn	narrowing of the descending portion of the aorta resulting in a limited flow of blood to the lower part of the body (Fig. 7.10)
patent ductus arteriosus pā′tĕnt dŭk′tŭs ăr-tĕr-ē-ō′sŭs	an abnormal opening between the pulmonary artery and the aorta caused by the failure of the fetal ductus arteriosus to close after birth (patent = open) (Fig. 7.11)

continued

Normal sinus rhythm (NSR)

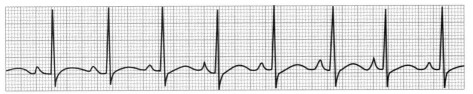

Bradycardia

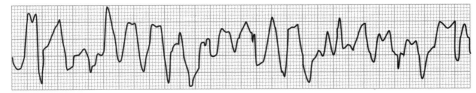

Fibrillation (ventricular)

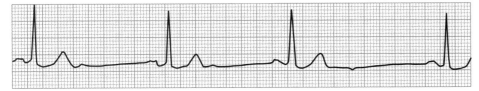

Flutter (atrial)

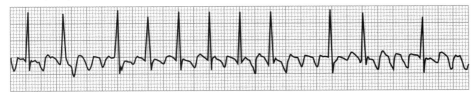

Heart block

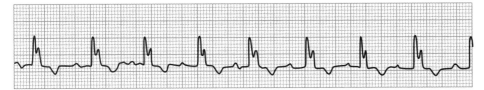

Premature ventricular contraction (PVC)

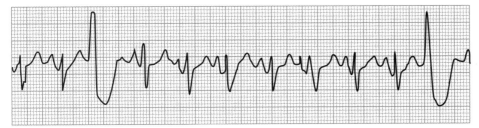

Tachycardia (sinus)

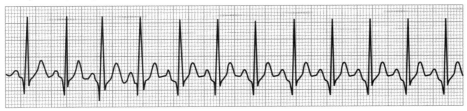

Figure 7.9. Electrocardiogram tracings showing common types of arrhythmia.

Term	Meaning
tetralogy of Fallot tet-ral′ō-jē făl-ō′	an anomaly that consists of four defects: pulmonary stenosis, ventricular septal defect, malposition of the aorta, and right ventricular hypertrophy—causes blood to bypass the pulmonary circulation so that deoxygenated blood goes into the systemic circulation resulting in cyanosis (tetra = four)
ventricular septal defect (VSD) ven-trik′yū-lăr sep′tăl dē′fekt	an opening in the septum separating the ventricles
congestive heart failure (CHF) kon-jes′tiv **left ventricular failure**	failure of the left ventricle to pump an adequate amount of blood to meet the demands of the body, resulting in a "bottleneck" of congestion in the lungs that may extend to the veins, causing edema in lower portions of the body

continued

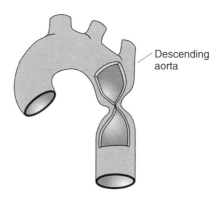

Descending aorta

Figure 7.10. Coarctation of the aorta.

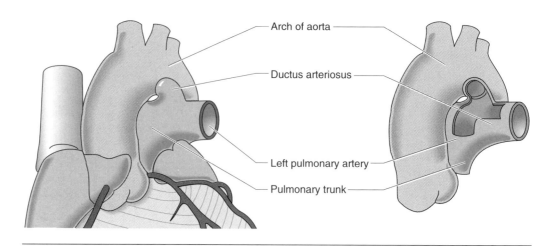

Arch of aorta

Ductus arteriosus

Left pulmonary artery

Pulmonary trunk

Figure 7.11. Patent ductus arteriosus.

Term	Meaning
cor pulmonale kōr pul-mō-nā′lē **right ventricular failure**	a condition of enlargement of the right ventricle as a result of chronic disease within the lungs that causes congestion within the pulmonary circulation and resistance of blood flow to the lungs (cor = heart)
coronary artery disease (CAD)	a condition affecting arteries of the heart that reduces the flow of blood and delivery of oxygen and nutrients to the myocardium—most often caused by atherosclerosis (Fig. 7.12)
hypertension (HTN) hī′per-ten′shŭn	persistently high blood pressure
essential hypertension ĕ-sen′shăl hī′per-ten′shŭn	high blood pressure attributed to no single cause, but risks include smoking, obesity, increased salt intake, hypercholesterolemia, and hereditary factors
secondary hypertension	high blood pressure caused by the effects of another disease (e.g., kidney disease)
mitral valve prolapse (MVP) mī′trăl	protrusion of one or both cusps of the mitral valve back into the left atrium during ventricular contraction, resulting in incomplete closure and backflow of blood
myocardial infarction (MI) mī-ō-kar′dē-ăl in-fark′shŭn	heart attack; death of myocardial tissue owing to loss of blood flow (ischemia) as a result of an occlusion (plugging) of a coronary artery—usually caused by atherosclerosis (Fig. 7.13)
myocarditis mī′o-kar-dī′tis	inflammation of myocardium most often caused by viral or bacterial infection
pericarditis per′i-kar-dī′tis	inflammation of the pericardium

continued

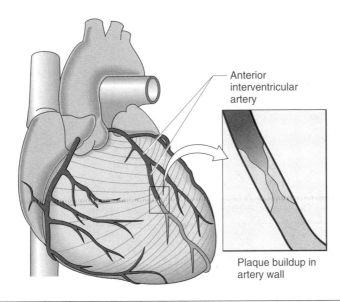

Anterior interventricular artery

Plaque buildup in artery wall

Figure 7.12. Coronary artery disease.

Term	Meaning
phlebitis flĕ-bī′tis	inflammation of a vein
rheumatic heart disease rū-mat′ik	damage to heart muscle and heart valves by rheumatic fever (a streptococcal infection)
thrombophlebitis throm′bō-flĕ-bī′tis	inflammation of a vein associated with a clot formation
varicose veins văr′ĭ-kōs	abnormally swollen twisted veins with defective valves, most often seen in the legs (Fig. 7.14)
deep vein thrombosis (DVT) throm-bō′sis	formation of a clot in a deep vein of the body, occurring most often in the femoral and iliac veins

Diagnostic Tests and Procedures

Test or Procedure	Explanation
auscultation aws-kŭl-tā′shŭn	a physical examination method of listening to sounds within the body with the aid of a stethoscope (e.g., auscultation of the chest for heart and lung sounds) (Fig. 7.15)
bruit brū-ē′	noise; an abnormal heart sound caused by turbulence within
gallop	an abnormal heart sound that mimics the gait of a horse; related to abnormal ventricular contraction
electrocardiogram (ECG or EKG) ē-lek-trō-kar′dē-ō-gram	an electrical picture of the heart represented by positive and negative deflections on a graph labeled with the letters P, Q, R, S, and T, corresponding to events of the cardiac cycle (Fig. 7.16)

continued

AUSCULTATION. The Latin root means to listen or hear with attention. Listening to the sound of the breathing and of the beating of the heart is an ancient art that was current in Hippocrates' time. It was accomplished by placing the ear directly on the chest wall—direct or immediate auscultation. Indirect or mediate auscultation has been utilized in modern times since the invention of the stethoscope.

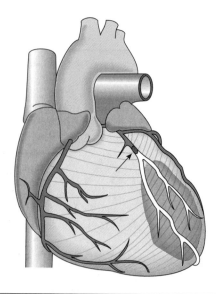

Figure 7.13. Anterolateral myocardial infarction, caused by occlusion of anterior descending branch of left coronary artery.

Test or Procedure	Explanation
stress electrocardiogram	an ECG of the heart recorded during the induction of controlled physical exercise using a treadmill or ergometer (bicycle), useful in detecting conditions, (e.g., ischemia, infarction, etc.) (Fig. 7.17)
Holter ambulatory monitor hōlt er am'byū-lă-tōr-ē mon'i-ter	a portable electrocardiograph worn by the patient that monitors electrical activity of the heart over 24 hours—useful in detecting periodic abnormalities
telephonic ECG monitoring	use of a portable ECG monitor, connected through telephone lines via a modem, that allows the patient to transmit ECG recordings to a staffed monitoring center for cardiac evaluation

continued

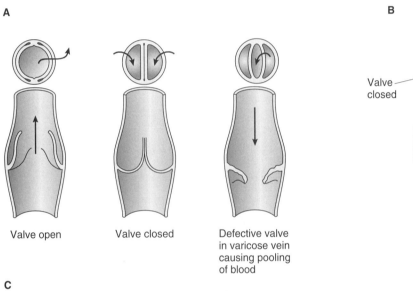

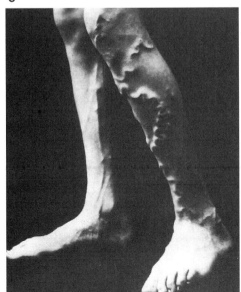

Figure 7.14. Varicose veins. **A.** Function of valves in venous system. **B.** Contraction of skeletal muscle causes valves to open and close, preventing backflow of blood returning to heart. **C.** Varicose veins.

Test or Procedure	Explanation
magnetic resonance angiography (MRA) rez'ō-nans an-jē-og'ră-fē	magnetic resonance imaging of the heart and blood vessels for evaluation of pathology
nuclear medicine imaging nū'klē-ar med'i-sin im'ă-jing	scan of the heart after administration of radioactive isotopes to visualize structures and analyze functions
positron emission tomography (PET) **scan** poz'i-tron ē-mish'shun tō-mog'ră-fē	use of nuclear isotopes and computed tomography to produce perfusion (blood flow) images and study the cellular metabolism of the heart
myocardial radionuclide perfusion scan mī-ō-kar'dē-ăl ră'dē-ō-nū'klīd per-fyū'zhŭn	a scan of the heart made after an intravenous injection of an isotope (e.g., as thallium) that is absorbed by myocardial cells in proportion to blood flow throughout the heart
myocardial radionuclide perfusion stress scan	nuclear scans of the heart taken before and after the induction of controlled physical exercise (treadmill or bicycle) or pharmaceutical agent that produces the effect of exercise stress in patients unable to ambulate
radiology	x-ray imaging
angiography an-jē-og'ră-fē	x-ray of a blood vessel after injection of contrast medium
angiogram an'jē-ō-gram	record obtained by angiography

continued

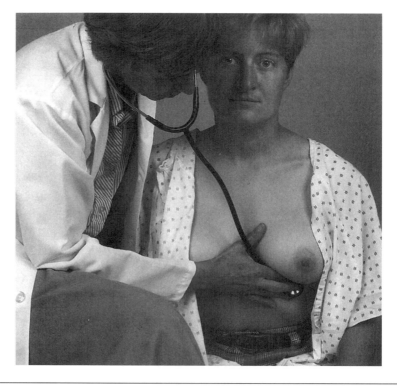

Figure 7.15. Auscultation.

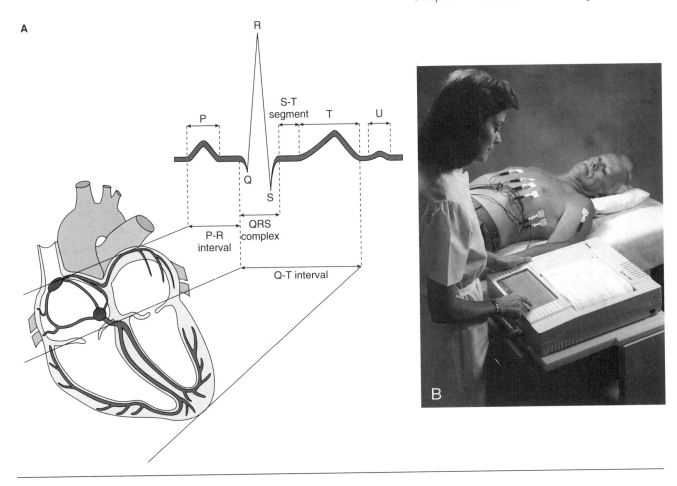

Figure 7.16. A. Electrocardiographic mapping of normal cardiac conduction. **B**. Resting electrocardiogram.

Test or Procedure	Explanation
coronary angiogram kōr'o-nār-ē an'jē-ō-gram	x-ray of the blood vessels of the heart (Fig. 7.18)
arteriogram ar-tēr'e-ō-gram	x-ray of a particular artery (e.g. coronary arteriogram, renal arteriogram)
aortogram ā-ōr'tō-gram	x-ray of the aorta
venogram vē'nō-gram	x-ray of a vein
cardiac catheterization kar'dē-ak kath'ĕ-ter-ī-zā'shŭn	introduction of a flexible, narrow tube or *catheter* through a vein or artery into the heart to withdraw samples of blood, measure pressures within the heart chambers or vessels, and inject contrast media for fluoroscopic radiography and cine film (motion picture) imaging of the chambers of the heart and coronary arteries — very often includes interventional procedures such as angioplasty, atherectomy, etc. (see endovascular procedures listed under "Operative Terms") (Fig. 7.19)

continued

Test or Procedure	Explanation
left heart catheterization	x-ray of the left ventricular cavity and coronary arteries
right heart catheterization	measurement of oxygen saturation and pressure readings of the right side of the heart

continued

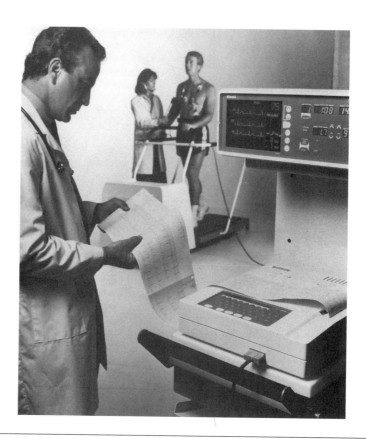

Figure 7.17. Stress electrocardiography.

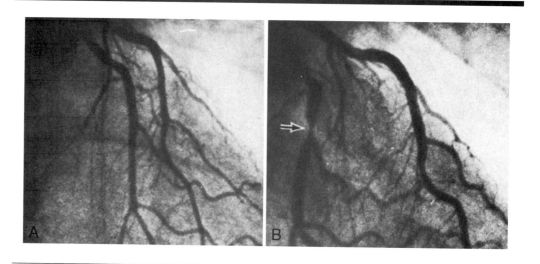

Figure 7.18. Coronary angiograms before (**A**) and after (**B**) drug-induced coronary artery spasm.

Test or Procedure	Explanation
ventriculogram ven-trik′ū-lō-gram	an x-ray visualizing the ventricles
stroke volume (SV)	measurement of amount of blood ejected from a ventricle in one contraction
cardiac output (CO)	measurement of amount of blood ejected from either ventricle of the heart per minute
ejection fraction ē-jek′shŭn frak′shŭn	measurement of volume percentage of left ventricular contents ejected with each contraction
sonography	sonographic imaging
echocardiography (ECHO) ek′ō-kar-dē-og′ră-fē	recording of sound waves through the heart to evaluate structure and motion (Fig. 7.20) (see Color Atlas, plate 11)

continued

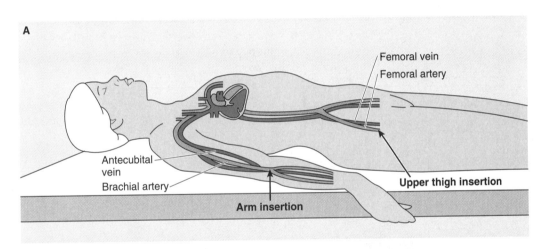

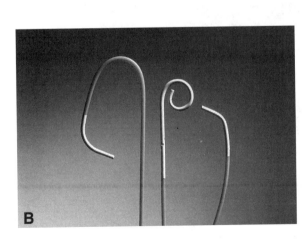

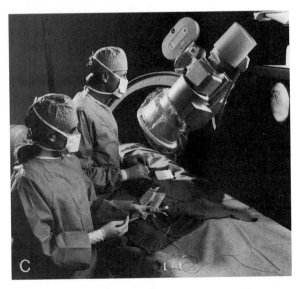

Figure 7.19. Cardiac catheterization. **A.** Possible insertion sites for cardiac catheterization. **B.** Cardiac catheterization catheters: *left,* 6 French JL4; *middle,* 6 French pigtail; *right,* 6 French JR4. **C.** Cardiac catheterization laboratory.

Test or Procedure	Explanation
stress echocardiogram (stress ECHO)	an echocardiogram of the heart recorded during the induction of controlled physical exercise (treadmill or bicycle) or a pharmaceutical agent that produces the effect of exercise stress in patients unable to ambulate—useful in detecting conditions such as ischemia, infarction, etc.
transesophageal echocardiogram (TEE) trans-ē-sof′ă-jē′ăl	an echocardiographic image of the heart after placement of an ultrasonic transducer at the end of an endoscope inside the esophagus
Doppler sonography dŏp′lĕr sŏ-nog′ră-fē	ultrasound technique used to evaluate blood flow to determine the presence of a deep vein thrombosis (DVT) or carotid insufficiency, or flow through the heart, chambers, valves, etc. (see Color Atlas, plates 13 and 14) (Fig. 7.21)
intravascular sonography in′tră-vas′kyū-lăr	ultrasound images made after a sonographic transducer is placed at the tip of a catheter within a blood vessel—done to evaluate pathological conditions such as build-up of plaque, etc.

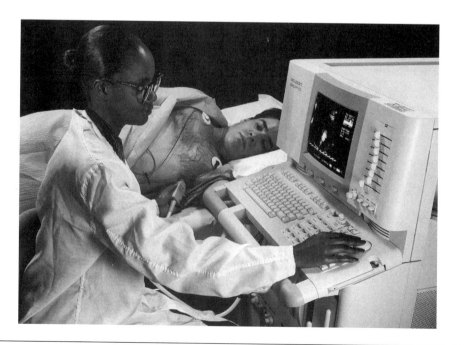

Figure 7.20. Echocardiography.

Operative Terms

Term	Meaning
coronary artery bypass graft (CABG)	grafting of a portion of a blood vessel retrieved from another part of the body (such as a length of saphenous vein from leg or mammary artery from the chest wall) to bypass an occluded coronary artery restoring circulation to myocardial tissue (Fig. 7.22)
anastomosis ă-nas'tō-mō'sis	opening; joining of two blood vessels to allow flow from one to the other
valve replacement	replacement of a diseased heart valve with an artificial one (Fig. 7.23)
valvuloplasty val'vyū-lō-plas-tē	repair of a heart valve
endovascular surgery	interventional procedures performed at the time of cardiac catheterization (Fig. 7.24)
angioscopy (vascular endoscopy) an-jē-os'kō-pē	use of a flexible fiberoptic angioscope accompanied by an irrigation system, camera, video recorder, and a monitor that is guided through a specific blood vessel to visually assess a lesion and select the mode of therapy
arteriotomy ăr-tēr-ē-ot'ō-mē	an incision into an artery
atherectomy ăth-er-ek'tō-mē	excision of atheromatous plaque from within an artery utilizing a device housed in a flexible catheter that selectively cuts away or pulverizes tissue buildup

continued

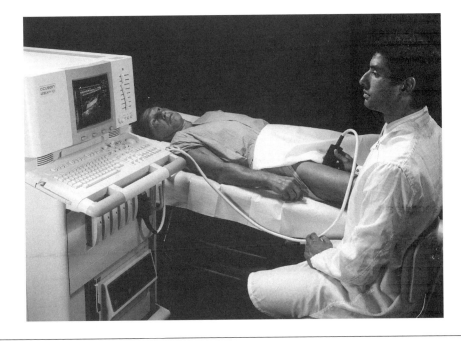

Figure 7.21. Doppler vascular imaging.

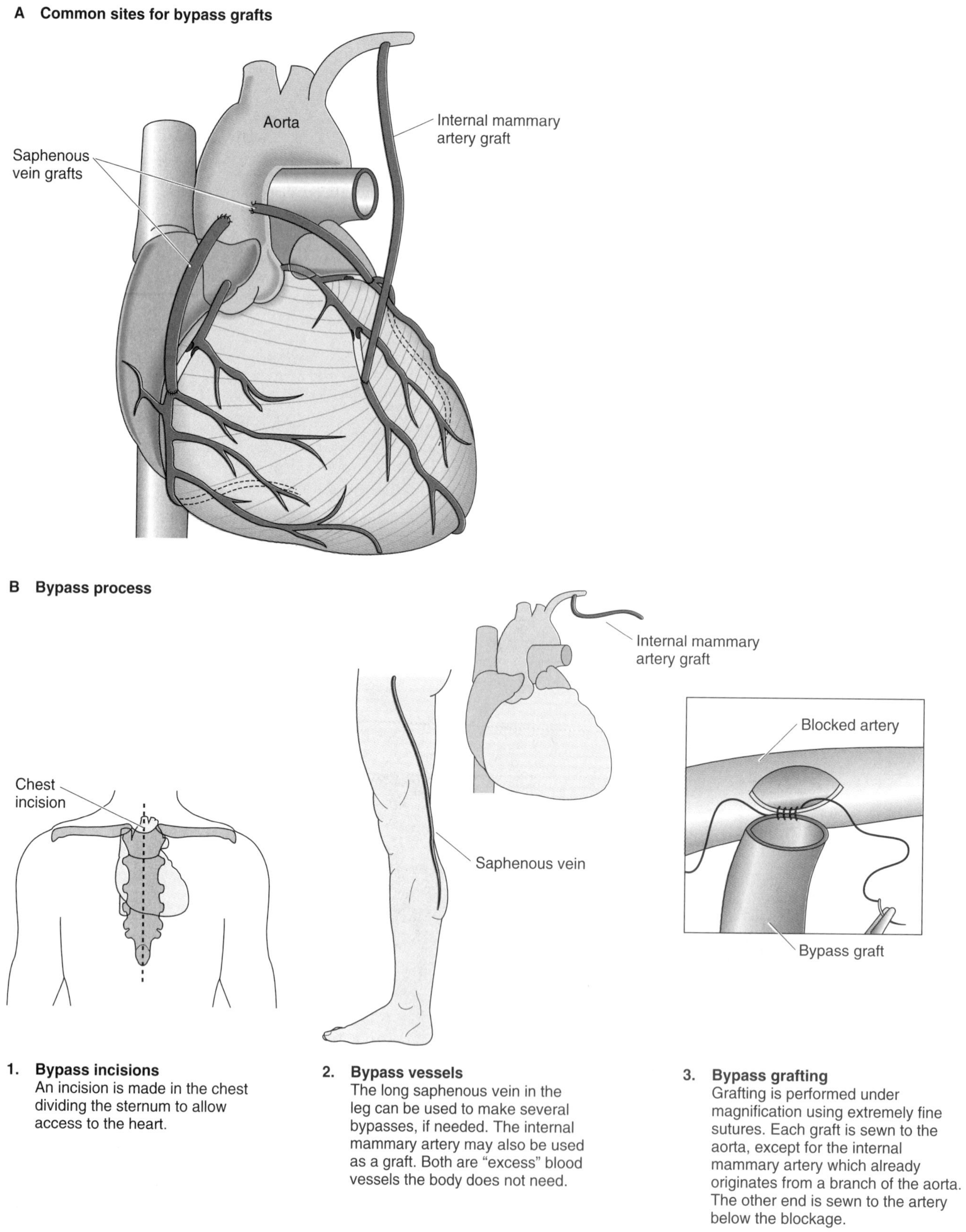

A Common sites for bypass grafts

Aorta

Internal mammary artery graft

Saphenous vein grafts

B Bypass process

Internal mammary artery graft

Chest incision

Saphenous vein

Blocked artery

Bypass graft

1. **Bypass incisions**
    An incision is made in the chest dividing the sternum to allow access to the heart.

2. **Bypass vessels**
    The long saphenous vein in the leg can be used to make several bypasses, if needed. The internal mammary artery may also be used as a graft. Both are "excess" blood vessels the body does not need.

3. **Bypass grafting**
    Grafting is performed under magnification using extremely fine sutures. Each graft is sewn to the aorta, except for the internal mammary artery which already originates from a branch of the aorta. The other end is sewn to the artery below the blockage.

Figure 7.22. Coronary artery bypass graft. **A.** Common sites for bypass grafts. **B.** Bypass process.

Term	Meaning
embolectomy em-bō-lek′tō-mē	incision into an artery for the removal of an embolus
thrombectomy throm-bek′tō-mē	incision into an artery for the removal of a thrombus
endarterectomy end-ar-ter-ek′tō-mē	coring of the lining of an artery to clear a blockage caused by a clot or atherosclerotic plaque buildup
percutaneous transluminal coronary angioplasty (PTCA) per-kyū-tā′nē-ŭs trăns-lū′mĭ-năl kōr′o-nār-ē an′jē-ō-plas-tē	a method of treating the narrowing of a coronary artery by inserting a specialized catheter with a balloon attachment, then inflating it to dilate and open the narrowed portion of the vessel and restore blood flow to the myocardium (see Color Atlas, plate 12)
intravascular stent in′tra-vas′kyū-lăr	implantation of a device used to reinforce the wall of a vessel and assure its patency (openness)—most often used to treat a stenosis or a dissection (a split or tear in the wall of a vessel)

Therapeutic Terms

Term	Meaning
defibrillation dē-fib-ri-lā′shŭn	termination of ventricular fibrillation by delivery of an electrical stimulus to the heart, most commonly by applying electrodes of the defibrillator externally to the chest wall but can be performed internally at the time of open heart surgery or via an implanted device (Fig. 7.25)

continued

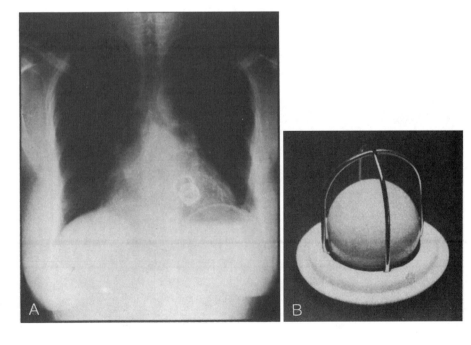

Figure 7.23. A. X-ray showing artificial replacement of mitral valve (Starr-Edwards). **B.** Starr-Edwards mitral valve.

ATHERECTOMY DEVICES

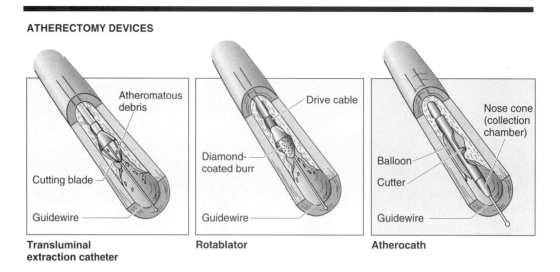

Transluminal
extraction catheter

Rotablator

Atherocath

INTRAVASCULAR STENT

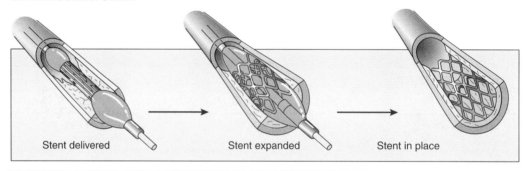

Figure 7.24. Examples of devices used in endovascular interventional procedures.

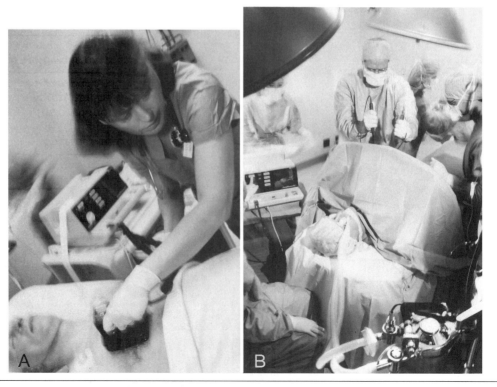

Figure 7.25. A. External defibrillation. **B.** Internal defibrillation performed in operating room.

Term	Meaning
defibrillator dē-fib-ri-lā-ter	device that delivers the electrical stimulus in defibrillation
cardioversion kar'dē-ō-ver'zhŭn	termination of tachycardia either by pharmaceutical means or by delivery of electrical energy
implantable cardioverter defibrillator (ICD) kar'de-o-ver'ter dē-fib-ri-lā'ter	an implanted, battery-operated device with rate sensing leads that monitors cardiac impulses and initiates an electrical stimulus as needed to stop ventricular fibrillation or tachycardia
pacemaker	a device used to treat slow heart rates by electrically stimulating the heart to contract, most often implanted with lead wires and battery circuitry under the skin but can be temporarily placed externally with lead wires inserted into the heart via a vein (Fig. 7.26)
thrombolytic therapy throm-bō-lit'ik	dissolution of thrombi using drugs [e.g., streptokinase or tissue plasminogen activator (TPA)]

continued

A

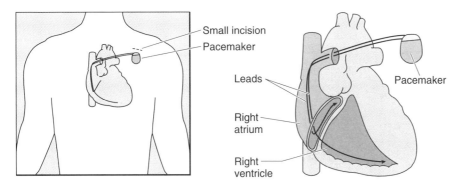

A small incision is made in the upper chest, below the clavicle, to access a large vein nearby.

The pacemaker leads are then guided through the vein and into the heart. After proper placement is determined, the leads are secured in position.

A small "pocket" to house the pacemaker is created just under the skin at the incision site. The leads are connected to the pacemaker that is secured in the "pocket." Finally the incision is closed with a few sutures.

B

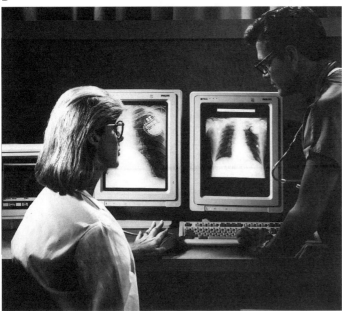

Figure 7.26. Pacemaker. **A.** Endocardial pacemaker; **B.** Teleradiology/critical care workstation chest x-rays on screen show pacemaker placement.

Term	Meaning

Common Therapeutic Drug Classifications

Term	Meaning
angiotensin-converting enzyme (ACE) inhibitor ăn′jē-ō-tĕn′sin kŏn-vĕr′ting ĕn′zīm	drug that suppresses the conversion of angiotensin in the blood by the angiotensin-converting enzyme; used in the treatment of hypertension
antianginal an′tē-an′ji-năl	a drug that dilates coronary arteries, restoring oxygen to the tissues to relieve the pain of angina pectoris
antiarrhythmic an′tē-ă-rith′mik	a drug that counteracts cardiac arrhythmia
anticoagulant an′tē-kō-ag′yū-lant	a drug that prevents clotting of the blood commonly used in treating thrombophlebitis
antihypertensive an′tē-hī-per-ten′siv	a drug that lowers blood pressure
beta-adrenergic blocking agents bā′tă ad-rĕ-ner′jik blok′ing **beta-blockers** bā′tă blok′ers	agents that inhibit responses to sympathetic adrenergic nerve activity causing a slowing of electrical conduction and heart rate and a lowering of the pressure within the walls of the vessels; used to treat angina pectoris and hypertension
calcium channel blockers kal′sē-ŭm chan′l blok′ers	agents that inhibit the entry of calcium ions in heart muscle cells causing a slowing of the heart rate, lessening the demand for oxygen and nutrients, and relaxing of the smooth muscle cells of the blood vessels to cause dilation; used to prevent or treat angina pectoris, some arrhythmias, and hypertension
cardiotonic kar′dē-ō-ton′ik	a drug that increases the force of myocardial contractions in the heart commonly used to treat congestive heart failure
diuretic dī-yū-ret′ik	a drug that increases the secretion of urine commonly prescribed in treating hypertension
hypolipidemic hī-pō-lip′i-dē′mik	a drug that reduces serum fat and cholesterol

PRACTICE EXERCISES

For the following terms, draw a line or lines to separate prefixes, combining forms, and suffixes. Then define the term.

1. angiography _____

2. varicosis_____

3. pectoral _____

4. vasospasm_____

5. venous _____

6. aortocoronary _____

7. thrombophlebitis _____

8. arteriosclerosis _____

9. vasculopathy _____

10. atherogenesis _____

11. cardiomyoliposis _____

12. atrial_____

13. stethoscope _____

14. arteriorrhexis _____

15. myocardium _____

16. aortoplasty _____

17. sphygmoid _____

18. venostomy_____

19. arteriostenosis_____

20. arteriotomy _____

21. thrombopoiesis_____

22. cardioaortic _____

23. ventriculogram _____

24. angiodystrophia _____

25. phlebitis _____

26. thrombophilia _____

27. angioplasty _____

28. venostasis _____

29. endarterectomy _____

30. cardiotoxic _____

31. arteriogram _____

32. atherectomy _____

33. thrombolysis _____

34. aortorrhaphy _____

35. cardiac _____

Match the following terms with their meanings:

36. atherosclerosis	____	a.	high blood pressure
37. infarct	____	b.	bulging of a vessel
38. hypotension	____	c.	stationary clot
39. vegetation	____	d.	cramp in leg muscle
40. embolus	____	e.	normal blood pressure
41. occlusion	____	f.	hard nonelastic condition
42. hypertension	____	g.	traveling clot
43. thrombus	____	h.	buildup of fat
44. constriction	____	i.	growth on tissue

45. normotension ____   j. a plugging

46. angina ____   k. loss of blood flow

47. claudication ____   l. narrowing

48. ischemia ____   m. cramp in heart muscle

49. arteriosclerosis ____   n. low blood pressure

50. aneurysm ____   o. scar left by necrosis

Write the correct medical term for each of the following:

51. _____ malformations of the heart present at birth

52. _____ thickening, loss of elasticity, and calcification of arterial walls

53. _____ irregularity or loss of rhythm of the heartbeat

54. _____ a general term for disease of the heart muscle

55. _____ joining of two blood vessels to allow flow from one to the other

56. _____ an abnormal heart sound that mimics the gait of a horse

57. _____ a recording of sound waves directed through the heart to evaluate structure and motion

58. _____ a condition of enlargement of the right ventricle as a result of chronic disease within the lungs

59. _____ an x-ray of the blood vessels of the heart made with the introduction of a catheter and release of a contrast medium

60. _____ electrocardiogram of the heart recorded during controlled physical exercise

Write the full medical term for the following abbreviations:

61. PVC _____

62. PDA _____

63. ASHD _____

64. ICD _____

65. CHF _____

66. CAD _____

67. HTN _____

68. MVP _____

69. MRA _____

70. VSD _____

Match the following abbreviations with their meanings:

71. ECG _____   a. balloon angioplasty

72. TPA _____   b. magnetic resonance of blood vessels

73. MRA _____   c. a clot in a vein

74. PTCA _____   d. heart bypass surgery

75. MI _____   e. electrical picture of heart

76. DVT _____   f. echocardiogram directed through the esophagus

77. ASD _____   g. left ventricular failure

78. CABG _____   h. thrombolytic drug

79. TEE _____   i. an abnormal opening in the atrial septum

80. CHF _____   j. heart attack

Medical Record Analyses

MEDICAL RECORD 7.1

Richard Stratten has had serious heart problems for more than 10 years. He has had two operations. During the last 6 months he has developed increasing pain in the chest and is having more trouble breathing. His cardiologist, Dr. Charles Feingold, has now admitted him to Central Medical Center for further tests.

Directions

Read Medical Record 7.1 for Richard Stratten (pages 192–195) and answer the following questions. This record is the history and physical examination dictated by Dr. Feingold after his examination of Mr. Stratten.

Questions about Medical Record 7.1

Write your answers in the spaces provided.

1. Below are medical terms used in this record you have not yet encountered in this text. Underline each where it appears in the record and define below.

   obtuse _____

   dyspnea (dyspneic) _____

   hiatal hernia_____

   basilar rales _____

   visceromegaly _____

   clubbing _____

2. In your own words, not using medical terminology, briefly describe why Mr. Stratten has been admitted to the hospital and what test will he be undergoing.

   _____

   _____

   _____

3. Name the diagnosis that underlies the nature of Mr. Stratten's heart conditions.

   _____

   _____

   Briefly describe this diagnosis using nonmedical language.

   _____

   _____

   _____

4. Identify the surgical procedure noted in the history that was *initially* performed to treat Mr. Stratten's heart disease.

   a. dilation of narrow occluded coronary arteries

   b. replacement of occluded arteries with transplanted portion of vein

   c. replacement of a diseased heart valve

   d. coring of the lining of an artery to remove a thrombus

   e. heart transplant

5. What were the patient's symptoms eight years later on May 15, 19xx?

   _____

   Using nonmedical language, briefly describe the diagnosis made at that time.

   _____

   _____

   _____

6. Describe the test that showed changes consistent with the diagnosis.

   _____

   _____

7. Spell out TPA and identify the reason why the drug was given to Mr. Stratten.

   _____

   _____

8. Which of the following were findings of the radiographic tests performed after the May 15 hospitalization? (Mark all that are appropriate.)

   a. hemorrhage of insertion site of obtuse marginal artery graft

   b. thromboembolism in the left anterior descending artery

   c. occluded circumflex artery

   d. torn sutures of the circumflex artery graft

   e. stenosis of left anterior descending artery graft

   f. total occlusion of the left internal mammary vein graft

   g. dilated right coronary artery graft

9. List the arteries that were grafted in *both* bypass operations.

   _____

   _____

10. Using nonmedical language, list the three symptoms Mr. Stratten is now experiencing?

    a. _____

    b. _____

    c. _____

11. Mr. Stratten is taking five different medications. Translate the medication instruction for these:

Drug Name	Dosage	Frequency of Dose
_____	_____	_____
_____	_____	_____
_____	_____	_____
_____	_____	_____
_____	_____	_____

12. What family members have had a medical history of problems in the same body system?

    _____

    _____

13. In addition to Mr. Stratten's heart problems, Dr. Feingold's physical examination revealed abnormal findings in what other areas?

    a. head

    b. abdomen

    c. extremities

    d. all of the above

    e. none of the above

14. What does "probable end-stage cardiomyopathy" mean? What treatment seems possible to Dr. Feingold, even though he had not yet performed the diagnostic tests for which he hospitalized Mr. Stratten?

    _____

    _____

    _____

    _____

CENTRAL MEDICAL CENTER
211 Medical Center Drive • Central City, US 90000-1234 • PHONE: (012) 125-6784 • FAX: (012) 125-9999

HISTORY

CHIEF COMPLAINT:
The patient is admitted for heart catheterization and coronary arteriography with a view of possible cardiac transplantation.

HISTORY OF PRESENT ILLNESS:
The patient is a 53-year-old Caucasian male who has had a known history of coronary artery disease. The patient had initial 4-vessel bypass surgery ten years ago on July 18, 199x, at which time the patient had a saphenous vein bypass graft to the left anterior descending, diagonal, obtuse marginal, and right coronary artery.

Eight years later, on May 15, 199x, the patient was rehospitalized at Central Medical Center because of acute chest pain with electrocardiogram changes consistent with acute inferior wall infarction for which the patient was given TPA. Following that, the patient had dramatic improvement in terms of electrocardiogram changes and symptoms and subsequently underwent reevaluation, including heart catheterization and coronary arteriography. This revealed the following findings:

> Native right coronary artery, left anterior descending, and circumflex were all totally occluded. The bypass graft to the left anterior descending had an 80% stenosis proximally and was totally occluded distally. Circumflex was previously totally occluded. Bypass graft to the obtuse marginal had a 70% occlusion followed by 90% occlusion at the insertion site of the graft. The right coronary artery graft had 95-98% stenosis. This diagonal graft was previously demonstrated to be totally occluded.

Because of this, the patient underwent a second bypass surgery on May 25, 199x, at which time the patient had a left internal mammary graft to the left anterior descending and right internal mammary graft to the diagonal. The patient also had a saphenous vein bypass graft to the obtuse marginal and right coronary artery.

Since that time, the patient has continued to have intermittent angina, particularly within the last six months or so. In addition, the patient has gotten progressively weaker and dyspneic.

(continued)

HISTORY AND PHYSICAL PAGE 1	PT. NAME: STRATTEN, R. ID NO: ROOM NO: ADM. DATE: October 15, 199x ATT. PHYS: C. FEINGOLD, M.D.

Medical Record 7.1.

CENTRAL MEDICAL CENTER
211 Medical Center Drive • Central City, US 90000-1234 • PHONE: (012) 125-6784 • FAX: (012) 125-9999

HISTORY

At the present time, the patient is taking Nitro-Bid 2.5 mg b.i.d., Capoten 6.25 mg t.i.d., Slow-K 1 tablet b.i.d, Procan SR 500 mg q 6 h, and Lasix 600 mg p.o. b.i.d.

Because of increasing symptoms, the patient is being evaluated for cardiac transplant. The patient is undergoing heart catheterization for evaluation.

PAST MEDICAL HISTORY:
PAST ILLNESSES: There is no prior history of hypertension or diabetes. See above regarding previous coronary bypass surgery and myocardial infarctions.

The patient has a known hiatal hernia, but it is asymptomatic at this time.

ALLERGIES: None known.

MEDICATIONS: See above.

PREVIOUS OPERATIONS: See above.

FAMILY HISTORY:
Father died of coronary artery disease at age 50. Paternal uncle also died of coronary artery disease. Maternal uncle and grandfather are both diabetic. The patient has no siblings. The remainder of family history is noncontributory.

SOCIAL HISTORY:
MARITAL HISTORY: Single.

HABITS: The patient is a nonsmoker and denies drinking ethanolic beverages.

INVENTORY BY SYSTEMS:
Noncontributory. There is no prior history of transient ischemic attack or claudication.

(continued)

HISTORY AND PHYSICAL PAGE 2	PT. NAME: STRATTEN, R. ID NO: ROOM NO: ADM. DATE: October 15, 199x ATT. PHYS: C. FEINGOLD, M.D.

Medical Record 7.1. *Continued.*

CENTRAL MEDICAL CENTER
211 Medical Center Drive • Central City, US 90000-1234 • PHONE: (012) 125-6784 • FAX: (012) 125-9999

PHYSICAL EXAMINATION

GENERAL:
The patient is a well-developed, well-nourished Caucasian male who is not in acute distress.

VITAL SIGNS:
Blood Pressure: 120/80. Pulse: 70 and regular.

HEENT:
HEAD: Normocephalic, atraumatic.

NECK: Neck veins are essentially normal. There are no carotid bruits.

CHEST:
HEART: Revealed cardiomegaly. There is no murmur. There is an equivocal third heart sound.

LUNGS: There are a few basilar rales.

ABDOMEN:
No visceromegaly. The bowel sounds are normal. No masses or tenderness.

RECTAL:
Deferred.

EXTREMITIES:
No clubbing, cyanosis, or peripheral edema. The peripheral pulses are intact.

NEUROLOGIC:
Physiologic.

IMPRESSION:
CORONARY ARTERY DISEASE WITH PREVIOUS ANTERIOR AND INFERIOR WALL INFARCTION STATUS POST PREVIOUS CORONARY BYPASS SURGERY x 2 WITH PROGRESSIVE INCREASE IN SYMPTOMATOLOGY IN TERMS OF ANGINA AND DYSPNEA WITH PROBABLE END-STAGE CARDIOMYOPATHY.

(continued)

HISTORY AND PHYSICAL PAGE 3	PT. NAME: STRATTEN, R.
	ID NO:
	ROOM NO:
	ADM. DATE: October 15, 199x
	ATT. PHYS: C. FEINGOLD, M.D.

Medical Record 7.1. *Continued.*

CENTRAL MEDICAL CENTER
211 Medical Center Drive • Central City, US 90000-1234 • PHONE: (012) 125-6784 • FAX: (012) 125-9999

HISTORY AND PHYSICAL

The details of heart catheterization and coronary angiography have been discussed with the patient, including the risks and potential complications. The patient understands and wishes to proceed. This will be performed on October 16, 199x.

C. Feingold, M.D.

CF:ti

D: 10/19/9x
T: 10/20/9x

HISTORY AND PHYSICAL Page 4	PT. NAME: STRATTEN, R. ID NO: ROOM NO: ADM. DATE: October 15, 199x ATT. PHYS: C. FEINGOLD, M.D.

Medical Record 7.1. *Continued.*

MEDICAL RECORD 7.2

William Smith woke in the middle of the night with substernal chest heaviness that radiated to both arms. After getting no relief from taking aspirin and antacids, he went to the emergency room and was seen by Dr. Roland Galasso. The chest pain subsided only after administration of intravenous nitroglycerin. Dr. Galasso decided to admit Mr. Smith for further cardiac evaluation and treatment. A cardiac catheterization was performed the next day.

Directions

Read Medical Record 7.2 for William Smith (pages 198–199) and answer the following questions. This record is a report of the cardiac catheterization performed by Dr. Galasso and transcribed by a cardiology department transcriptionist.

Questions about Medical Record 7.2

Write your answers in the spaces provided:

1. Below are medical terms used in this record you have not yet encountered in this text. Underline each where it appears in the record and define below.

   ostium _____

   hemodynamic _____

   mitral regurgitation _____

   focal _____

2. In your own words, not using medical terminology, briefly describe the *indications* for performing the cardiac catheterization. _____

   _____

3. Put the following actions in correct order by numbering them 1 to 14.

   ____ pigtail catheter advanced to the left ventricle

   ____ hemostasis obtained by C-clamp pressure

   ____ right coronary arteriography performed

   ____ pigtail catheter exchanged for left coronary artery catheter

   ____ informed consent signed

   ____ arterial pressures were recorded

   ____ right groin prepped and draped

   ____ left coronary arteriography performed

   ____ right femoral artery entered and Cordis sheath inserted

   ____ right coronary catheter and femoral artery sheath removed

   ____ pigtail catheter inserted through sheath and guided to descending thoracic aorta

   ____ left coronary catheter exchanged for right coronary catheter

_____ left ventriculography performed

_____ heparin was administered

4. Briefly describe conclusions of the procedure in nonmedical language:

a. _____

b. _____

5. From the recommendations, describe the test that will be performed right away.

_____

6. Identify the possible complications likely to occur in the future.

_____

_____

_____

Describe the procedure that is recommended should these complications occur.

_____

_____

_____

CENTRAL MEDICAL CENTER
211 Medical Center Drive • Central City, US 90000-1234 • PHONE: (012) 125-6784 • FAX: (012) 125-9999

CARDIAC CATHETERIZATION

DATE OF PROCEDURE: November 3, 199x

PROCEDURE PERFORMED: Left heart catheterization with left ventriculography, left and right coronary arteriography.

INDICATIONS: Recent onset of angina pectoris.

CATHETERS USED: 6 French pigtail Cordis, 6 French JL4, 6 French JR4.

CONTRAST: Optiray-320.

MEDICATIONS GIVEN: None.

PROCEDURE IN DETAIL:
Informed consent was obtained. The patient was brought to the Cardiac Catheterization Laboratory where the right groin was prepped and draped in the usual sterile fashion. The skin was anesthetized with 1% Xylocaine. The right femoral artery was entered by Seldinger technique and a 7 French Cordis sheath was inserted through which a 7 French angled pigtail catheter was inserted and advanced under fluoroscopic guidance to the descending thoracic aorta. Heparin was administered. Arterial pressures were recorded. The pigtail catheter was then advanced across the aortic valve to the left ventricle. Pressures were recorded, and left ventriculography was performed by power injection of 40 cc of contrast at 12 cc per second with cine in the RAO projection. Post ventriculography pressures were recorded, and pullback across the aortic valve was performed. The pigtail catheter was exchanged for a left coronary catheter as listed above which was advanced to the ostium of the left coronary artery. Left coronary arteriography was performed by hand injections of 8-10 cc of contrast with cine in multiple views. The left coronary catheter was exchanged for the right coronary catheter, as listed above, and it was then advanced to the ostium of the right coronary artery. Right coronary arteriography was performed by hand injections of 8-10 cc of contrast with cine in multiple views. The right coronary catheter and femoral artery sheath were removed, and hemostasis was obtained by C-clamp pressure for 30-45 minutes. Complications: None. Fluoro time: 2.2 minutes. Contrast dose: 76 cc.

(continued)

CARDIAC CATHETERIZATION Page 1	PT. NAME: SMITH, W. ID NO: ROOM NO: ATT. PHYS: R. GALASSO, M.D.

Medical Record 7.2.

CENTRAL MEDICAL CENTER
211 Medical Center Drive • Central City, US 90000-1234 • PHONE: (012) 125-6784 • FAX: (012) 125-9999

CARDIAC CATHETERIZATION

FINDINGS:

1. HEMODYNAMICS:
   Left ventricle: 182/0; end-diastolic: 16 mm Hg. Aorta: 190/70; mean: 110 mm Hg.

2. LEFT VENTRICULOGRAPHY:
   The left ventricle is normal in configuration, dimensions, and segmental wall motion with ejection fraction computed at 58% by area-length method. There is no evidence of mitral regurgitation.

3. CORONARY ARTERIOGRAPHY:
   Left Main: Normal.

   Left Anterior Descending: Seventy percent focal stenosis immediately after the first septal perforator branch. The remainder of the left anterior descending is within normal limits.

   Ramus Intermedius: Normal.

   Left Circumflex: Nondominant vessel with one marginal branch, all free of disease.

   Right Coronary Artery: Large dominant vessel free of disease.

CONCLUSIONS:

1. MODERATE STENOSIS OF THE LEFT ANTERIOR DESCENDING CORONARY ARTERY.

2. NORMAL LEFT VENTRICULAR FUNCTION WITH EJECTION FRACTION 56%.

RECOMMENDATIONS:
The patient will be managed medically at this time. Radionuclide perfusion stress testing will be performed. If the patient has progressive anginal symptoms or has marked reversible ischemia in the distribution of the left anterior descending coronary artery, angioplasty of this vessel would be considered.

CARDIAC CATHETERIZATION Page 2	PT. NAME: SMITH, W. ID NO: ROOM NO: ATT. PHYS: R. GALASSO, M.D.

Medical Record 7.2. *Continued.*

Blood and Lymph Systems

OBJECTIVES

After completion of this chapter you will be able to

1. Define common combining forms used in relation to the blood and lymph system

2. Define the basic anatomical terms referring to blood and lymph

3. Define common symptomatic, diagnostic, operative, and therapeutic terms referring to blood and lymph

4. List common diagnostic tests and procedures related to the blood and lymph systems

5. Explain terms and abbreviations used in documenting medical records involving the blood or lymph

Combining Forms

Combining Form	Meaning	Example
blast/o	germ or bud	erythroblastemia ĕ-rith'rō-blas-tē'mē-ă
-blast (also a suffix)		megaloblast meg'ă-lō-blast
chrom/o	color	chromic krō'mik
chyl/o	juice	chylemia kī-lē'mē-ă
hem/o	blood	hemostat hē'mo-stat
hemat/o		hematopoiesis hē'mă-tō-poy-ē'sis
immun/o	safe	immunology im'yū-nol'ō-jē
lymph/o	clear fluid	lymphogenous lim-foj'ĕ-nŭs
phag/o	eat or swallow	phagocytosis fag'ō-sī-tō'sis
plas/o	formation	aplastic ā-plas'tik
reticul/o	a net	reticulocyte re-tik'yū-lō-sīt
splen/o	spleen	splenomegaly splē-nō-meg'ă-lē
thromb/o	clot	thrombocyte throm'bō-sīt
thym/o	thymus gland	thymic thī'mik

Blood System Overview

The blood circulates through the blood vessels to transport oxygen, nutrients, and hormones to body cells and to carry away wastes. The liquid portion of the blood is called *plasma*. The cellular components suspended in the plasma are the *erythrocytes*, *leukocytes*, and *platelets*. The portion of the plasma that remains after the clotting process is called *serum* (see Color Atlas, plate 15)

Anatomical Terms

Term	Meaning
Terms Related to Blood Fluid	
plasma plaz'mah	liquid portion of the blood and lymph containing water, proteins, salts, nutrients, hormones, vitamins, and cellular components (leukocytes, erythrocytes, and platelets)

continued

Term	Meaning
serum sēr′ŭm	liquid portion of the blood left after the clotting process

Cellular Components of Blood

Term	Meaning
erythrocyte ĕ-rith′rō-sīt	red blood cell that transports oxygen and carbon dioxide within the bloodstream (see Color Atlas, plate 15)
hemoglobin hē-mō-glō′bin	protein-iron compound contained in the erythrocyte that has bonding capabilities for the transport of oxygen and carbon dioxide
leukocyte lu′kō-sīt	white blood cell that protects the body from invasion of harmful substances (see Color Atlas, plate 15)
granulocytes gran′yū-lō-sīts	a group of leukocytes containing granules in their cytoplasm
neutrophil nū′trō-fil	a granular leukocyte, named for the neutral stain of its granules, that fights infection by swallowing bacteria (phagocytosis) (neutro = neither; phil = attraction for)
polymorphonuclear leukocyte (PMN) pol-ē-mōr′fō-nū′klē-ăr	another term for neutrophil, named for the many segments present in its nucleus (poly = many; morpho = form; nucleus = kernel)
band	an immature neutrophil
eosinophil ē-ō-sin′ō-fil	a granular leukocyte, named for the rose-color stain of its granules, that increases with allergy and some infections (eos = dawn-colored (rosy); phil = attraction for)
basophil bā′sō-fil	a granular leukocyte, named for the dark stain of its granules, that brings anticoagulant substances to inflamed tissues (baso = base; phil = attraction for)
agranulocytes ă-gran′yū-lō-sīts	a group of leukocytes without granules in their nuclei
lymphocyte lim′fō-sīt	an agranulocytic leukocyte that is active in the process of immunity—there are three categories of lymphocytes: T cells (thymus dependent), B cells (bone marrow-derived), and NK (natural killer) cells
monocyte mon′ō-sīt	an agranulocytic leukocyte that performs phagocytosis to fight infection (mono = one)
platelets plāt′lets	thrombocytes; cell fragments in the blood essential for blood clotting

SERUM. Serum is Latin for whey, the watery part of curdled milk, which looks similar to the watery part of clotted blood. The term was first recorded in English in 1672.

Lymphatic System Overview

The lymphatic system is made up of an intricate network of capillaries, vessels, valves, ducts, nodes, and organs. It protects the body by filtering microorganisms and foreign particles from the lymph and supporting the activities of the lymphocytes in the immune response. It also serves to maintain the body's internal fluid environment by acting as an intermediary between the blood in the capillaries and tissue cells. It is also responsible for carrying fats away from the digestive organs (Fig. 8.1).

Anatomical Terms

Term	Meaning
Lymph Organs	
thymus thī′mŭs	primary gland of the lymphatic system, located within the mediastinum, helps maintain the body's immune response by producing T lymphocytes
spleen splēn	organ between stomach and diaphragm that filters out aging blood cells, removes cellular debris by performing phagocytosis, and provides the environment for the initiation of immune responses by lymphocytes

continued

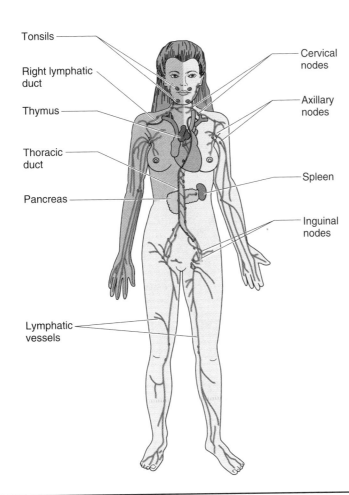

Figure 8.1. Lymphatic system.

Term	Meaning

Lymph Structures

Term	Meaning
lymph limf	fluid originating in the organs and tissues of the body that is circulated through the lymph vessels
lymph capillaries limf kap'i-lār-ē	microscopic vessels that draw lymph from the tissues to the lymph vessels
lymph vessels limf ves'ĕlz	vessels that receive lymph from the lymph capillaries and circulate it to the lymph nodes
lacteals lak'tē-ălz	specialized lymph vessels in the small intestine that absorb fat into the bloodstream (lacteus = milky)
chyle kīl	white or pale yellow substance of the lymph that contains fatty substances absorbed by the lacteals
lymph nodes limf nōdz	many small oval structures that filter the lymph received from the lymph vessels—major locations include the cervical region, axillary region, and inguinal region
lymph ducts limf dŭktz	collecting channels that carry lymph from the lymph nodes to the veins
right lymphatic duct lim-fat'ik dŭkt	receives lymph from the right upper part of the body
thoracic duct thō-ras'ik dŭkt	receives lymph from the left side of the head, neck, chest, abdomen, left arm, and lower extremities

Immunity

Term	Meaning
immunity i-myū'ni-tē	process of disease protection induced by exposure to an antigen
antigen an'ti-jen	a substance that, when introduced into the body, causes formation of antibodies against it
antibody an'tē-bod-ē	substance produced by the body that destroys or inactivates an antigen that has entered the body
active immunity ak'tiv i-myū'ni-tē	an immunity that protects the body against a future infection, as the result of antibodies that develop *naturally* after contracting an infection or *artificially* after administration of a vaccine
passive immunity pas'iv i-myū'ni-tē	an immunity resulting from antibodies that are conveyed *naturally* through the placenta to a fetus or *artificially* by injection of a serum containing antibodies

Symptomatic and Diagnostic Terms

Term	Meaning

Symptomatic

Term	Meaning
anisocytosis an-ī'sō-sī-tō'sis	presence of red blood cells of unequal size (aniso = unequal)

continued

Term	Meaning
pancytopenia pan′sī-tō-pē′nē-ă	an abnormally reduced number of all cellular components in the blood
erythropenia ĕ-rith-rō-pē′nē-ă	an abnormally reduced number of red blood cells
hemolysis hē-mol′i-sis	breakdown of the red blood cell membrane
immunocompromised im′yū-nō-kom′pro-mīzd	impaired immunologic defenses caused by an immunodeficiency disorder or therapy with immuno-suppressive agents
immunosuppression im′yū-nō-sŭ-presh′ŭn	impaired ability to provide an immune response
lymphadenopathy lim-fad-ĕ-nop′ă-thē	presence of enlarged lymph nodes
lymphocytopenia lim′fō-sī-tō-pē′nē-ă	an abnormally reduced number of lymphocytes
macrocytosis mak′rō-sī-tō′sis	presence of large red blood cells
microcytosis mī-krō-sī-tō′sis	presence of small red blood cells
neutropenia nū-trō-pē′nē-ă	a decrease in the number of neutrophils
poikilocytosis poy′ki-lō-sī-tō′sis	presence of large, irregularly shaped red blood cells (poikilo = irregular)
reticulocytosis re-tik′yū-lō-sī-tō′sis	an increase of immature erythrocytes in the blood
splenomegaly splē-nō-meg′ă-lē	enlargement of the spleen

Diagnostic

acquired immunodeficiency syndrome (AIDS) ă-kwīrd′ i-myūn′o-dē-fish′en-sē sin′drōm	a syndrome caused by the human immunodeficiency virus (HIV) that renders immune cells ineffective, permitting opportunistic infections, malignancies, and neurologic diseases to develop; it is transmitted sexually or through exposure to contaminated blood
anemia ă-nē′mē-ă	a condition in which there is a reduction in the number of red blood cells, the amount of hemoglobin, or the volume of packed red cells in the blood, resulting in a diminished ability of the red blood cells to transport oxygen to the tissues; common types follow:
iron deficiency anemia i′ern dē-fish′en-sē	a microcytic-hypochromic type of anemia characterized by a lack of iron, affecting production of hemoglobin and small red blood cells containing low amounts of hemoglobin (Fig. 8.2)

continued

Term	Meaning
pernicious anemia per-nish′ŭs	a macrocytic normochromic type of anemia characterized by an inadequate supply of vitamin B_{12}, causing red blood cells to become large, varied in shape, and reduced in number (Fig. 8.3)
aplastic anemia ā-plas′tik	a normocytic-normochromic type of anemia characterized by the failure of bone marrow to produce red blood cells
erythroblastosis fetalis ĕ-rith′rō-blas-tō′sis fē′tă′lis	a disorder that results from the incompatibility of a fetus with an Rh positive blood factor and a mother who is Rh negative, causing red blood cell destruction in the fetus; necessitates a blood transfusion to save the fetus
Rh factor	presence, or lack, of antigens on the surface of red blood cells that may cause a reaction between the blood of the mother and fetus, resulting in fetal anemia
Rh positive	presence of antigens
Rh negative	absence of antigens
hemochromatosis hē′mō-krō-mă-tō′sis	hereditary disorder that results in an excessive buildup of iron deposits in the body
hemophilia hē-mō-fil′ē-ă	group of hereditary bleeding disorders in which there is a defect in clotting factors necessary for coagulation of blood
leukemia lū-kē′mē-ă	chronic or acute malignant disease of the blood-forming organs, marked by abnormal leukocytes in the blood and bone marrow; classified according to the types of white cells affected, e.g., myelocytic, lymphocytic, etc.

continued

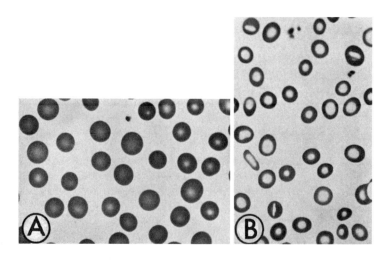

Figure 8.2. A blood smear showing normal erythrocytes (**A**) compared with a blood smear revealing microcytic-hypochromic erythrocytes in a patient with iron deficiency anemia (**B**).

Term	Meaning
myelodysplasia mī′ĕ-lō-dis-plā′zē-ă	disorder within the bone marrow characterized by the proliferation of abnormal stem cells (cells that give rise to the different types of blood cells); usually develops into a specific type of leukemia
lymphoma lim-fō′mă	any neoplastic disorder of lymph tissue, usually malignant, as in Hodgkin's disease
metastasis mĕ-tas′tă-sis	process by which cancer cells are spread by blood or lymph circulation to distant organs
mononucleosis mon′ō-nū-klē-ō′sis	viral condition characterized by an increase in mononuclear cells (monocytes and lymphocytes) in the blood along with enlarged lymph nodes (lymphadenopathy), fatigue, and sore throat (pharyngitis)
polycythemia pol′ē-sī-thē′mē-ă	increase in the number of erythrocytes and hemoglobin in the blood
septicemia sep-ti-sē′mē-ă	systemic disease caused by the infection of microorganisms and their toxins in the circulating blood
thrombocytopenia throm′bō-sī-tō-pē′nē-ă	bleeding disorder characterized by an abnormal decrease in the number of platelets in the blood that impairs the clotting process

Diagnostic Tests and Procedures

Test or Procedure	Explanation
Blood Studies	
phlebotomy flĕ-bot′ō-mē **venipuncture** ven-i-pŭnk-chūr	incision into or puncture of a vein to withdraw blood for testing (Fig. 8.4)

continued

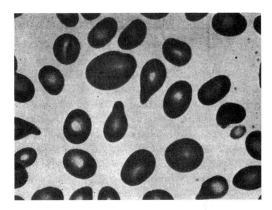

Figure 8.3. Photomicrograph of a blood smear from a patient with pernicious anemia reveals macrocytosis, anisocytosis, and poikilocytosis.

Test or Procedure	Explanation
blood chemistry blŭd kem′is-trē	test of the fluid portion of blood to measure the presence of a chemical constituent (e.g., glucose, cholesterol, etc.)
biochemistry panel (BCP) **chem profile** bī-ō-kem′is-trē	battery of automated blood chemistry tests performed on a single sample of blood; used as a general screen for disease or to target specific organs such as a heart profile, thyroid panel, etc. (Fig. 8.5)
sequential multiple analyzer (SMA)	trade name of the instrument first used to perform automated blood chemistry testing; the abbreviation is sometimes used to identify a chemistry panel
blood culture blŭd kŭl′chŭr	test to determine infection in the bloodstream by isolating a specimen of blood in an environment that encourages the growth of microorganisms; the specimen is observed and the organisms that grow in the culture are identified
erythrocyte sedimentation rate (ESR) ĕ-rith′trō-sīt sed′i-men-tā′shŭn rāt	timed test to measure the rate at which red blood cells settle or fall through a given volume of plasma
partial thromboplastin time (PTT)	test to determine coagulation defects such as platelet disorders
thromboplastin throm-bō-plas′tin	substance present in tissues, platelets, and leukocytes that is necessary for coagulation
prothrombin time (PT)	test to measure activity of prothrombin in the blood
prothrombin prō-throm′bin	protein substance in the blood that is essential to the clotting process
complete blood count (CBC)	one of the most common laboratory blood tests performed as a screen of general health or for diagnostic purposes; the following is a listing of the component tests included in a CBC (Fig. 8.6)

continued

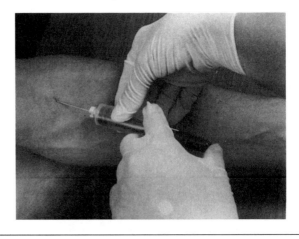

Figure 8.4. Common venipuncture site for withdrawal of blood for testing purposes.

Test or Procedure	Explanation
	(note: CBC results are usually reported with normal values so that the clinician can interpret the results based on the instrumentation utilized by the laboratory; normal ranges also may vary depending on the region, climate, etc.)
white blood count (WBC)	a count of the number of white blood cells per cubic millimeter obtained by manual or automated laboratory methods
red blood count (RBC)	a count of the number of red blood cells per cubic millimeter obtained by manual or automated laboratory methods
hemoglobin (HGB or Hgb) hē-mō-glō′bin	a test to determine the blood level of hemoglobin (expressed in grams)
hematocrit (HCT or Hct) hē′mă-tō-krit	a measurement of the percentage of packed red blood cells in a given volume of blood
blood indices in′di-sēz	calculations of RBC, HGB, and HCT results to determine the average size, hemoglobin concentration, and content of red blood cells for classification of anemia
mean corpuscular (cell) volume (MCV) kōr-pŭs′kyū-lăr	calculation of the volume of individual cells in cubic microns using HCT and RBC results: MCV = HCT/RBC
mean corpuscular (cell) hemoglobin (MCH) kōr-pŭs′kyū-lăr hē-mō-glō′bin	calculation of the content in weight of hemoglobin in the average red blood cell using HGB and RBC results: MCH = HGB/RBC
mean corpuscular (cell) hemoglobin concentration (MCHC) hē-mō-glō′bin kon-sen-trā′shŭn	calculation of the average hemoglobin concentration in each red blood cell using HGB and HCT results: MCHC = HGB/HCT
differential count	determination of the number of each type of white blood cell (leukocyte) seen on a stained blood smear; each type is counted and reported as a percentage of the total examined

Type of Leukocyte	Normal Range
lymphocytes	25–33%
monocytes	3–7%
neutrophils	54–75%
eosinophils	1–3%
basophils	0–1%

Test or Procedure	Explanation
red cell morphology mōr-fol′ō-jē	as part of identifying and counting the WBCs, the condition of the size and shape of the red blood cells in the background of the smeared slide is noted (e.g., anisocytosis, poikilocytosis)

continued

CENTRAL MEDICAL CENTER

211 Medical Center Drive · Central City, US 90000-1234 · PHONE: (012) 125-6784 · FAX: (012) 125-9999

11//02/9x
14:27

NAME   :   TEST, PATIENT   LOC: TEST   DOB: 02/03/9x   AGE: 38Y
MR#   :   TEST-221   SEX: M
ACCT # :   H111111111

M63561 COLL: 11/02/9x 13:24   REC: 11/02/9x 13:25

BIOCHEM PANEL

Blood Urea Nitrogen	*30	[5 - 25]	mg/dl
Sodium	139	[135 - 153]	mEq/L
Potassium	4.2	[3.5 - 5.3]	mEq/L
Chloride	105	[101 - 111]	mEq/L
CO_2	27	[24 - 31]	mmol/L
Glucose, Random	*148	[70 - 110]	mg/dl
Creatinine	*1.5	[< 1.5]	mg/dl
SGOT (AST)	18	[10 - 42]	U/L
CPK, Total	45	[22 - 269]	U/L
LDH	134	[91 - 180]	U/L
SGPT (ALT)	*8	[10 - 60]	U/L
GGT	34	[7 - 64]	U/L
Alkaline Phosphatase	58	[42 - 121]	U/L
Total Protein	6.5	[6.0 - 8.0]	G/dl
Albumin	3.7	[3.5 - 5.0]	G/dl
Amylase	33	[< 129]	U/L
Bilirubin, Total	0.7	[< 1.5]	mg/dl
Calcium, Total	9.7	[8.6 - 10.6]	mg/dl
Phosphorus	3.9	[2.7 - 4.5]	mg/dl
Uric Acid	7.1	[1.2 - 7.5]	mg/dl
Cholesterol	184	[< 200]	mg/dl
Triglycerides	159	[46 - 236]	mg/dl

TEST, PATIENT   TEST-221   END OF REPORT   PAGE 1
11/02/9x 14:27   INTERIM REPORT

INTERIM REPORT COMPLETED

Figure 8.5. Biochemistry panel report.

CENTRAL MEDICAL CENTER

211 Medical Center Drive • Central City, US 90000-1234 • PHONE: (012) 125-6784 • FAX: (012) 125-9999

11//02/9x
14:27

NAME :	TEST, PATIENT	LOC: TEST	DOB: 07/14/9x	AGE: 27Y
MR# :	TEST-221			SEX: M
ACCT # :	H111111111			

M63558 COLL: 11/02/9x 13:23   REC: 11/02/9x 13:24

CBC

WBC	*11.5	[4.5 - 10.5]	K/UL
RBC	5.84	[4.6 - 6.2]	M/UL
HGB	17.2	[14.0 - 18.0]	G/DL
HCT	50.8	[42.0 - 52.0]	%
MCV	87	[82 - 92]	FL
MCH	29.5	[27 - 31]	PG
MCHC	33.9	[32 - 36]	G/DL
PLT	202	[150 - 450]	K/UL
Auto Lymph %	15	[20 - 40]	%
Auto Mono %	2	[1 - 11]	%
Auto Neutro %	82	[50 - 75]	%
Auto Eos %	1	[0 - 6]	%
Auto Baso %	0	[0 - 2]	%
Auto Lymph #	1.7	[1.5 - 4.0]	K/UL
Auto Mono #	0.2	[0.2 - 0.9]	K/UL
Auto Neutro #	9.4	[1.0 - 7.0]	K/UL
Auto Eos #	0.1	[0 - 0.7]	K/UL
Auto Baso #	0.0	[0 - 0.2]	K/UL

TEST, PATIENT TEST-221	END OF REPORT	PAGE 1
11/02/9x 14:27		INTERIM REPORT

INTERIM REPORT COMPLETED

Figure 8.6. Complete blood count (CBC) report.

Test or Procedure	Explanation
platelet count (PLT) plăt′let	calculation of the number of thrombocytes in the blood: normal range 150,000–450,000/cubic millimeters

Bone and Lymph Studies

bone marrow aspiration bōn mar′ō as-pi-rā′shŭn	needle aspiration of bone marrow tissue for pathological examination
lymphangiogram lim-fan′jē-ō-gram	an x-ray image of a lymph node or vessel taken after injection of a contrast medium (Fig. 8.7)

Operative Terms

Term	Meaning
bone marrow transplant bōn mar′ō tranz′plant	transplantation of healthy bone marrow from a compatible donor to a diseased recipient to stimulate blood cell production
lymphadenectomy lim-fad-ĕ-nek′tō-mē	removal of a lymph node
lymphadenotomy lim-fad-ĕ-not′ă-mē	incision into a lymph node

continued

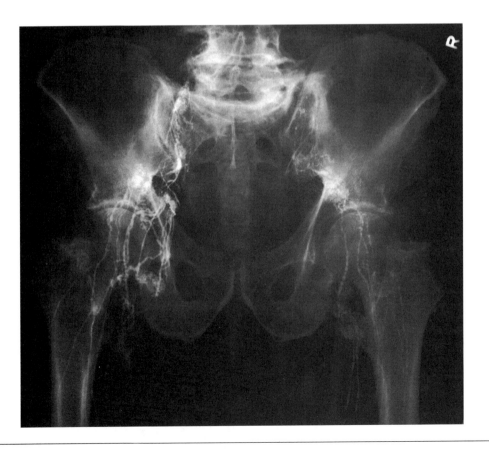

Figure 8.7. Lymphangiogram of the pelvic region. Contrast was used to image the lymph vessels and nodes.

Term	Meaning
lymph node dissection limf nōd di-sek′shŭn	removal of possible cancer-carrying lymph nodes for pathological examination
splenectomy splē-nek′tō-mē	removal of the spleen
thymectomy thī-mek′tō-mē	removal of the thymus gland

Therapeutic Terms

Term	Meaning
blood transfusion	introduction of blood products into the circulation of a recipient whose blood volume is reduced or is deficient in some manner
autologous blood aw-tol′ŏ-gŭs blud	blood donated by, and stored for, a patient for future personal use (e.g., upcoming surgery)
homologous blood hŏ-mol′ō-gŭs blud	blood voluntarily donated by any person for transfusion to a compatible recipient
blood component therapy	transfusion of specific blood components such as packed red blood cells, platelets, plasma, etc.
crossmatching	a method of matching a donor's blood to the recipient by mixing a sample in a test tube to determine compatibility
chemotherapy kem′ō-thēr-ă-pē	treatment of malignancies, infections, and other diseases with chemical agents that destroy selected cells or impair their ability to reproduce
plasmapheresis plaz′mă-fĕ-rē′sis	removal of plasma from the body with separation and extraction of specific elements (such as platelets) followed by reinfusion (apheresis = a withdrawal)

Common Therapeutic Drug Classifications

Term	Meaning
anticoagulant an′tē-kō-ag′yū-lant	a drug that prevents clotting of the blood
hemostatic hē-mō-stat′ik	a drug that stops the flow of blood within the vessels
vasoconstrictor vā′sō-kon-strik′ter	a drug that causes a narrowing of blood vessels, decreasing blood flow
vasodilator vā′sō-dī-lā′ter	a drug that causes dilation of blood vessels, increasing blood flow

PRACTICE EXERCISES

For the following terms, draw a line or lines to separate prefixes, combining forms, and suffixes. Then define the term.

1. erythroblastosis _____

2. chylopoiesis _____

3. hemocytometer _____

4. splenorrhagia _____

5. lymphadenitis _____

6. erythrochromia _____

7. reticulocytosis _____

8. thymopathy _____

9. leukocytic _____

10. lymphangiogram _____

11. splenomalacia _____

12. erythrocytorrhexis _____

13. reticular _____

14. lymphoid _____

15. promyelocyte _____

16. metamyelocyte _____

17. chromophilic _____

18. leukocytopenia _____

19. splenectomy _____

20. immunologic _____

21. chylorrhea _____

22. hemodialysis_____

23. lymphoma_____

24. cytomorphology_____

25. hemolysis_____

26. lymphadenectomy_____

27. metastasis _____

28. anemia _____

29. splenomegaly _____

30. immunotoxic_____

Name the blood studies that are part of the blood indices:

31. _____

32. _____

33. _____

Fill in the blanks with the appropriate medical terms and abbreviations:

34. The procedure of counting the number of leukocytes in the blood is called a _____ _____ _____ and is abbreviated _____.

35. The blood study that determines the amount of pigment present in RBCs is called a _____ and is abbreviated _____.

36. The blood study that determines packed red blood cell volume is called a _____ and is abbreviated _____.

37. The classification of WBCs is performed in a _____ _____.

Write the full medical term for the following abbreviations:

38. PT _____

39. ESR _____

40. PTT _____

41. CBC _____

Match the following terms with their meanings:

42. microcytosis _____   a. large red blood cells

43. poikilocytosis _____   b. thrombocyte

44. neutrophil _____   c. WBC with rose-stained granules

45. monocyte _____   d. RBC

46. eosinophil _____   e. an agranulocyte active in immunity

47. lymphocyte _____   f. WBC with dark stained granules

48. basophil _____   g. WBC termed "one cell"

49. platelet _____   h. RBCs of unequal size

50. erythrocyte _____   i. WBC with granules

51. granulocyte _____   j. large, irregular RBCs

52. anisocytosis _____   k. a polymorphonuclear WBC

53. macrocytosis _____   l. small red blood cells

Write the correct medical term for each of the following:

54. a decrease in the number of neutrophils _____

55. blood donated by a person, and stored, for his or her future use _____

56. impaired ability to provide an immune response _____

57. test tube method of matching a donor's blood to the recipient _____

58. syndrome caused by HIV _____

59. removal of plasma from the body, extraction of specific elements, then reinfusion

_____

60. blood voluntarily donated by any person for transfusion _____

Medical Record Analyses

MEDICAL RECORD 8.1

Henry Lin went to his personal physician after a period of generally not feeling well, losing his appetite, and starting to lose weight. His doctor then admitted him to Central Medical Center hospital for additional tests after conducting a physical examination and blood tests. He is now being treated as an outpatient by his internist, Dr. Bradley, and an oncologist, Dr. Ellison, to whom he was referred for consultation and concurrent care.

Directions

Read Medical Record 8.1 for Mr. Lin (pages 219–220) and answer the following questions.

The progress note is the oncology/hematology progress note dictated by Dr. Ellison, the oncologist treating Mr. Lin, at the time of a follow-up visit two weeks after Mr. Lin's hospitalization. The second document is a hematology lab report, submitted before a second follow-up with Dr. Ellison two weeks later.

Questions about Medical Record 8.1

Write your answers in the spaces provided.

1. Below are medical terms used in the progress note you have not yet encountered in this text. Underline each where it appears in the record and define below.

   edema _____

   scaphoid _____

   anorexia _____

2. In your own words, not using medical terminology, translate Mr. Lin's diagnosis:

   _____

3. Name the diagnostic test that confirmed this diagnosis:

   _____

4. Write the medical term for Mr. Lin's enlarged spleen:

   _____

5. Dr. Ellison's March 31 record includes the results of two CBC component tests from the earlier March 23 lab report, as well as results from the same tests for March 31. The April 15 lab report also contains the CBC component tests. In the spaces below, write the name of the tests and their results at these three times. Do not use abbreviations. Be sure to include units of measure.

Test	Result		
	March 23	March 31	April 15
_____	_____	_____	_____
_____	_____	_____	_____

6. What are the three elements Dr. Ellison includes in Mr. Lin's treatment plan?

   a. _____

   b. _____

   c. _____

7. Study the April 15 laboratory report carefully and complete the following table of selected test results. Write the name of the component that is abbreviated and an N if the result for Mr. Lin is within the normal range or an A (abnormal) if the result is outside the normal range.

   a. WBC _____

   b. RBC _____

   c. HGB _____

   d. HCT _____

   e. MCV _____

   f. MCH _____

   g. MCHC _____

   h. PLT _____

   i. lymph _____

   j. mono _____

   k. neutro _____

   l. eos _____

   m. baso _____

CENTRAL MEDICAL GROUP, INC.

Department of Oncology/Hematology

201 Medical Center Drive • Central City, US 90000-1234 • PHONE: (012) 125-8888 • FAX: (012) 125-3434

PROGRESS NOTE

PATIENT: LIN, HENRY N.

DATE: March 31, 199x

Mr. Lin is a 69-year-old man seen for myelodysplasia while hospitalized on March 17, 199x. He was transfused with 4.0 U of packed cells during that hospitalization. A bone marrow revealed histology consistent with chronic myelomonocytic leukemia (myelodysplasia).

A follow-up blood count was obtained through Dr. Bradley's office on March 23, 199x, and revealed a hemoglobin of 11.0 G/DL and a hematocrit of 31.0%.

There have been no fevers, sweats, or anorexia; but he has noted some weight loss. There has been no bleeding. There has been no nausea, vomiting, or dark and bloody stools.

Exam: Weight: 172 lb. Blood Pressure: 120/50. Temperature: 98.6°F. Pulse: 88. Respirations: 18.

HEENT: Mild gum atrophy and inflammation. NECK: Supple. LYMPH NODES: There is no cervical or supraclavicular adenopathy. LUNGS: Clear. CARDIOVASCULAR: Normal. ABDOMEN: Scaphoid, soft, and nontender. The spleen is enlarged. EXTREMITIES: Without edema or petechiae.

TODAY'S LAB: Complete blood count reveals a total leukocyte count of 6600/cu mm, a hemoglobin of 8.0 G/DL, a hematocrit of 23.0%, and a platelet count of 149,000/cu mm.

CLINICAL DIAGNOSIS:
Chronic myelomonocytic leukemia (myelodysplastic syndrome). The patient is transfusion dependent.

The patient will be typed and crossmatched today and will be transfused with 2.0 U of packed red blood cells through the Oncology Day Facility tomorrow on April 1, 199x.

I have asked the patient to follow up with Dr. Bradley next week and with me in two weeks.

A. Ellison, M.D.

AE:gds
cc: Blair Bradley, M.D.

D: 3/31/9x
T: 4/3/9x

Medical Record 8.1.

CENTRAL MEDICAL CENTER

211 Medical Center Drive • Central City, US 90000-1234 • PHONE: (012) 125-6784 • FAX: (012) 125-9999

04/15//9x
14:27

NAME	:	Lin, Henry	LOC: TEST	DOB: 02/02/xx	AGE: 69Y
MR#	:	TEST-226			SEX: M
ACCT #	:	168946701			

M63558 COLL: 04/15/9x 13:23   REC: 04/15/9x 13:25

CBC

WBC	4.1	[4.5 - 10.5]	K/UL
RBC	2.93	[4.6 - 6.2]	M/UL
HGB	9.1	[14.0 - 18.0]	G/DL
HCT	25.3	[42.0 - 52.0]	%
MCV	86.2	[82 - 92]	FL
MCH	31.1	[27 - 31]	PG
MCHC	36.0	[32 -36]	G/DL
PLT	90	[150 - 450]	K/UL
Auto Lymph %	8.3	[20 -40]	%
Auto Mono %	32.6	[1 - 11]	%
Auto Neutro %	57.8	[50 - 75]	%
Auto Eos %	1.0	[0 - 6]	%
Auto Baso %	0.3	[0 - 2]	%
Auto Lymph #	0.3	[1.5 - 4.0]	K/UL
Auto Mono #	1.3	[0.2 - 0.9]	K/UL
Auto Neutro #	2.4	[1.0 - 7.0]	K/UL
Auto Eos #	0.0	[0 - 0.7]	K/UL
Auto Baso #	0.0	[0 - 0.2]	K/UL

Lin, Henry   CBC   END OF REPORT   PAGE 1
04/15/9x 14:27   INTERIM REPORT

INTERIM REPORT COMPLETED

Medical Record 8.1. *Continued.*

MEDICAL RECORD 8.2

Susan Hall has been experiencing fatigue and a loss of energy in recent months that has also been noticed by her family and friends, so she saw her doctor for an evaluation.

Directions

Read Medical Record 8.2 for Ms. Hall (pages 224–225) and answer the following questions. The record represents the handwritten chart notes made by Ms. Hall's family practitioner, Dr. Robert Evans.

Questions about Medical Record 8.2

Write your answers in the spaces provided.

1. Below are medical terms or abbreviations you have not yet encountered in this text. Underline each where it appears in the record and define below.

    Fe _____

    clubbing _____

    menses _____

    edema _____

    hypothyroidism _____

2. List the two elements of the patient's complaint:

    a. _____

    b. _____

3. Which of the following is *not* mentioned in this history? (*Circle your answer choice.*)

    a. type of treatment Ms. Hall received for mononucleosis

    b. Ms. Hall's consumption of alcohol

    c. health status of the patient's sister

    d. how long Ms. Hall has been married

4. In your own words, not using medical terminology, briefly summarize Ms. Hall's past medical history:

5. In your own words, not using medical terminology, give the health status of Ms. Hall's family members:

   mother _____

   father _____

   sister _____

6. Which of the following describes the findings of the physical examination:

   a. swollen lymph glands

   b. blue condition of extremities

   c. normal exam

   d. slow heart rate

   e. fast heart rate

7. Dr. Evans' assessment of the cause of Ms. Hall's symptoms is _____. She may have _____ but he also wants to make sure she does *not* have _____.

8. Dr. Evans' treatment plan involves a blood workup. Identify the three laboratory tests ordered:

   a. _____

   b. _____

   c. _____

9. When does Dr. Evans want Ms. Hall to return for lab results?

   _____

10. Describe the patient's diagnosis in your own words:

    _____

    _____

    _____

    _____

11. What is the underlying cause of her condition?

    _____

12. Dr. Evans' treatment plan involves three areas. List the specific plan for each.

    Drug prescribed (how much and when):

    _____

    Suggestion for the patient to consider:

    _____

    Recheck of blood tests in the future (which tests):

    _____

13. When would Dr. Evans like to see Ms. Hall again?

    _____

PROGRESS NOTES

Patient Name: *HALL, Susan*

DATE	FINDINGS
2/3/9x	CC: 33 y.o. ♀ c/o feeling run down c̄ lack of energy off and on x past 6 mo.
	S denies fever/chills, nausea/vomiting diarrhea/constipation - no wt loss She reports very heavy menstrual periods lasting 5 days ever since DC of birth control pills about 1yr ago PMH: T+A, age 4 Mononucleosis at age 16 ALERGIES: Penicillin causes urticarial eruption SH: married x 5 yr - no children OH: works as accountant for law firm Habits Tobacco - none ETOH - occasional glass of wine. Drugs - none. Recreation - exercises 3x/wk on bike. FH: mother, age 59, has HTN father died at 60, MI sister, age 30, L+W
	O VS BP 130/74 P70 R15 T 98.8° PE WD WN ♀ in no acute distress HEENT - WNL neck s̄ adenopathy Heart RRR s̄ (m) abdomen - normal extremities - ø clubbing, cyanosis or edema GYN - deferred to gynecologist
	A Etiology of ↑fatigue and ↓ energy unclear Consider Fe deficiency in light of heavy menses. Also consider hypothyroidism although PE findings of this are absent
	P Blood workup to include Biochem-20 CBC c̄ differential and thyroid function panel pt to RTC in 1 wk for discussion of lab results .
	R Evans, MD

PROGRESS NOTES

Patient Name: _HALL, SUSAN_

DATE	FINDINGS
2/10/9X	S pt returns today for LAb results
	O Significant findings follow: Thyroid function studies — WNL Biochem-20 WNL except for Serum Iron 50 (75-175) CBC HGB 10.8 (12-16) HCT 32.4 (37-47) MCV 75 (80-95)
	A microcytic/hypochromic Anemia c̄ low serum Fe representing classic case of iron deficiency anemia due to excessively heavy menses
	P start oral iron supplements Rx Feosol tAb #100 ī tid pc RTO in ī mo for repeat CBC and serum Fe. Consider restart of birth control pills to decrease amount of menstrual flow
	R Evans, MD

Respiratory System

OBJECTIVES

After completion of this chapter you will be able to

1. Define common combining forms used in relation to the respiratory system

2. Define the basic anatomical terms referring to the respiratory system

3. Define common symptomatic, diagnostic, operative, and therapeutic terms referring to the respiratory system

4. List the common diagnostic tests and procedures related to the respiratory system

5. Explain the terms and abbreviations used in documenting medical records involving the respiratory system

Combining Forms

Combining Form	Meaning	Example
alveol/o	alveolus (air sac)	**alveolar** al-vē′ō-lăr
bronch/o	bronchus (airway)	**bronchoscope** brong′kō-skōp
bronchi/o		**bronchiocele** brong′kē-ō-sēl
bronchiol/o	bronchiole (little airway)	**bronchiolitis** brong-kē-ō-lī′tis
capn/o	carbon dioxide	**hypercapnia** hī-per-kap′nē-ă
carb/o		**hypocarbia** hī-pō-kar′bē-ă
laryng/o	larynx (voice box)	**laryngospasm** lă-ring′gō-spazm
lob/o	lobe (a portion)	**lobectomy** lō-bek′tō-mē
nas/o	nose	**nasal** nā′zăl
rhin/o		**rhinorrhea** rī-nō-rē′ă
or/o	mouth	**oropharyngeal** ōr-ō-fă-rin′jē-ăl
ox/o	oxygen	**hypoxemia** hī-pok-sē′mē-ă
pharyng/o	pharynx (throat)	**pharyngitis** far-in-jī′tis
phren/o	diaphragm (also mind)	**phrenospasm** fren′ō-spazm
pleur/o	pleura	**pleurisy** plūr′i-sē
pneum/o	air or lung	**pneumonia** nū-mō′nē-ă
pneumon/o		**pneumonectomy** nū′mō-nek′tō-mē
pulmon/o	lung	**pulmonologist** pŭl′mō-nol′ō-jist
sinus/o	sinus (cavity)	**sinusitis** sī-nŭ-sī′tis
spir/o	breathing	**spirometry** spī-rom′ĕ-trē
thorac/o	chest	**thoracotomy** thōr-ă-kot′ō-mē
pector/o		**pectoralgia** pek-tō-ral′jē-ă
steth/o		**stethoscope** steth′ō-skōp

continued

Combining Form	Meaning	Example
tonsill/o	tonsil (almond)	**tonsillitis** ton'si-lī'tis
trache/o	trachea (windpipe)	**trachea** trā'kē-ă
-pnea (additional suffix)	breathing	**dyspnea** disp-nē'ă

Respiratory System Overview

The respiratory system is composed of the organs and structures that function to exchange gases within the body. The exchange of gases, called respiration, occurs when oxygen from the air is inhaled into the lungs and passes into the blood and carbon dioxide diffuses from the blood into the lungs and is exhaled into the air. Respiration is also known as *breathing* or *ventilation*. Intake of air is called *inspiration* or *inhalation*, and outflow of air is called *expiration* or *exhalation* (see Color Atlas, plates 17 and 18) (Fig. 9.1).

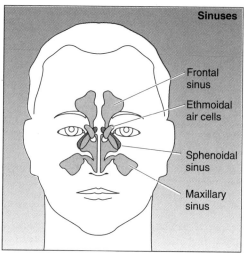

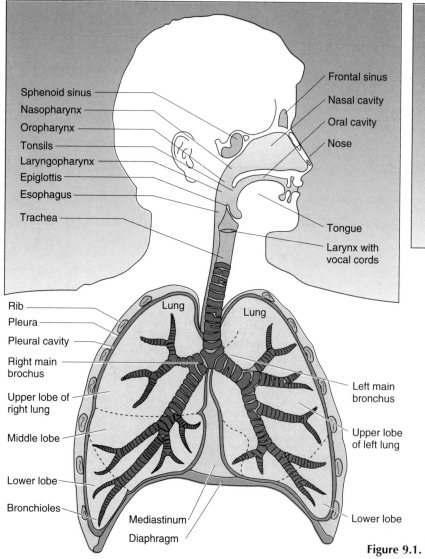

Figure 9.1. Respiratory tract.

Anatomical Terms

Term	Meaning
nose nōz	structure that warms, moistens, and filters air as it enters the respiratory tract and houses the olfactory receptors for the sense of smell
sinuses sī′nŭs-ĕz	air-filled spaces in the skull that open into the nasal cavity
pharynx far′ingks	throat; passageway for food to the esophagus and air to the larynx
nasopharynx nā-zō-far-ingks	part of the pharynx directly behind the nasal passages
oropharynx ŏr′ō-far-ingks	central portion of the pharynx between the roof of the mouth and upper edge of the epiglottis
laryngopharynx lă-ring′gō-far-ingks	lower part of the pharynx just below the oropharynx opening into the larynx and esophagus
tonsils ton′silz	oval lymphatic tissues on each side of the pharynx that filter air to protect the body from bacterial invasion— also called palatine tonsils
adenoid ad′ĕ-noyd	lymphatic tissue on the back of the pharynx behind the nose—also called pharyngeal tonsil
larynx lar′ingks	voice box; passageway for air moving from pharynx to trachea; contains vocal cords
glottis glot′is	opening between the vocal cords in the larynx
epiglottis ep-i-glot′is	a lid-like structure that covers the larynx during swallowing to prevent food from entering the airway
trachea tră′kē-ă	windpipe; passageway for air from the larynx to the area of the carina where it splits into right and left bronchus
right and left bronchus brong′kŭs	two primary airways branching from the area of the carina into the lungs
bronchial tree brong′kē-ăl	branched airways that lead from the trachea to the microscopic air sacs
bronchioles brong′kē-ōl	progressively smaller tubular branches of the airways
alveoli al-vē′ō-lī	thin-walled microscopic air sacs that exchange gases (see Color Atlas, plate 17)
lungs lŭngz	two spongy organs, located in the thoracic cavity enclosed by the diaphragm and rib cage, responsible for respiration
lobes lōbz	subdivisions of the lung, two on the left and three on the right
pleura plūr′ă	membranes enclosing the lung (visceral pleura) and lining the thoracic cavity (parietal pleura)

continued

Term	Meaning
pleural cavity plūr'ăl kav'i-tē	potential space between visceral and parietal layers of the pleura
diaphragm dī'ă-fram	muscular partition that separates the thoracic cavity from the abdominal cavity and aids in respiration by moving up and down
mediastinum me'dē-as-tī'nŭm	partition that separates the thorax into two compartments (that contain the right and left lungs) and encloses the heart, esophagus, trachea, and thymus gland
mucous membranes myū'kŭs mem'brān	thin sheets of tissue that line respiratory passages and secrete mucus, a viscid (sticky) fluid
cilia sil'ē-ă	hair-like processes from the surface of epithelial cells, such as those of the bronchi, that provide upward movement of mucus cell secretions
parenchyma pă-reng'ki-mă	functional tissues of any organ such as the tissues of the bronchioles, alveoli, ducts, and sacs that perform respiration

Symptomatic and Diagnostic Terms

Term	Meaning
Symptomatic	
Breathing (Fig. 9.2)	
eupnea yūp-nē'ă	normal breathing
bradypnea brad-ip-nē'ă	slow breathing
tachypnea tak-ip-nē'ă	fast breathing
hypopnea hī-pop'nē'ă	shallow breathing

continued

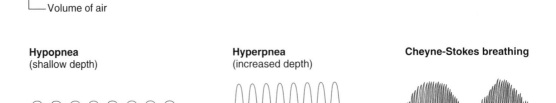

Figure 9.2. Examples of breathing patterns.

Term	Meaning
hyperpnea hī-perp′nē-ă	deep breathing
dyspnea disp-nē′ă	difficulty breathing
apnea ap′nē-ă	inability to breathe
orthopnea ōr-thop-nē′ă	ability to breathe only in an upright position (Fig. 9.3)
Cheyne-Stokes respiration res-pi-rā′shŭn	pattern of breathing characterized by a gradual increase of depth and sometimes rate to a maximum level, followed by a decrease, resulting in apnea
Lung Sounds	
crackles krak′ĕlz **rales** rahlz	popping sounds heard on auscultation of the lung when air enters diseased airways and alveoli—occurs in disorders such as bronchiectasis or atelectasis
wheezes hwēz′ez **rhonchi** rong′kī	high-pitched, musical sounds heard on auscultation of the lung as air flows through a narrowed airway—occurs in disorders such as asthma or emphysema
stridor strī′dōr	a high-pitched crowing sound that is a sign of obstruction in the upper airway (trachea or larynx)
General Symptomatic Terms	
dysphonia dis-fō′nē-ă	hoarseness

continued

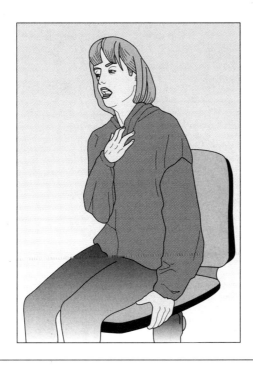

Figure 9.3. Orthopnea.

Term	Meaning
epistaxis ep′i-stak′sis	nosebleed (epi = upon; stazo = to drip)
expectoration ek-spek-tō-rā′shŭn	coughing up and spitting out of material from the lungs
sputum spū′tŭm	material expelled from the lungs by coughing
hemoptysis hē-mop′ti-sis	coughing up and spitting out blood originating in the lungs (ptysis = to spit)
hypercapnia hī-per-kap′nē-ă **hypercarbia** hī-per-kar′bē-ă	excessive level of carbon dioxide in the blood (capno = smoke; (carbo = coal)
hyperventilation hī′per-ven-ti-lā′shŭn	excessive movement of air in and out of the lungs causing hypocapnia
hypoventilation hī′pō-ven-ti-lā′shŭn	deficient movement of air in and out of the lungs causing hypercapnia
hypoxemia hī-pok-sē′mē-ă	deficient amount of oxygen in the blood
hypoxia hī-pok′sē-ă	deficient amount of oxygen in tissue cells
obstructive lung disorder lŭng dis-ōr′der	condition blocking flow of air moving out of the lungs (Fig. 9.4)
restrictive lung disorder	condition limiting the intake of air into the lungs (Fig. 9.4)
caseous necrosis kā′sē-ŭs nĕ-krō′sis	degeneration and death of tissue with a cheese-like appearance
pulmonary edema pŭl′mō-nār-ē e-dē′mă	fluid filling of the spaces around the alveoli eventually flooding into the alveoli
pulmonary infiltrate pŭl′mō-nār-ē in-fil′trāt	density on an x-ray representing solid material within the air spaces of the lungs, usually indicating inflammatory changes
rhinorrhea rī-nō-rē′ă	thin, watery discharge from the nose

continued

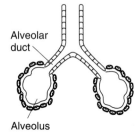

A Normal
Bronchioles and alveolar ducts are open, allowing air to reach alveoli and alveolar capillaries; alveoli and ducts are elastic, pushing air out of the lungs during expiration

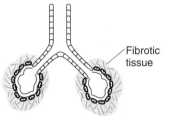

B Pneumoconiosis
Chronic inhalation of dust particles results in the formation of fibrotic tissue surrounding the alveoli, limiting their ability to stretch and restricting the intake of air

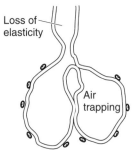

C Emphysema
Alveoli lose their elasticity, making it difficult to push air out of the lungs and obstructing exhalation of air

Figure 9.4. Comparison of normal alveoli (**A**) with alveoli in restrictive (**B**) and obstructive (**C**) lung disorders.

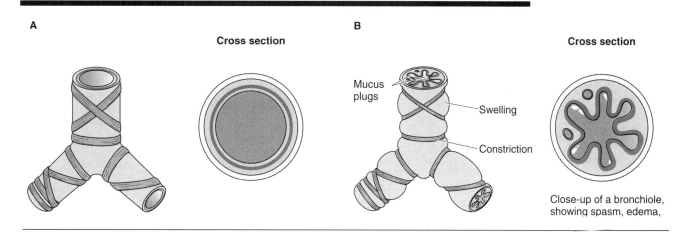

A   Cross section   B   Cross section

Mucus plugs

Swelling

Constriction

Close-up of a bronchiole, showing spasm, edema,

Figure 9.5. Constricted bronchial tubes in asthma. **A.** Normal. **B.** Asthma.

Term	Meaning
Diagnostic	
asthma az′mă	panting; obstructive pulmonary disease caused by a spasm of the bronchial tubes or by swelling of their mucous membrane, characterized by paroxysmal (sudden, periodic) attacks of wheezing, dyspnea, and cough (Fig. 9.5)
atelectasis at-ĕ-lek′tă-sis	collapse of lung tissue (alveoli) (atele = imperfect)
bronchitis brong-kī′tis	inflammation of the bronchi
bronchogenic carcinoma brong-kō-jen′ik kar-si-nō′mă	lung cancer
bronchospasm brong′kō-spazm	constriction of bronchi caused by spasm of the peribronchial smooth muscle
bronchiectasis brong-kē-ek′tă-sis	abnormal dilation of the bronchi with accumulation of mucus (Fig. 9.6)
emphysema em-fi-sē′mă	obstructive pulmonary disease characterized by overexpansion of the alveoli with air with destructive changes in their walls resulting in loss of lung elasticity and gas exchange (emphysan = to inflate) (Fig. 9.4C)
chronic obstructive pulmonary disease (COPD) kron′ik pŭl′mō-nār-ē di-zēz′	permanent, destructive pulmonary disorder that is a combination of chronic bronchitis and emphysema
laryngitis lar-in-jī′tis	inflammation of larynx
laryngotracheobronchitis (LTB) lăr-ing′gō-trā′kē-o-brong-kī′tis **croup** krūp	inflammation of the upper airways with swelling that creates a funnel-shaped elongation of tissue causing a distinct "seal bark" cough

continued

Term	Meaning
laryngospasm lă-ring′gō-spazm	spasm of laryngeal muscles causing constriction
nasal polyposis nā′zăl pol′i-pō′sis	presence of numerous polyps in the nose (a polyp is a tumor on a stalk)
pharyngitis far-in-jī′tis	inflammation of the pharynx
coryza kŏ-rī′ză	head cold; inflammation of the nasal mucous membranes
pleural effusion plŭr′ăl e-fū′zhŭn	accumulation of fluid within the pleural cavity (Fig. 9.7)
empyema em-pī-ē′mă **pyothorax** pī-ō-thōr′aks	accumulation of pus in the pleural cavity
hemothorax hē-mō-thōr′aks	blood in pleural cavity
pleuritis plū-rī′tis **pleurisy** plūr′i-sē	inflammation of pleura
pneumoconiosis nū′mō-kō-nē-ō′sis	chronic restrictive pulmonary disease resulting from prolonged inhalation of fine dusts such as coal, asbestos (asbestosis) or silicone (silicosis) (conio = dust) (Fig. 9.4B)

continued

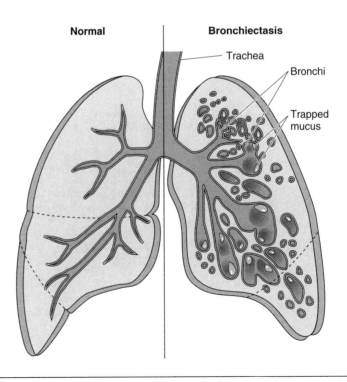

Figure 9.6. Bronchiectasis.

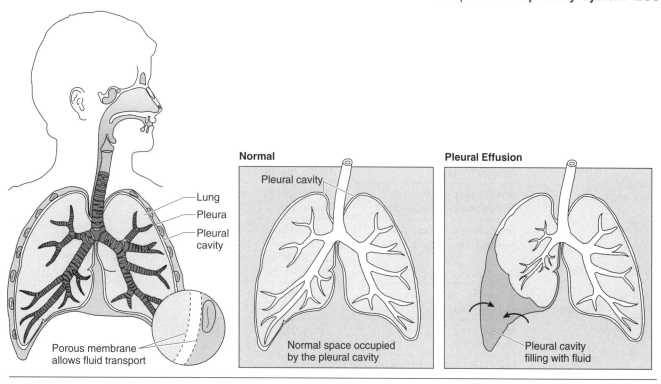

Figure 9.7. Pleural effusion.

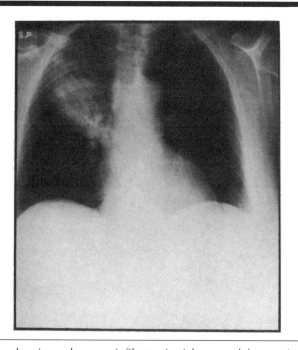

Figure 9.8. Chest x-ray showing pulmonary infiltrates in right upper lobe consistent with lobar pneumonia. Dense material (inflammatory exudate) absorbs radiation, whereas normal alveoli do not.

Term	Meaning
pneumonia nū-mō′nē-ă	infection of the lung caused primarily by bacteria, viruses, or chemicals (Fig. 9.8)
pneumocystis pneumonia nū-mō-sis′tis nū-mō′nē-ă	pneumonia caused by the *Pneumocystis carinii* organism—a common opportunistic infection seen in those with positive human immunodeficiency virus

continued

Term	Meaning
pneumothorax nū-mō-thōr'aks	air in the pleural cavity caused by a puncture of the lung or chest wall (Fig. 9.9)
pneumohemothorax nū'mō-hē-mō-thōr'aks	air and blood in the pleural cavity
pneumonitis nū-mō-nī'tis	inflammation of the lung often caused by hypersensitivity to chemicals or dusts
pulmonary embolism pŭl'mō-nar-ē em'bō-lizm	occlusion in the pulmonary circulation, most often caused by a blood clot
pulmonary tuberculosis (TB) pŭl'mō-nar-ē tū-ber-kyū-lō'sis	disease caused by the presence of *Mycobacterium tuberculosis* in the lungs characterized by the formation of tubercles, inflammation, and necrotizing caseous lesions (Fig. 9.10)
sinusitis sī-nŭ-sī'tis	inflammation of the sinuses
tonsillitis ton'si-lī'tis	acute or chronic inflammation of the tonsils
upper respiratory infection (URI) res'pi-ră-tōr-ē in-fek'shŭn	infectious disease of the upper respiratory tract involving the nasal passages, pharynx, and bronchi

Diagnostic Tests and Procedures

Test or Procedure	Explanation
arterial blood gases (ABGs) ar-tē'rē-ăl	analysis of arterial blood to determine adequacy of lung function in the exchange of gases

continued

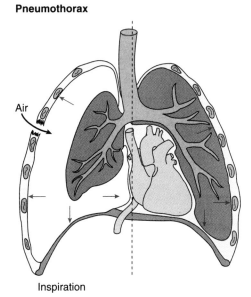

Normal

Pneumothorax

Air

Inspiration

Air entering through a wound in the chest causes a collapse of the lung; contents of the thoracic cavity shift to the opposite side, compressing the other lung

Figure 9.9. Simple pneumothorax.

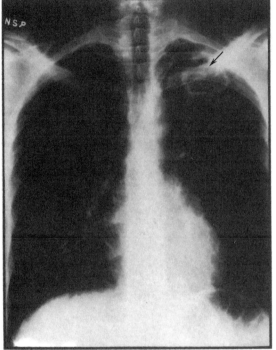

Figure 9.10. Chest x-ray showing presence of tuberculosis in left upper lobe (*arrow*).

STETHOSCOPE. The Greek word stethos means chest and skopeo means to view. The stethoscope was invented by René Laënnec in 1816. He is said to have first thought of it when watching children playing; some of them listening at one end of a beam of wood could hear a pin scratching at the other end. He applied this principle to auscultation of the chest, which was then performed by placing the ear directly on the patient's chest. The first stethoscope was made of wood.

Test or Procedure	Explanation
pH	a measure of blood acidity or alkalinity
PaO$_2$	partial pressure of oxygen measuring the amount of oxygen in the blood
PaCO$_2$	partial pressure of carbon dioxide measuring the amount of carbon dioxide in the blood
auscultation aws-kŭl-tā′shŭn	to listen; a physical examination method of listening to the sounds within the body with the aid of a stethoscope, such as auscultation of the chest for heart and lung sounds
endoscopy en-dos′kŏ-pē	examination of a body cavity with a flexible endoscope to examine within for diagnostic or treatment purpose
bronchoscopy brong-kos′kŏ-pē	use of a flexible endoscope, called a bronchoscope, to examine the airways (see Color Atlas, plate 18)
nasopharyngoscopy nā′zō-far′ing-gos′kŏ-pē	use of a flexible endoscope to examine the nasal passages and the pharynx (throat) to diagnose structural abnormalities such as obstructions, growths, cancers
lung biopsy (Bx) lŭng bī′op-sē	removal of a small piece of lung tissue for pathological examination
lung scan lŭng skan	nuclear scan of the lung to detect abnormalities of perfusion (blood flow) or ventilation (respiration), commonly called a V/Q (ventilation/perfusion) scan (Fig. 9.11)

continued

Test or Procedure	Explanation
magnetic resonance image (MRI) mag-net'ic rez'ō-nans im'ij	nonionizing image of the lung to visualize lung lesions
percussion per-kŭsh'ŭn	a physical examination method of tapping over the body to elicit vibrations and sounds to estimate the size, border, or fluid content of a cavity such as the chest
pulmonary function testing (PFT) pŭl'mō-nār-ē fŭngk'shŭn	direct and indirect measurements of lung volumes and capacities
spirometry spī-rom'ĕ-trē	a portion of pulmonary function testing that is a direct measurement of lung volume and capacity (Fig. 9.12)
tidal volume (TV or V_T) tī'dăl vol'yŭm	amount of air exhaled after a normal inspiration
vital capacity (VC) vīt-ăl kă-pas'i-tē	amount of air exhaled after a maximal inspiration

continued

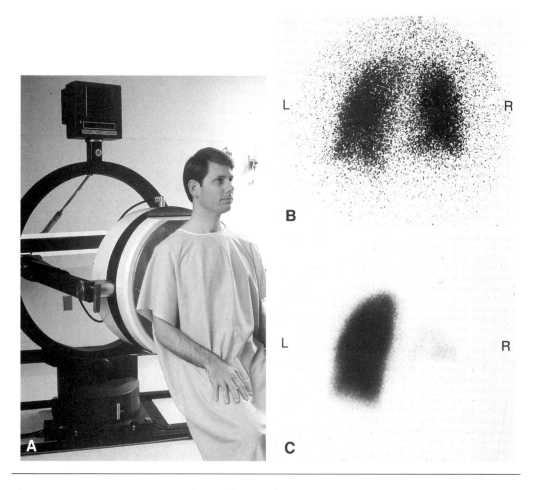

Figure 9.11. A. Gamma-camera used to produce nuclear lung scan. **B.** and **C.** Posterior lung scan in a patient with an embolus in the right lung. Ventilation image (**B**) shows a normal pattern. Absence of bloodflow to the right lung is apparent on perfusion scan (**C**). *L*, left; *R*, right.

A

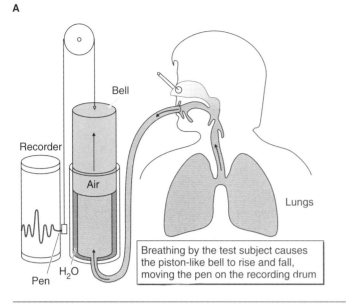

B

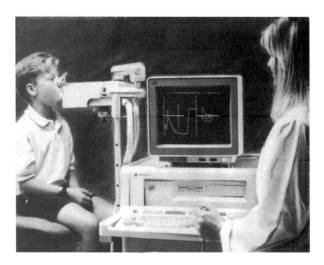

Recorder

Bell

Air

Lungs

Pen H₂O

Breathing by the test subject causes the piston-like bell to rise and fall, moving the pen on the recording drum

Figure 9.12. A. Principle of spirometry. **B.** Modern spirometry.

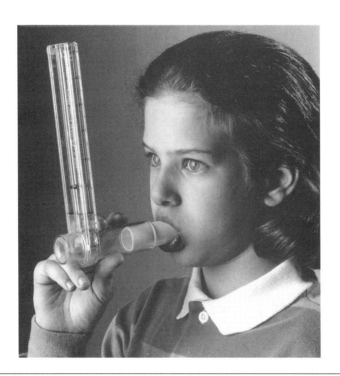

Figure 9.13. Routine peak flow monitoring by asthmatic adolescent female is performed to predict signs of oncoming attack.

Test or Procedure	Explanation
peak flow (PF) **peak expiratory flow rate** (PEFR) ek-spī′ră-tō-rē flō rāt	measure of the fastest flow of exhaled air after a maximal inspiration (Fig. 9.13)

continued

Test or Procedure	Explanation
radiology rā-dē-ol'ō-jē	x-ray imaging
chest x-ray (CXR)	x-ray image of the chest to visualize the lungs
computed tomography (CT) tō-mog'ră-fē	computed x-ray imaging of the head is used to visualize the structures of the nose and sinuses; CT of the thorax is used to detect lesions in the lung
pulmonary angiography pŭl'mō-nār-ē an-jē-og'ră-fē	x-ray of the blood vessels of lungs after injection of contrast material (Fig. 9.14)

Operative Terms

Term	Meaning
adenoidectomy ad'ĕ-noy-dek'tō-mē	excision of adenoids
lobectomy lō-bek'tō-mē	removal of a lobe of a lung
nasal polypectomy nā'zăl pol-i-pek'tō-mē	removal of a nasal polyp

continued

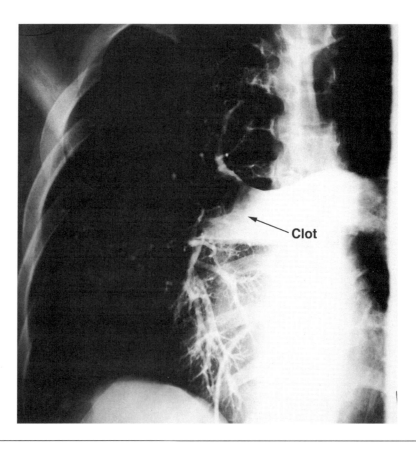

Figure 9.14. Pulmonary angiogram: embolus obstructing pulmonary circulation (*arrow*).

Term	Meaning
pneumonectomy nū′mō-nek′tō-mē	removal of an entire lung
thoracentesis thōr′ă-sen-tē′sis	puncture for aspiration of the chest (Fig. 9.15)
thoracoplasty thōr′ă-kō-plas-tē	repair of the chest involving fixation of the ribs
thoracoscopy thōr-ă-kos′kŏ-pē	endoscopic examination of the pleural cavity using a thoracoscope
thoracostomy thōr-ă-kos′tō-mē	creation of an opening in the chest usually for insertion of a tube (Fig. 9.15)
thoracotomy thōr-ă-kot′ō-mē	incision into chest
tonsillectomy ton′si-lek′tō-mē	excision of palatine tonsils
tonsillectomy and **adenoidectomy** (T & A) ad′ĕ-noy-dek′tō-mē	excision of tonsils and adenoids
tracheostomy trā′kē-os′tō-mē	creation of an opening in the trachea most often to insert a tube (Fig. 9.16)
tracheotomy trā′kē-ot′ō-mē	incision into trachea (Fig. 9.16)

Therapeutic Terms

Term	Meaning
cardiopulmonary resuscitation (CPR) kar′dē-ō-pŭl′mo-nār-ē rē-sŭs′i-tā′shŭn	a method of artificial respiration and closed chest massage used to restore breathing and cardiac output after cardiac arrest

continued

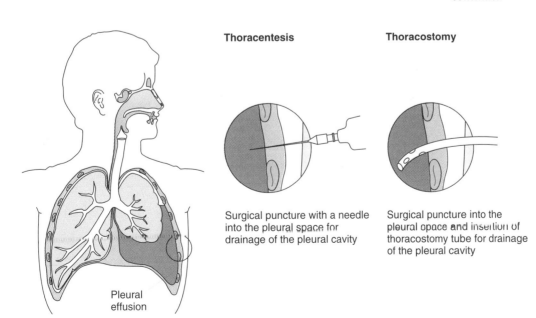

Thoracentesis

Thoracostomy

Surgical puncture with a needle into the pleural space for drainage of the pleural cavity

Surgical puncture into the pleural space and insertion of thoracostomy tube for drainage of the pleural cavity

Pleural effusion

Figure 9.15. Common treatments of pleural effusion.

Tracheotomy
Incision of the trachea for exploration, for removal of a foreign body, or for obtaining a biopsy specimen

Tracheostomy
Incision of the trachea and insertion of a tube to facilitate passage of air or removal of secretions

Sagittal view, with tracheostomy tube in place

Incision

Placement of tracheostomy tube

Tracheostomy tube

Figure 9.16. Operative procedures related to the trachea.

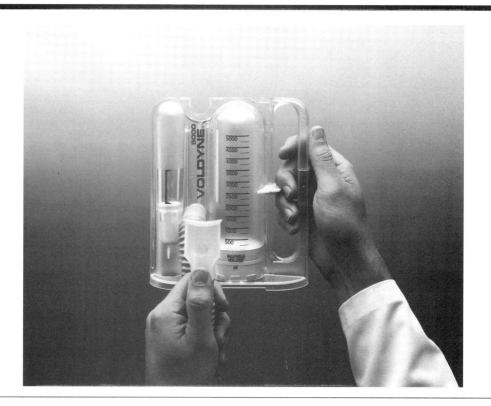

Figure 9.17. Incentive spirometer.

Term	Meaning
endotracheal intubation en′dō-trā′kē-ăl in-tū-bā′shŭn	passage of a tube into the trachea via the nose or mouth to open the airway for delivering gas mixtures to the lungs (e.g., oxygen, anesthetics, or air)
incentive spirometry in-sen′tiv spī-rom′ĕ-trē	a common postoperative breathing therapy using a specially designed spirometer to encourage the patient to inhale and repeatedly sustain an inspiratory volume to exercise the lungs and prevent pulmonary complications (Fig. 9.17)

continued

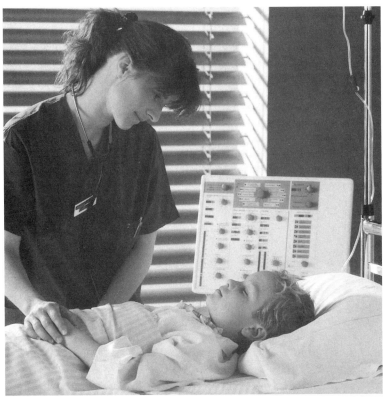

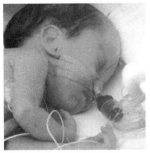
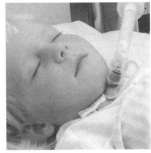
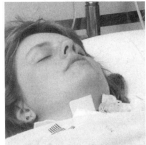

Neonate   Pediatric   Adult

Figure 9.18. Mechanical ventilation.

Term	Meaning
mechanical ventilation mĕ-kan'i-kăl ven-ti-lā'shŭn	mechanical method performed by a respiratory therapist to provide assisted breathing using a ventilator (Fig. 9.18)

Common Therapeutic Drug Classifications

antibiotic an'tē-bī-ot'ik	a drug that kills or inhibits growth of microorganisms
anticoagulant an'tē-kō-ag'yū-lant	drug that dissolves, or prevents the formation of, thrombi or emboli in the blood vessels (e.g., heparin)
antihistamine an-tē-his'tă-mēn	a drug that neutralizes or inhibits the effects of histamine
histamine his'tă-mēn	a compound in the body that is released by injured cells in allergic reactions, inflammation, etc., causing constriction of bronchial smooth muscle, dilation of blood vessels, etc.

continued

Term	Meaning
bronchodilator brong-kō-dī-lā′ter	a drug that dilates the muscular walls of the bronchi
expectorant ek-spek′tō-rănt	a drug that breaks up mucus and promotes coughing

PRACTICE EXERCISES

For the following terms, draw a line or lines to separate prefixes, combining forms, and suffixes. Then define the term.

1. bronchostomy _____

2. tracheopyosis _____

3. hyperpnea _____

4. thoracentesis _____

5. rhinostenosis _____

6. hypoxia _____

7. sinusitis _____

8. hypoxemia _____

9. pleuritis _____

10. hypercarbia _____

11. tracheotomy _____

12. dysphonia _____

13. bronchoscope _____

14. oropharyngeal _____

15. hypopnea _____

16. pneumonectomy _____

17. rhinorrhea _____

18. thoracostomy _____

19. eupnea _____

20. tonsillectomy _____

21. pharyngitis _____

22. bronchospasm _____

23. laryngostenosis _____

24. tracheobronchitis _____

25. rhinophonia _____

26. phrenoptosis _____

27. peripleural _____

28. stethoscope _____

29. rhinoscleroma _____

30. pneumonic _____

31. bronchorrhea _____

32. nasopharyngoscopy _____

33. bronchiectasis _____

34. rhinitis _____

35. sinusotomy _____

36. lobectomy _____

37. pectoral _____

38. rhinoplasty _____

39. alveolitis _____

Write the correct medical term for each of the following:

40. air in pleural space _____

41. pus in pleural space _____

42. blood in pleural space _____

43. listening to sounds within the body _____

44. endoscope used to examine the airways _____

45. coughing up and spitting out material from lungs _____

46. inflammation of the pleura_____

47. to elicit sounds or vibrations by tapping _____

48. deficient movement of air in and out of the lungs_____

49. puncture for aspiration of the chest _____

50. type of technology used in a lung scan _____

51. hoarseness_____

52. inflammation of the voice box _____

53. deficient amount of oxygen in tissue cells_____

54. disease characterized by overexpansion of the alveoli with air_____

_____

55. nosebleed_____

56. cancer originating in the bronchus _____

57. head cold _____

58. a collapse of lung tissue _____

59. material expelled from the lungs by coughing _____

60. a high-pitched crowing sound that is a sign of obstruction in the upper airway

_____

61. blood clot in the lungs_____

62. surgical creation of an opening in the trachea _____

63. disease characterized by paroxysmal wheezing, dyspnea, and cough_____

64. excessive movement of air in and out of lungs _____

65. common lung infection seen in those with positive HIV _____

66. name referring to a combination of emphysema and chronic bronchitis_____

_____

Complete the medical term by writing the missing part:

67. _____ coni _____ = lung condition caused by prolonged dust inhalation

68. bronchi _____ = dilation of bronchus

69. _____ plasty = surgical repair of the chest

70. _____ itis = inflammation of the lung

71. _____ metry = measured breathing

72. _____ pnea = normal breathing

73. _____ pnea = slow breathing

74. _____ pnea = difficulty breathing

75. _____ pnea = inability to breathe except in an upright position

76. _____ pnea = inability to breathe

77. _____ pnea = fast breathing

Write the full medical term for the following abbreviations:

78. PEFR _____

79. VC _____

80. TB _____

81. CPR _____

82. COPD _____

83. $PaCO_2$ _____

84. URI _____

85. V_T _____

86. PFT _____

Write the standard abbreviations for the following:

87. chest x-ray _____

88. analysis of blood to determine the adequacy of lung function in exchange of gases

_____

89. surgical removal of the tonsils and adenoids _____

Match the following terms with the appropriate right column term:

90. crackles   _____   a. naso

91. wheezes   _____   b. hyperventilation

92. pleurisy   _____   c. hypercarbia

93. pneumoconiosis _____   d. thoraco

94. empyema   _____   e. rales

95. hemothorax   _____   f. asbestosis

96. stetho   _____   g. pleuritis

97. hypercapnia   _____   h. rhonchi

98. hyperpnea   _____   i. pyothorax

99. rhino   _____   j. thoracentesis

Medical Record Analyses

MEDICAL RECORD 9.1

Richard Puma, a heavy smoker until recently, had been treated for pneumonia in the last month. Even though his condition deteriorated in the last few days, he refused to be hospitalized. Today, May 18, having much trouble breathing, he came to Central Medical Center and was seen by Dr. Theresa Cunningham.

Directions

Read Medical Record 9.1 for Richard Puma (pages 253–256) and answer the following questions. This record includes the history, physical examination, and discharge summary dictated by Dr. Cunningham and transcribed the next day.

Questions about Medical Record 9.1

Write your answers in the spaces provided.

1. Below are medical terms used in these records you have not yet encountered in this text. Underline each where it appears in the record and define below.

   hepatosplenomegaly _____

   precordial _____

   fulminant _____

   respiratory acidosis _____

   cardiac arrest _____

2. In your own words, not using medical terminology, describe Mr. Puma's chief complaint to Dr. Cunningham.

   _____

   _____

   _____

3. Following are various elements from the history of Mr. Puma's present illness. Put them in correct chronological order by numbering them 1 to 8, starting with the event that occurred first.

   _____ progressive worsening with shortness of breath

   _____ refusal to be hospitalized

   _____ intermittent fever and chills for past month

   _____ administration of Cipro began

   _____ administration of Cipro started a second time

_____ presentation to Bradford Emergiclinic

_____ diagnosis of pneumonia

_____ productive cough with show of blood

4. In your own words, not using medical terminology, describe how Mr. Puma looked in general at the time of examination.

_____

_____

_____

5. Although examination of the abdomen produced no negative findings, Dr. Cunningham's auscultation of the lungs and heart was more significant. In your own words, what were her findings?

_____

_____

_____

6. Dr. Cunningham concluded her examination with a diagnosis and treatment plan. Although the cause of Mr. Puma's condition is unclear, the diagnosis statement itself is definite. Describe it in your own words.

_____

_____

_____

7. In the history and physical examination, Dr. Cunningham's treatment plan called for what immediate action?

_____

_____

_____

8. As noted in the discharge summary, Dr. Anderson was next to see Mr. Puma. In your own words describe Dr. Anderson's specialty:

_____

9. What diagnostic test was first to be performed on admission to CCU?

_____

10. During the CCU examination, what happened to Mr. Puma?

    _____

    How did Dr. Anderson respond?

    _____

11. Put Dr. Cunningham's final three diagnoses in your own words (do not include history or treatment information).

    a. _____

    b. _____

    c. _____

CENTRAL MEDICAL CENTER
211 Medical Center Drive • Central City, US 90000-1234 • PHONE: (012) 125-6784 • FAX: (012) 125-9999

HISTORY

CHIEF COMPLAINT:
Marked respiratory distress.

HISTORY OF PRESENT ILLNESS:
The patient is a 62-year-old white male who had a history of pneumonia four weeks ago. This was treated with Cipro which responded after two weeks of medication; however, after being off the medication for one day, he developed problems. He was restarted on half a dose for five more days with some improvement. This was finished 1½ weeks ago. The patient had hemoptysis and yellow sputum at that time. It cleared with the Cipro; however, it has returned intermittently. Over the past ten days, he has become progressively worse with marked increase in his shortness of breath as well as an inability to lie down for the past two to three weeks. Until one month ago, he states he felt relatively well with normal activities, although he has been febrile with intermittent chills. At this time, there is no history of angina. He was seen initially at the Bradford Emergiclinic because of the progressive nature of his shortness of breath. Then, two days ago, he was seen there again because of pneumonia and the treatment. At that time, hospitalization was recommended, but the patient refused.

PAST MEDICAL HISTORY:
The patient states there is no prior history of heart disease, although he says an electrocardiogram showed a possible old heart attack in the past; this was noted approximately 14 years ago. He has a history of possible hypertension in the past.

ALLERGIES: He has no known allergies.

HABITS: He smoked two packs of cigarettes per day for 35 years; he stopped one month ago. He drinks approximately one beer a month.

SURGERIES: He had several hernia surgeries in the past.

FAMILY HISTORY: The patient's father died at age 42 of heart problems.

REVIEW OF SYSTEMS:
Noncontributory to the present illness.

(continued)

HISTORY AND PHYSICAL
Page 1

PT. NAME: PUMA, RICHARD G.
ID NO: 077321
ADM. DATE: May 18, 19xx
ATT. PHYS. T. CUNNINGHAM, M.D.

Medical Record 9.1.

CENTRAL MEDICAL CENTER

211 Medical Center Drive • Central City, US 90000-1234 • PHONE: (012) 125-6784 • FAX: (012) 125-9999

PHYSICAL EXAMINATION

GENERAL APPEARANCE:
Markedly tachypneic, thin, cyanotic white male in marked respiratory distress. VITAL SIGNS:
Blood pressure: 90/50.

HEENT:
Eyes: Pupils are equal and reactive to light and accommodation. Extraocular movements are
normal. Ears, nose, and throat are negative.

NECK: Supple. Jugular venous pulsations are normal. Carotids are 2+ and equal bilaterally
without bruit.

CHEST:
LUNGS: There is a very rapid rate with a few basilar rales and decreased breath sounds in the
bases.

HEART: It was difficult to auscultate because of the marked tachypnea and respiratory noises.
There were no obvious murmurs heard.

ABDOMEN: Soft and nontender. No hepatosplenomegaly or masses were noted.

GENITALIA/RECTAL:
Normal male. The rectal examination was not performed due to the acute nature of the patient's
illness.

EXTREMITIES:
There was no edema. Peripheral pulses are barely palpable. There was no marked cyanosis.

LABORATORY AND X-RAY DATA:
An electrocardiogram shows regular sinus rhythm with PVCs and fusion beats, nonspecific interior
ventricular conduction delay, right axis deviation, poor precordial R-wave progression, and
nonspecific ST-T wave changes.

(continued)

HISTORY AND PHYSICAL Page 2	PT. NAME: PUMA, RICHARD G. ID NO: 077321 ADM. DATE: May 18, 19xx ATT. PHYS. T. CUNNINGHAM, M.D.

Medical Record 9.1. *Continued.*

CENTRAL MEDICAL CENTER

211 Medical Center Drive • Central City, US 90000-1234 • PHONE: (012) 125-6784 • FAX: (012) 125-9999

PHYSICAL EXAMINATION

IMPRESSION:

1. MARKED, SEVERE RESPIRATORY DISTRESS WITH CYANOSIS DUE TO UNKNOWN ETIOLOGY. RULE OUT FULMINANT PNEUMONIA, RULE OUT CONGESTIVE HEART FAILURE. RULE OUT OTHER CAUSES.

2. CHRONIC OBSTRUCTIVE PULMONARY DISEASE.

3. POSSIBLE HISTORY OF HYPERTENSION, PRESENTLY HYPOTENSIVE.

PLAN:

The patient is admitted to the CCU immediately after being seen in the office. Upon admission, he will be seen by Dr. Anderson in pulmonary consult. Further evaluation and treatment will depend upon the results of the studies.

T. Cunningham, M.D.

T. Cunningham, M.D.

TC:ti

D: 5/18/9x
T: 5/19/9x

HISTORY AND PHYSICAL PAGE 3	PT. NAME: PUMA, RICHARD G. ID NO: 077321 ADM. DATE: May 18, 19xx ATT. PHYS. T. CUNNINGHAM, M.D.

Medical Record 9.1. _Continued._

CENTRAL MEDICAL CENTER

211 Medical Center Drive • Central City, US 90000-1234 • PHONE: (012) 125-6784 • FAX: (012) 125-9999

DISCHARGE SUMMARY

DATE OF ADMISSION: May 18, 199x   **DATE OF DISCHARGE:** May 18, 199x

DIAGNOSES:
1. ACUTE SEVERE RESPIRATORY DISTRESS, WITH RESPIRATORY FAILURE, TREATED, DIED.
2. CARDIAC ARREST, DUE TO UNKNOWN ETIOLOGY, PROBABLY SECONDARY TO MARKED PULMONARY DISEASE, TREATED WITH CARDIOPULMONARY RESUSCITATION, UNSUCCESSFUL.
3. CHRONIC OBSTRUCTIVE PULMONARY DISEASE WITH A LONG HISTORY OF TOBACCO ABUSE.

SUMMARY:
This patient was seen in the office on the morning of admission in marked respiratory distress. He was markedly tachypneic and cyanotic, and he had a history of pneumonia which was treated one month ago with progressive symptoms over the past week.

The patient was admitted immediately to the CCU where he was met by M. Anderson, M.D., a pulmonologist, who saw him in consultation. During the initial evaluation, while the patient was getting ready for a CXR in the CCU, he suddenly had a cardiac arrest.

Resuscitation was begun immediately. The patient was seen by me at that time; however, he did not respond to any measures. An arterial line was placed. He had marked respiratory acidosis, and after no response to resuscitation, he was pronounced dead.

T. Cunningham, M.D.

TC:ti

D: 5/18/9x
T: 5/19/9x

DISCHARGE SUMMARY	PT. NAME:	PUMA, RICHARD G.
	ID NO:	077321
	ROOM:	CCU
	ATT. PHYS.	T. CUNNINGHAM, M.D.

Medical Record 9.1. _Continued._

MEDICAL RECORD 9.2

Angelica Torrance, a retired painter who for years has boasted to friends that she has the good health of a 30-year-old, suffered a broken ankle when she slipped off a footstool in her basement. The surgical repair of her fracture at Central Medical Center was routine, but soon after surgery Ms. Torrance developed other problems, and a pulmonologist was eventually called in for a consultation.

Directions

Read Medical Record 9.2 for Ms. Torrance (pages 259–261) and answer the following questions. This record is the history and physical examination report from Dr. Carl Brownley, the pulmonologist who consulted with Ms. Torrance's doctors after she developed breathing problems.

Questions about Medical Record 9.2

Write your answers in the spaces provided.

1. Below are medical terms used in this record you have not yet encountered in this text. Underline each where it appears in the record and define below.

   morphine _____

   heparin _____

   obese _____

2. In your own words, not using medical terminology, describe what surgery Ms. Torrance had for her broken ankle.

   _____

   _____

   _____

3. Describe in your own words the four symptoms that Ms. Torrance developed post-surgically:

   a. _____

   b. _____

   c. _____

   d. _____

4. Before Ms. Torrance's acute "sense of suffocating," she was being treated with what three pharmacological treatments?

   a. _____

   b. _____

   c. _____

5. Immediately after her reported "sense of suffocating," she was given what two treatments?

   a. _____

   b. _____

6. Put the following events that occurred in the hospital in correct order by numbering them 1 to 8:

_____ postoperative pulmonary symptoms

_____ transport to intensive care

_____ sense of suffocation

_____ episode of tachycardia

_____ nuclear lung scan showing high probability of embolus

_____ evaluation for complications in the lungs

_____ open reduction, internal fixation

_____ intravenous drugs first administered

7. In your own words, not using medical terminology, describe the two diagnostic imaging studies performed the morning of 10/24:

a. _____

b. _____

8. Name and describe the test that was performed to monitor Ms. Torrance's heparin therapy.

_____

_____

_____

9. Translate into lay language Dr. Brownley's first four assessments from the examination:

a. _____

b. _____

c. _____

d. _____

10. Dr. Brownley's recommendations include requests for certain tests to be run (or run again) and certain other actions to be taken while Ms. Torrance stays in the hospital. Without using abbreviations, list the tests to be performed and the actions to be taken.

Tests:

a. _____

b. _____

c. _____

d. _____

e. _____

f. _____

Actions:

g. _____

h. _____

CENTRAL MEDICAL CENTER

211 Medical Center Drive • Central City, US 90000-1234 • PHONE: (012) 125-6784 • FAX: (012) 125-9999

HISTORY

DATE OF CONSULTATION:
October 24, 199x

HISTORY:
The patient is a 75-year-old woman who is admitted to this hospital on October 18, 199x, after having fractured her right ankle. She underwent an ORIF of this lesion. Upon emerging from surgery, it was noted that she was quite wheezy and was having copious, purulent secretions. She was started on antibiotics; however, fever, cough, and breathlessness persisted. Finally, she was evaluated on October 20, 199x, for possible pulmonary complications. A V/Q scan at that time showed a high probability for pulmonary emboli, and she was started on IV Heparin along with her antibiotics and bronchodilators. The patient did well with resolution of symptoms and fever and was progressing to the point of discharge.

Late yesterday evening, however, the patient developed the acute onset of "a sense of suffocating." This lasted for about 20-30 minutes and did resolve somewhat with the application of nasal oxygen and morphine sulfate 2 mg. The patient denies any cough, mucus, or actual chest pressure or pain. She denies any wheezing during this episode. Her heart rate went as high as 115-120; however, she was normotensive.

She was transported to ICU for further evaluation and management. An ECG obtained at that time revealed slight ST segment depression and T wave flattening at V4-6 with sinus tachycardia. Arterial blood gases done during the episode on 7 L O_2 showed a PaO_2 of 78, a pH of 7.44, and a $PaCO_2$ of 35. This morning, a chest x-ray revealed continuing resolution of the right upper and right lower lobe infiltrates. A V/Q scan showed evidence of resolving multiple perfusion defects on the right that appeared to actually match the defects noted on the chest x-ray. PTT, which had been continually in control during her Heparin therapy, was as high as 150 on 7 units of Heparin per hour.

PAST MEDICAL HISTORY:
The patient denies a past history of chronic respiratory disease but did have severe pneumonia about 30 years ago. The patient is a nonsmoker who has never smoked, and she has an essentially negative past medical history.

ALLERGIES:
The patient denies any personal allergies, but her family all suffer from chronic post nasal drip.

(continued)

PULMONARY CONSULTATION Page 1	PT. NAME: TORRANCE, ANGELICA W. ID NO: IP-228904 ROOM NO: 663 ATT. PHYS. C. BROWNLEY, M.D.

Medical Record 9.2.

CENTRAL MEDICAL CENTER

211 Medical Center Drive • Central City, US 90000-1234 • PHONE: (012) 125-6784 • FAX: (012) 125-9999

PHYSICAL EXAMINATION

GENERAL:
Well-nourished, somewhat overweight woman in no acute distress, having recently come back from x-ray with no undue dyspnea.

VITAL SIGNS:
BP: 110/70. Respirations: 16. Heart Rate: 80 and regular. Temperature: 99°.

CHEST:
LUNGS: Fair expansion bilaterally. Percussion node is normal. There are rare, distant end inspiratory rales at both bases but no wheezes or rhonchi.

HEART: No clinical cardiomegaly. There are no murmurs or gallops.

ABDOMEN:
Obese, soft, nontender.

EXTREMITIES:
1+ pretibial edema on the left with a cast on the right.

ASSESSMENT:
1. ACUTE ONSET OF SHORTNESS OF BREATH OF UNCLEAR ETIOLOGY.
2. HYPOXIA.
3. HYPOTHROMBINEMIA (PATIENT ON HEPARIN).
4. STATUS POST PULMONARY EMBOLISM WITH RESOLUTION AND NO EVIDENCE OF RECURRENCE.
5. STATUS POST OPEN REDUCTION INTERNAL FIXATION OF TRIMALLEOLAR FRACTURE ON THE RIGHT.
6. RULE OUT ACUTE MYOCARDIAL INFARCTION VERSUS ISCHEMIA.
7. POSSIBLE MUCOUS PLUG.

(continued)

PULMONARY CONSULTATION Page 2	PT. NAME: TORRANCE, ANGELICA W. ID NO: IP-228904 ROOM NO: 663 ATT. PHYS. C. BROWNLEY, M.D.

Medical Record 9.2. *Continued.*

CENTRAL MEDICAL CENTER

211 Medical Center Drive • Central City, US 90000-1234 • PHONE: (012) 125-6784 • FAX: (012) 125-9999

PHYSICAL EXAMINATION

RECOMMENDATIONS:
Cardiac enzymes should be obtained, and the ECG should be repeated as well. Recheck ABGs. Recheck PTT and discontinue Heparin until PTT diminishes to the 60s. Check CBC and Biochem Panel-20. Continue to observe in the ICU.

It is somewhat unclear as to what is the etiology of the episode of dyspnea. A possibility might be a mucous plug which has mobilized into the central airway and momentarily caused increased respiratory distress.

Thank you for the opportunity to assist in the management of this patient.

C. Brownley

C.Brownley, M.D.
Pulmonologist

CB:im

D: 10/24/9x
T: 10/25/9x

PULMONARY CONSULTATION Page 3	PT. NAME: TORRANCE, ANGELICA W. ID NO: IP-228904 ROOM NO: 663 ATT. PHYS. C. BROWNLEY, M.D.

Medical Record 9.2. *Continued.*

10 Nervous System

OBJECTIVES

After completion of this chapter you will be able to

1. Define common combining forms used in relation to the nervous system

2. Define the basic anatomical terms referring to the nervous system

3. Define common symptomatic, diagnostic, operative, and therapeutic terms referring to the nervous system

4. List the common diagnostic tests and procedures related to the nervous system

5. Explain the terms and abbreviations used in documenting medical records involving the nervous system

Combining Forms

Combining Form	Meaning	Example
cerebr/o	brain	cerebrospinal ser′ĕ-brō-spī-năl
encephal/o		encephalography en-sef-ă-log′ră-fē
cerebell/o	cerebellum (little brain)	cerebellar ser-e-bel′ar
crani/o	skull	cranium krā′nē-ŭm
esthesi/o	sensation	hyperesthesia hī′per-es-thē′zē-ă
gangli/o	ganglion (knot)	ganglioneuroma gang′glē-ō-nū-rō′mă
gli/o	glue	glial glī′ăl
gnos/o	knowing	gnosia nō′sēă
kinesi/o	movement	kinesiology ki-nē-sē-ol′ō-jē
mening/o	meninges (membrane)	meningocele mĕ-ning′gō-sēl
meningi/o		meningitis men-in-jī′tis
myel/o	spinal cord or bone marrow	myeloma mī-ĕ-lō′mă
narc/o	stupor	narcotic nar-kot′ik
neur/o	nerve	neuralgia nū-ral′jē-ă
phas/o	speech	dysphasia dis-fā′zē-ă
somat/o	body	psychosomatic sī′kō-sō-mat′ik
somn/o	sleep	polysomnography pol′ē-som-nog′ră-fē
spin/o	spine (thorn)	spinal spī′năl
spondyl/o	vertebra	spondylosyndesis spon′di-lō-sin-dē′sis
vertebr/o		vertebral ver′te-brăl

continued

Combining Form	Meaning	Example
stere/o	three dimensional or solid	**stereotaxic** ster′ē-ō-tak′sik
tax/o	order or coordination	**ataxic** ă-tak′sik
thalam/o	thalamus (a room)	**thalamotomy** thal-ă-mot′ō-mē
top/o	place	**topesthesia** top′es-thē′-zē-ă
ventricul/o	ventricle (belly or pouch)	**ventriculostomy** ven-trik-yū-lot′ō-mē

Suffixes

-asthenia	weakness	**neurasthenia** nūr-as-thē′nē-ă
-lepsy	seizure	**narcolepsy** nar′kō-lep-sē
-paresis	slight paralysis	**hemiparesis** hem′-ē-pa-rē′sis
-plegia	paralysis	**paraplegia** par-ă-plē′jē-ă

Nervous System Overview

The nervous system is an intricate communication network of structures that activates and controls all functions of the body and receives all input from the environment (see Color Atlas, plates 19–21).

There are two major classes of cells that make up the nervous system: the *neuron*, the basic structure, and the *neuroglia*, the supporting cells (Fig. 10.1).

Each neuron is made up of a *soma* (the body of the neuron), *dendrites* (the afferent branches of the soma), and an *axon* (the efferent branch of the soma), which are linked via terminals called *synapses*. At the synapse, chemicals known as *neurotransmitters* are released to effect changes that inhibit or excite cells. They function within the vast complex of impulse-carrying fibers called *nerves*. A ganglion is a collection of somas in the peripheral nervous system, and a nucleus is a collection of somas in the central nervous system.

Four types of neuroglia perform essential functions in the nervous system: *ependymal cells* make the cerebrospinal fluid that circulates in and around the brain and spinal cord. The star-shaped *astrocytes* have the responsibility of passing nutrients from blood to neurons. *Myelin*, the lipid that surrounds nerve fibers and helps to conduct neuronal impulses, is produced by the *oligodendroglia*. The small, branching *microglia* perform phagocytosis.

The nervous system has three divisions: (*a*) central nervous system, (*b*) peripheral nervous system, and (*c*) autonomic nervous system.

Anatomical Terms

Term	Meaning
central nervous system (CNS)	brain and spinal cord

continued

NEURON

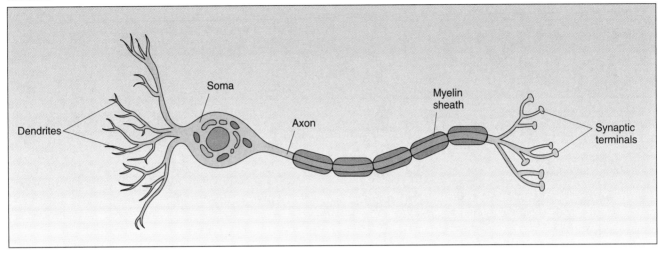

GLIAL CELLS

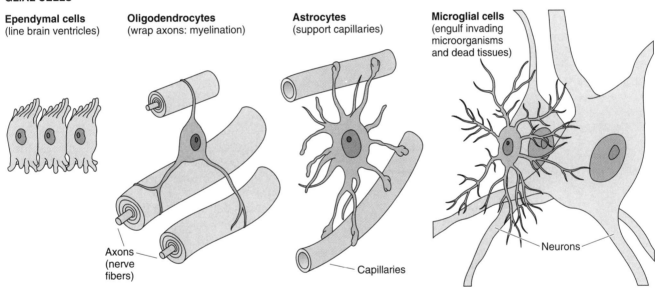

Figure 10.1. Basic components of the nervous system.

Term	Meaning
brain	portion of the central nervous system contained within the cranium (Fig. 10.2)
cerebrum sĕr-e′brum	largest portion of the brain; it is divided into right and left halves known as *cerebral hemispheres* that are connected by a bridge of nerve fibers called the *corpus callosum*; lobes of the cerebrum are named after the skull bones they underlie
frontal lobe frŭn′tăl lōb	anterior section of each cerebral hemisphere responsible for voluntary muscle movement and personality

continued

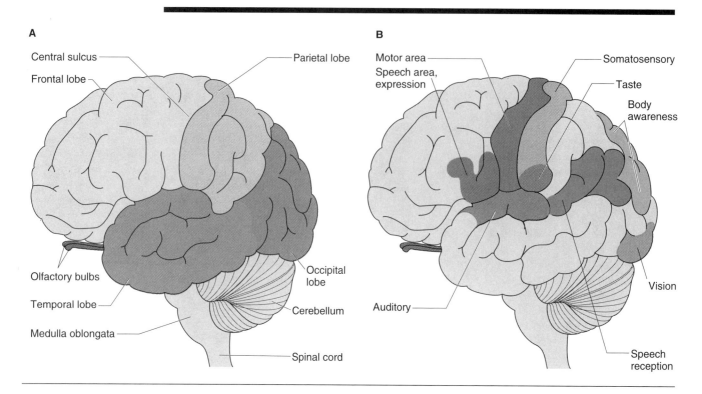

Figure 10.2. A. Lobes of the brain. **B.** Localized functions of the cerebrum.

Term	Meaning
parietal lobe pă-rī′ĕ-tăl lōb	portion posterior to the frontal lobe, responsible for sensations such as pain, temperature, touch
temporal lobe tem′pŏ-răl lōb	portion that lies below the frontal lobe, responsible for hearing, taste, and smell
occipital lobe ok-sip′i-tăl lōb	portion posterior to the parietal and temporal lobes, responsible for vision
cerebral cortex ser′ĕ-brăl kōr′teks	outer layer of the cerebrum consisting of gray matter, responsible for higher mental functions (cortex = bark)
thalamus (diencephalon) thal′ă-mŭs dī-en-sef′ă-lon	two gray matter nuclei deep within the brain responsible for relaying sensory information to the cortex
gyri jī′rī	ring or circle; convolutions (mounds) of the cerebral hemispheres
sulci sŭl′sī	ditch; shallow grooves that separate gyri
fissures fish′ŭrz	splitting crack; deep grooves in the brain
cerebellum ser-ĕ-bel′ŭm	portion of the brain located below the occipital lobes of the cerebrum, responsible for control and coordination of skeletal muscles (Fig. 10.3)

continued

Term	Meaning
brainstem brān'stem	region of the brain that serves as a relay between the cerebrum, cerebellum, and spinal cord, responsible for breathing, heart rate, and body temperature; there are three levels: mesencephalon (midbrain); pons; medulla oblongata

continued

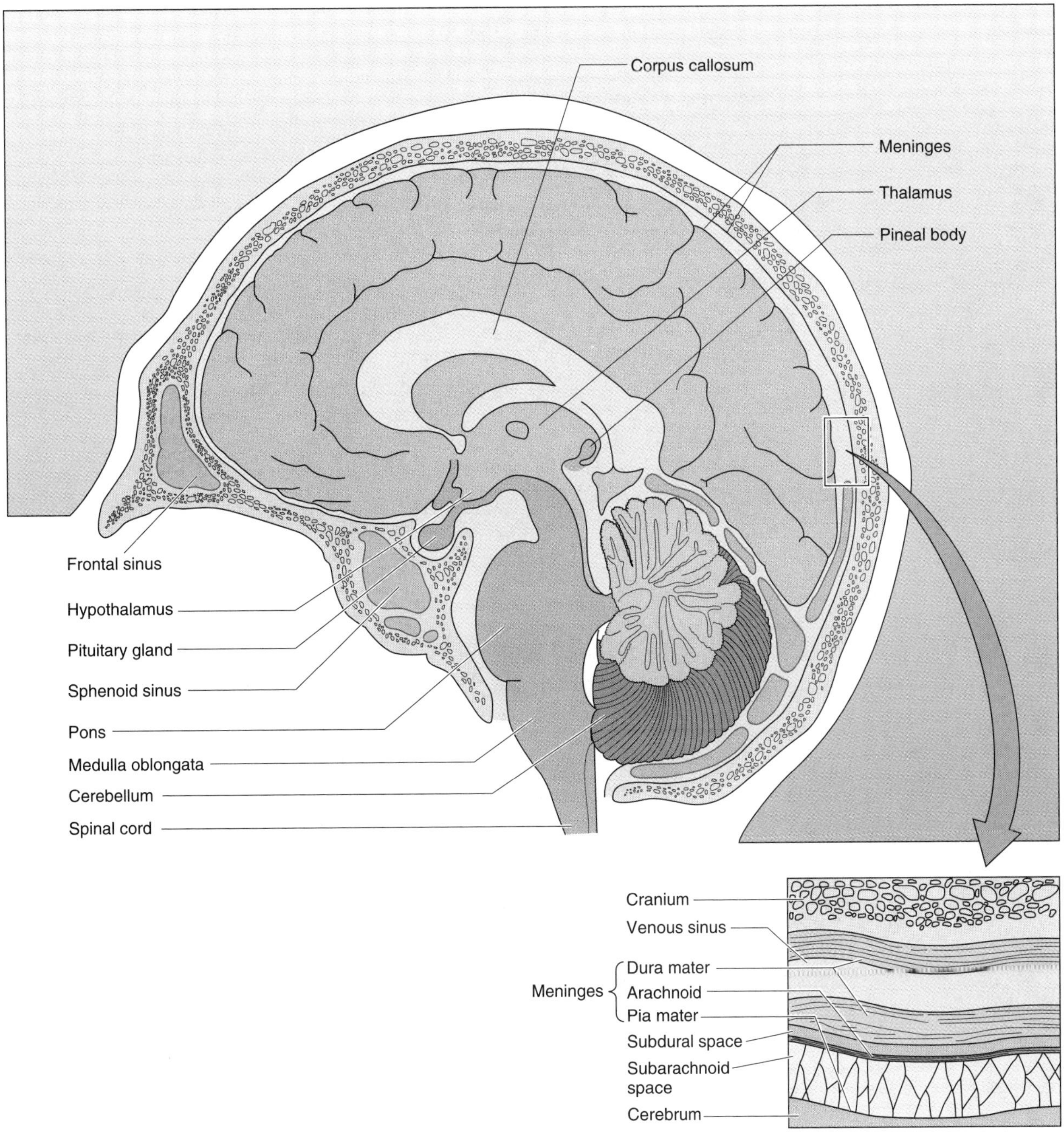

Figure 10.3. Midsagittal view of the brain.

Term	Meaning
ventricles ven′tri-klz	series of interconnected cavities within the cerebral hemispheres and brainstem filled with cerebrospinal fluid (see Color Atlas, plate 20)
cerebrospinal fluid (CSF) ser′ĕ-brō-spī-năl flū′id	plasma-like clear fluid circulating in and around the brain and spinal cord
spinal cord spī-năl kōrd	column of nervous tissue from the brainstem through the vertebrae, responsible for nerve conduction to and from the brain and the body
meninges mĕ-nin′jēz	three membranes that cover the brain and spinal cord, consisting of the dura mater, pia mater, and arachnoid
peripheral nervous system (PNS)	nerves that branch from the central nervous system, including nerves of the brain (cranial nerves) and spinal cord (spinal nerves) (see Color Atlas, plate 21)
cranial nerves krā′nē-ăl nervz	12 pairs of nerves arising from the brain
spinal nerves	31 pairs of nerves arising from the spinal cord
sensory nerves sen′sŏ-rē nervz	nerves that conduct impulses from body parts and carry sensory information to the brain—also called afferent nerves (ad = toward; ferre = carry)
motor nerves	nerves that conduct motor impulses from the brain to muscles and glands; also called efferent nerves (e = out; ferre = carry)
autonomic nervous system (ANS)	nerves that carry involuntary impulses to smooth muscle, cardiac muscle, and various glands
hypothalamus hī′pō-thal′ă-mŭs	control center for the autonomic nervous system located below the thalamus (diencephalon)
sympathetic nervous system sim-pă-thet′ik	division of the ANS concerned primarily with preparing the body in stressful or emergency situations
parasympathetic nervous system par-ă-sim-pă-thet′ik	division of the ANS that is most active in ordinary conditions; it counterbalances the effects of the sympathetic system by restoring the body to a restful state after a stressful experience

Symptomatic and Diagnostic Terms

Term	Meaning
Symptomatic	
aphasia ă-fā′zē-ă	inability to speak

continued

Term	Meaning
dysphasia dis-fā′zē-ă	difficulty speaking
coma kō′mă	a deep sleep; a general term referring to levels of decreased consciousness with varying responsiveness; a common method of assessment is the Glasgow coma scale
delirium dē-lir′ē-ŭm	a state of mental confusion due to disturbances in cerebral function—many causes including fever, shock, or drug overdose (deliro = to draw the furrow awry in ploughing, i.e., to go off the rails)
dementia dē-men′shē-ă	an impairment of intellectual function characterized by memory loss, disorientation, and confusion (dementio = to be mad)
motor deficit mō′ter def′i-sit	loss or impairment of muscle function
sensory deficit sen′sŏ-rē def′i-sit	loss or impairment of sensation
neuralgia nū-ral′jē-ă	pain along the course of a nerve
paralysis	to disable; temporary or permanent loss of motor control
flaccid paralysis flas′sid pă-ral′i-sis	defective (flabby) or absent muscle control caused by a nerve lesion
spastic paralysis spas′tik pă-ral′i-sis	stiff and awkward muscle control caused by a central nervous system disorder
hemiparesis hem-ē-pa-rē′sis	partial paralysis of the right or left half of the body
sciatica sī-at′i-kă	pain that follows the pathway of the sciatic nerve caused by compression or trauma of the nerve or its roots
seizure sē′zher	sudden, transient disturbances in brain function resulting from abnormal firing of nerve impulses (that may or may not be associated with convulsion)
convulsion kon-vŭl′shŭn	to pull together; type of seizure that causes a series of sudden, involuntary contractions of muscles
syncope sin′kŏ-pē	fainting
tactile stimulation tak′til	evoking a response by touching
hyperesthesia hī′per-es-thē′zē-ă	increased sensitivity to stimulation such as touch or pain
paresthesia par-es-thē′zē-ă	abnormal sensation of numbness and tingling without objective cause

COMA. Coma is derived from a Greek word meaning a deep sleep, a state of unconsciousness from which one cannot be roused. In Greek mythology Comus was the guardian of banquets who indulged in nightly orgies that resulted in a state of profound insensibility caused by a drunken stupor. The ingestion of a toxin such as alcohol intoxication is only one of many causes of coma. The words comic and comical share the same origin with coma.

Term	Meaning
Diagnostic	
agnosia ag-nō′sē-ă	any of many types of loss of neurological function associated with interpretation of sensory information
astereognosis ă-stēr′ē-og-nō′sis	inability to judge the form of an object by touch (e.g., a coin from a key)
atopognosis ă-top-og-nō′sis	inability to locate a sensation properly, such as to locate a point touched on the body
Alzheimer's disease	disease of structural changes in the brain resulting in an irreversible deterioration that progresses from forgetfulness and disorientation to loss of all intellectual functions; total disability, and death
cerebral palsy (CP) ser′ĕ-brăl pawl′zē	condition of motor disfunction caused by damage to the cerebrum during development or injury at birth characterized by partial paralysis and lack of muscle coordination (palsy = paralysis)
cerebrovascular disease	disorder resulting from a change within one or more blood vessels of the brain
cerebral arteriosclerosis ar-tēr′ē-ō-skler-ō′sis	hardening of the arteries of the brain
cerebral atherosclerosis ath′er-ō-skler-ō′sis	condition of lipid buildup within the blood vessels of the brain
cerebral aneurysm an′yū-rizm	dilation of a blood vessel in the brain
cerebral thrombosis throm-bō′sis	presence of a stationary clot in a blood vessel of the brain
cerebral embolism em′bō-lizm	presence of a floating clot in a blood vessel of the brain
cerebrovascular accident (CVA) **stroke**	damage to the brain caused by cerebrovascular disease such as occlusion of a blood vessel by an embolus or thrombus or intracranial hemorrhage after rupture of an aneurysm (Fig 10.4)
transient ischemic attack (TIA) tran′zē-ĕnt is-kē′mik	brief episode of loss of blood flow to the brain usually caused by a partial occlusion that results in temporary neurologic deficit (impairment)—often precedes a CVA (Fig. 10.5)
carotid TIA ka-rot′id	ischemia of the anterior circulation of the brain

continued

Cerebral thrombosis

Cerebral embolism

Intracranial hemorrhage

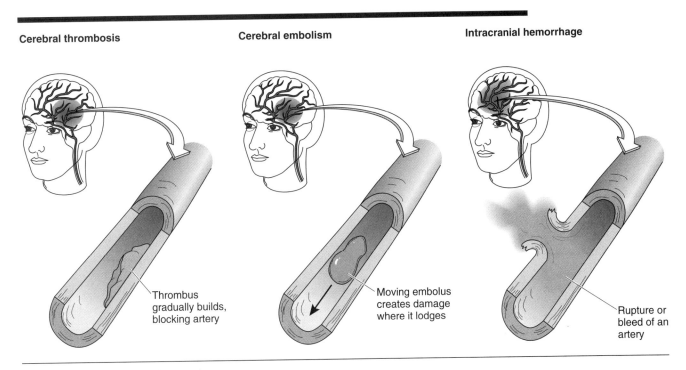

Thrombus gradually builds, blocking artery

Moving embolus creates damage where it lodges

Rupture or bleed of an artery

Figure 10.4. Cerebrovascular accident.

Frontal view

Circle of Willis
view from underneath the brain

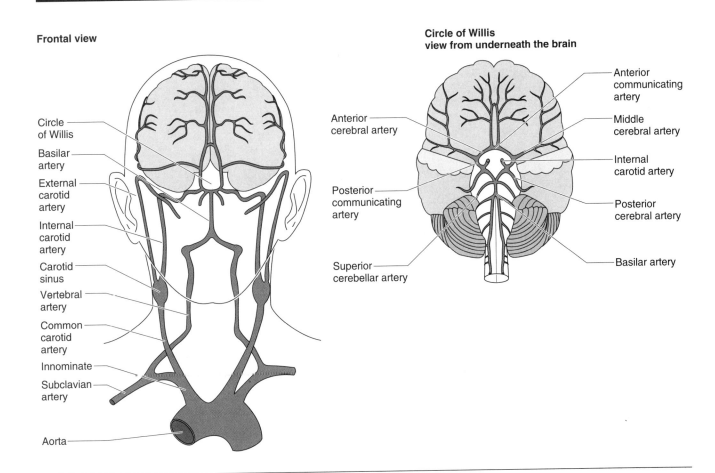

Circle of Willis

Basilar artery

External carotid artery

Internal carotid artery

Carotid sinus

Vertebral artery

Common carotid artery

Innominate

Subclavian artery

Aorta

Anterior cerebral artery

Posterior communicating artery

Superior cerebellar artery

Anterior communicating artery

Middle cerebral artery

Internal carotid artery

Posterior cerebral artery

Basilar artery

Figure 10.5. Sites of transient ischemic attack: carotid and vertebrobasilar circulation.

EPILEPSY. Epilepsy comes from a Greek word for seizure. The word was used by Aristotle for a convulsive seizure, a condition that came to be called epilepsy. It was regarded in ancient times as an infliction from the gods, hence the Roman term, morbus sacer (sacred disease). Many other terms were applied to epilepsy such as "disease of Hercules" because sufferers seemed to have superhuman strength.

Term	Meaning
vertebrobasilar TIA ver'tĕ-brō-bas'i-lăr	ischemia of the posterior circulation of the brain
encephalitis en-sef-ă-lī'tis	inflammation of the brain
epilepsy ep'i-lep'sē	disorder affecting the central nervous system characterized by recurrent seizures (Fig. 10.6)
tonic-clonic ton'ik-klon'ik	stiffening-jerking; a major motor seizure involving all muscle groups—previously termed grand mal (big bad)
absence ab'sens	seizure involving a brief loss of consciousness without motor involvement—previously termed petit mal (little bad)
partial	seizure involving only limited areas of the brain with localized symptoms
glioma glī-ō'mă	tumor of glial cells graded by degree of malignancy
herpes zoster her'pēz zos'ter	viral disease affecting the peripheral nerves characterized by painful blisters that spread over the skin following the affected nerves, usually unilateral—also known as shingles (Fig. 10.7)

continued

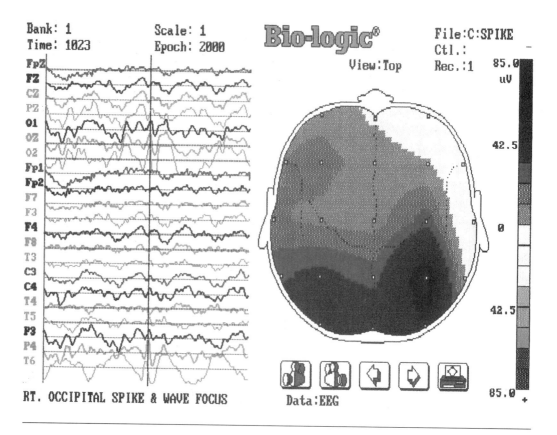

Figure 10.6. Right occipital spike and wave focus. An electroencephalogram wave form diagnostic of epilepsy.

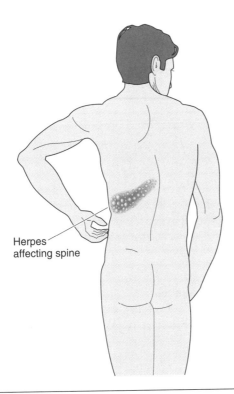

Figure 10.7. Herpes zoster: typical eruption site.

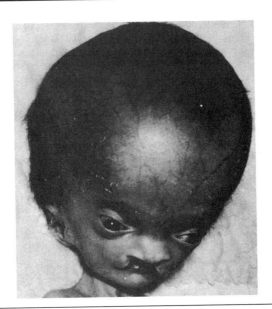

Figure 10.8. Hydrocephalus.

Term	Meaning
Huntington's disease (HD) **Huntington's chorea** kor-e'ă	hereditary disease of the central nervous system characterized by bizarre involuntary body movements and progressive dementia (choros = dance)
hydrocephalus hı-dro-sef'ă-lŭs	abnormal accumulation of cerebrospinal fluid in the ventricles of the brain as a result of developmental anomalies, infection, injury, or tumor (Fig. 10.8)

continued

Term	Meaning
meningioma mĕ-nin′jē-ō′mă	benign tumor of the coverings of the brain (meninges)
meningitis men-in-jī′tis	inflammation of the meninges
migraine headache mī′grān	paroxysmal attacks of mostly unilateral headache often accompanied by disordered vision, nausea, and/or vomiting, lasting hours or days and caused by dilation of arteries
multiple sclerosis (MS) sklĕ-rō′sis	disease of the central nervous system characterized by the demyelination (deterioration of the myelin sheath) of nerve fibers, with episodes of neurologic dysfunction (exacerbation) followed by recovery (remission) (Fig. 10.9)
myasthenia gravis mī-as-thē′nē-ă gra′văs	autoimmune disorder that affects the neuromuscular junction causing a progressive decrease in muscle strength with activity and a return of strength after a period of rest
myelitis mī-ĕ-lī′tis	inflammation of the spinal cord
narcolepsy nar′kō-lep-sē	sleep disorder characterized by sudden, uncontrollable need to sleep, attacks of paralysis (cataplexy), and dreams intruding while awake (hypnagogic hallucinations)

continued

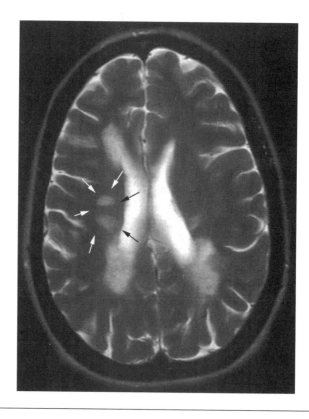

Figure 10.9. Magnetic resonance image of the brain. *Arrows,* plaque formation in patient with multiple sclerosis.

Term	Meaning
Parkinson's disease	slowly progressive degeneration of nerves in the brain characterized by tremor, rigidity of muscles, and slow movements (bradykinesia), usually occurring later in life (Fig. 10.10)
plegia plē′jē-ă	paralysis
hemiplegia hem-ē-plē′jē-ă	paralysis on one side of the body
paraplegia par-ă-plē′jē-ă	paralysis from the waist down
quadriplegia kwah′dri-plē′jē-ă	paralysis of all four limbs
poliomyelitis po′lē-ō-mı′ĕ-lī′tis	inflammation of the gray matter of the spinal cord caused by a virus, often resulting in spinal and muscle deformity and paralysis (polio = gray)
polyneuritis pol′ē-nū-rī-tis	inflammation involving two or more nerves, often owing to a nutritional deficiency such as lack of thiamine
sleep apnea ap′nē-ă	periods of breathing cessation that occur during sleep, often causing snoring
spina bifida spī′nă bi′fă-dă	congenital defect in the spinal column characterized by the absence of vertebral arches, often resulting in pouching of spinal membranes or tissue (Fig. 10.11)

continued

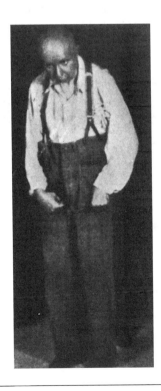

Figure 10.10. Patient with Parkinson's disease.

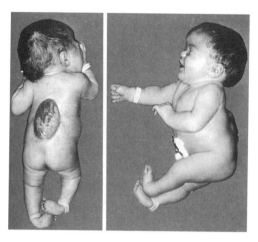

Figure 10.11. Spina bifida with myelocele.

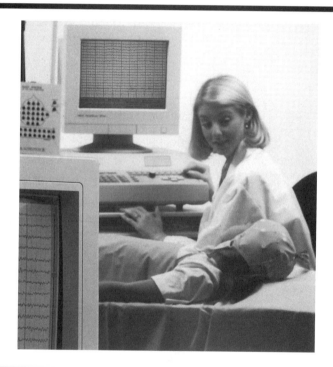

Figure 10.12. Electroencephalography procedure.

Diagnostic Tests and Procedures

Test or Procedure	Explanation
electrodiagnostic procedures ē-lek′trō-dī-ag-nō′sis	
electroencephalogram (EEG) ē-lek′trō-en-sef ′ă-lō-gram	record of the minute electrical impulses of the brain used to identify neurologic conditions that affect brain function and level of consciousness (Fig. 10.12) (see Color Atlas, plate 22)

continued

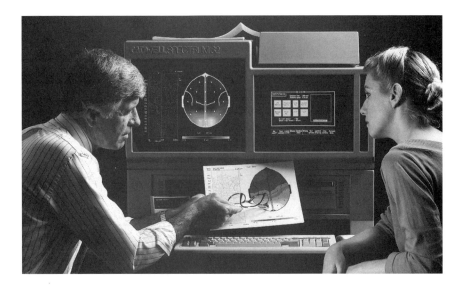

Figure 10.13. Evaluation of evoked potentials.

SOMNUS. "Somnus" is a Latin word for sleep that was derived from ancient mythology. Somnus was the poetical god of sleep, the son of Nox (night), who lived with his brother Thanatos (death) in a palace at the western end of the world.

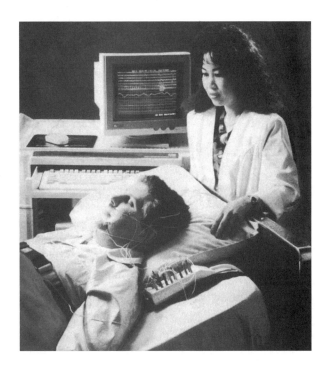

Figure 10.14. Polysomnography.

Test or Procedure	Explanation
evoked potentials ē vokt′ pō-ten′shăls	minute electrical waves that are sorted out of ongoing EEG activity to diagnose auditory, visual, and sensory pathway disorders (Fig. 10.13)
nerve conduction velocity (NCV) nerv kon-dŭk′shŭn	electrical shock of peripheral nerves to record time of conduction; used to diagnose various peripheral nervous system diseases
polysomnography (PSG) pol′ē-som-nog′ră-fē	various aspects of sleep (eye and muscle movements, respiration, EEG patterns) are recorded for diagnosis of sleep disorders (Fig. 10.14)

continued

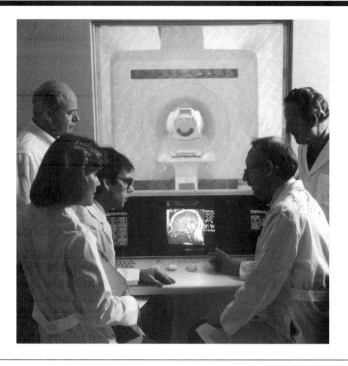

Figure 10.15. Magnetic resonance imaging unit.

Test or Procedure	Explanation
lumbar puncture (LP) lŭm'bar pŭnk'chur	spinal tap; introduction of a specialized needle into the spine in the lumbar region for diagnostic or therapeutic purpose, e.g., to obtain cerebrospinal fluid for testing
magnetic resonance imaging (MRI) magnet'ic rez'o-nans im'ă-jing	nonionizing imaging technique using magnetic fields and radio frequency waves to visualize anatomical structures (especially soft tissue) such as the tissues of the brain and spinal cord (Fig. 10.15) (see Color Atlas, plates 19 and 20)
magnetic resonance angiography (MRA) magnet'ic rez'o-nans an-je-og'ră-fe	use of magnetic resonance in imaging of the blood vessels—useful in detecting pathological conditions such as thrombosis, atherosclerosis, etc.
intracranial MRA in'tră-kra'ne-ăl	magnetic resonance image of the head to visualize the vessels of the circle of Willis (common site of cerebral aneurysm, stenosis or occlusion) (Fig. 10.16A)
extracranial MRA eks-tră-kra'ne-ăl	magnetic resonance image of the neck to visualize the carotid artery (Fig. 10.16B)
nuclear medicine imaging	radionuclide organ imaging
SPECT brain scan (single photon emission computed tomography)	scan combining nuclear medicine and computed tomography to produce images of the brain after administration of radioactive isotopes

continued

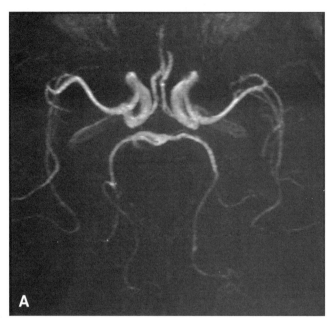
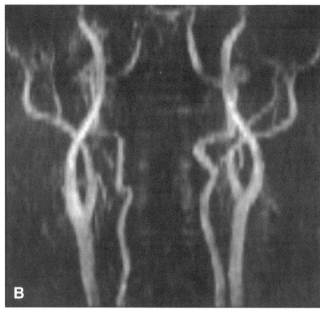

Figure 10.16. A. Normal intracranial magnetic resonance angiography showing circulation of the circle of Willis. **B.** Normal extracranial magnetic resonance angiography showing carotid circulation.

Test or Procedure	Explanation
positron emission tomography (PET) poz'i-tron ē-mish'ŭn tō-mog'ră-fē	technique combining nuclear medicine and computed tomography to produce images of brain anatomy and corresponding physiology—used to study stroke, Alzheimer's disease, epilepsy, metabolic brain disorders, chemistry of nerve transmissions in the brain, etc.; it provides greater accuracy than SPECT but is used less often because of cost and limited availability of the radioisotopes (Fig. 10.17) (see Color Atlas, plate 22)
radiography rā'dē-og'ră-fē	x-ray imaging
cerebral angiogram ser'ĕ-brăl an'jē-ō-gram	x-ray of blood vessels in the brain after intracarotid injection of contrast medium
computed tomography (of the head)	computed tomographic x-ray images of the head used to visualize abnormalities within; i.e., brain tumors, malformations, etc.
myelogram	x-ray of the spinal cord made after intraspinal injection of contrast medium
reflex testing	test performed to observe the body's response to a stimulus
deep tendon reflexes (DTR)	involuntary muscle contraction after percussion at a tendon (e.g., patella, Achilles, etc.) indicating function; positive findings are noted when there is either no reflex response or an exaggerated response to stimulus; numbers are often used to record responses:

continued

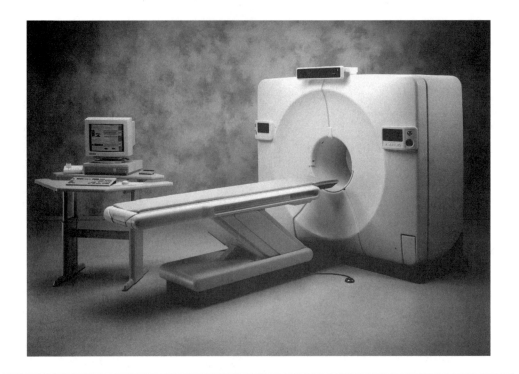

Figure 10.17. Positron emission tomography scanner.

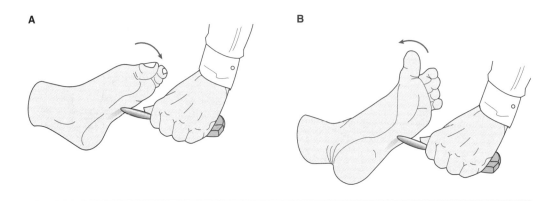

Figure 10.18. Reflex testing. **A.** Normal plantar reflex. **B.** Babinski's sign.

Test or Procedure	Explanation
	no response 1+ diminished response 2+ normal response 3+ more brisk than average response 4+ hyperactive response
Babinski's sign or reflex	pathological response to stimulation of the plantar surface of the foot; a positive sign is indicated when the toes dorsiflex (curl upward) (Fig. 10.18)
transcranial sonogram trans-krā′nē-ăl	image made by sending ultrasound beams through the skull to assess blood flow in intracranial vessels—used in diagnosis and management of stroke and head trauma (Fig. 10.19)

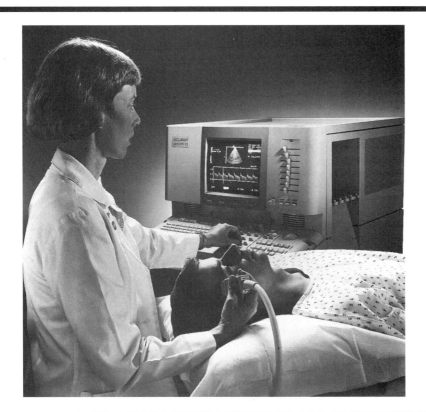

Figure 10.19. Transcranial sonography procedure.

Operative Terms

Term	Meaning
craniectomy kra′ne-ek′to-me	excision of part of the skull to approach the brain
craniotomy kra-ne-ot′o-me	incision into the skull to approach the brain
discectomy (diskectomy) dis-ek′to-me	removal of a herniated disc often done percutaneously (Fig. 10.20)
laminectomy lam′i-nek′to-me	excision of one or more laminae of the vertebrae to approach the spinal cord
vertebral lamina	flattened posterior portion of the vertebral arch (see Color Atlas, plate 8)
microsurgery mi-kro-ser′jer-e	utilization of a microscope to dissect minute structures during surgery (Fig. 10.21)
neuroplasty nur′o-plas-te	surgical repair of a nerve
spondylosyndesis spon′di-lo-sin-de′sis	spinal fusion (Fig. 10.22)

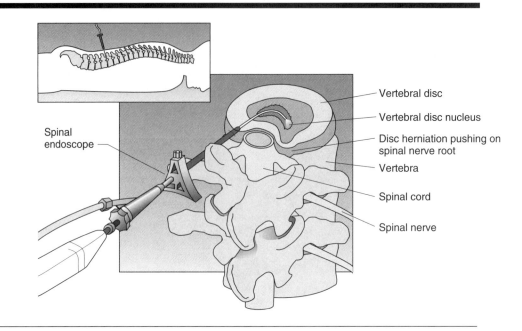

Spinal endoscope

Vertebral disc

Vertebral disc nucleus

Disc herniation pushing on spinal nerve root

Vertebra

Spinal cord

Spinal nerve

Figure 10.20. Discectomy.

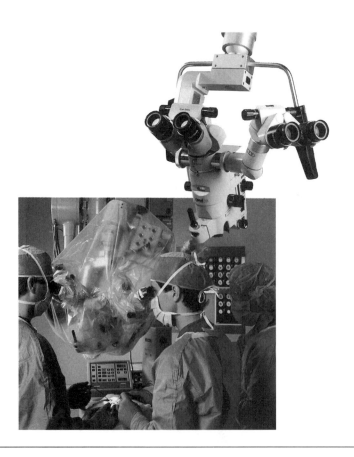

Figure 10.21. Microscope designed for neurological surgery.

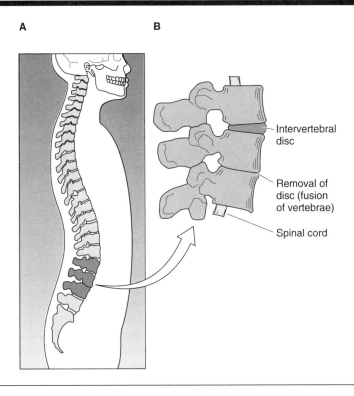

Figure 10.22. Spondylosyndesis. **A.** Spinal column. **B.** Spinal fusion.

Therapeutic Terms

Term	Meaning
chemotherapy kem′ō-thār-ă-pē	treatment of malignancies, infections, and other diseases with chemical agents that destroy selected cells or impair their ability to reproduce
radiation therapy rā′dē-ā′shŭn thār′ă-pē	treatment of neoplastic disease using ionizing radiation to impede proliferation of malignant cells (Fig. 10.23)
stereotactic (stereotaxic) radiosurgery ster′ē-ō-tak′tik (ster′ē-ō-tak′sik) rā′dē-ō-ser′jer-ē	radiation treatment to inactivate malignant lesions involving the focus of multiple, precise external radiation beams on a target with the aid of a stereotactic frame and imaging such as CT, MRI, or angiography; used to treat inoperable brain tumors, etc.
stereotactic (stereotaxic) frame	mechanical device used to localize a point in space targeting a precise site (Fig. 10.24)

Common Therapeutic Drug Classifications

analgesic an-ăl-jē′zik	agent that relieves pain
anticonvulsant an′tē-kon-vŭl′sant	agent that prevents or lessens convulsion
antidepressant an′tē-dē-pres′ănt	agent that counteracts depression

continued

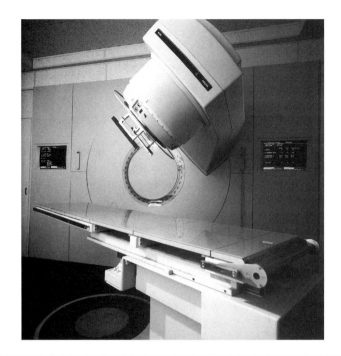

Figure 10.23. Radiation therapy: linear accelerator.

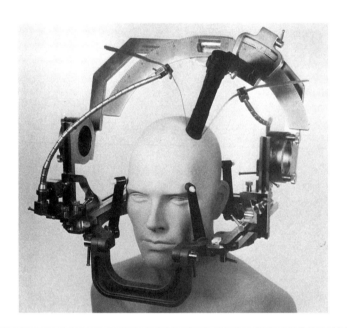

Figure 10.24. Stereotactic frame.

Term	Meaning
sedative sed′ă-tiv	agent that quiets nervousness
hypnotic hip-not′ik	agent that induces sleep

PRACTICE EXERCISES

For the following terms, draw a line or line to separate prefixes, combining forms, and suffixes. Then define the term.

1. ganglioma _____

2. neurogenic _____

3. encephalocele _____

4. dystaxia _____

5. ventriculitis _____

6. myelorrhaphy _____

7. esthesioneurosis _____

8. cerebral angiogram _____

9. spondylosyndesis _____

10. hemiplegia _____

11. craniotomy _____

12. topoanesthesia _____

13. neuroglial _____

14. neurocytolysis _____

15. somnipathy _____

16. myelopathy _____

17. hydrocephalic _____

18. polyneuritis _____

19. neuralgia _____

20. encephalitis _____

21. parasomnia _____

22. narcolepsy _____

23. stereotaxy _____

24. hemiparesis _____

25. neurasthenia _____

26. glioma _____

27. intracranial _____

28. aphasic _____

29. agnosia _____

30. cerebrospinal _____

Write the correct medical term for each of the following:

31. an x-ray of the spinal cord made after injection of a contrast medium

    _____

32. inflammation of the meninges _____

33. excision of a herniated disc _____

34. inability to locate a sensation properly, such as to locate a point touched on the body

    _____

35. a slowly progressive, degeneration of nerves in the brain characterized by tremor, rigidity of muscles, and slow movements

    _____

36. a pathological response to stimulation of the plantar surface of the foot indicated by dorsiflexion of the toes

    _____

37. numbness and tingling _____

38. state of unconsciousness _____

39. a type of seizure that causes a series of sudden, involuntary contractions of muscles

    _____

40. congenital defect of the spinal column resulting in pouching of spinal membranes

_____

41. a type of agnosia indicating an inability to judge the form of an object by touch, e.g., a coin from a key

_____

Complete the medical term by writing the missing part:

42. electro_____gram = record of electrical brain impulses

43. _____syndesis = spinal fusion

44. crani_____ = excision of part of the skull

45. cerebral_____sclerosis = fat build-up in blood vessel of brain

46. hyper_____ = increased sensations

47. dys_____ = difficulty speaking

48. _____algesia = loss of sense of pain

Match the following terms with the appropriate terms in the right column:

49. herpes zoster _____   a. tonic-clonic

50. spinal tap _____   b. CVA

51. faint _____   c. Alzheimer's disease

52. grand mal _____   d. PSG

53. petit mal _____   e. flaccid

54. cerebral thrombus _____   f. absence

55. flabby _____   g. clot

56. stroke _____   h. LP

57. dementia _____   i. shingles

58. sleep study _____   j. syncope

Write the full medical term for the following abbreviations:

59. CT _____

60. MRI _____

61. NCV _____

62. PET _____

63. MS _____

64. CNS _____

65. CP _____

66. TIA _____

67. EEG _____

68. DTR _____

69. SPECT _____

70. PSG _____

71. ANS _____

72. PNS _____

73. CSF _____

74. MRA _____

75. CVA _____

Medical Record Analyses

MEDICAL RECORD 10.1

Mary Clarke came into the living room where her father, Bob Clarke, had been watching television and found him slumped back in his chair, apparently asleep. When she could not wake him she realized he was unconscious and called 911. The ambulance rushed him to the Central Medical Center emergency room, where he was seen by Dr. Gregory Kincaid.

Directions

Read Medical Record 10.1 for Mr. Clarke (pages 291–293) and answer the following questions. This record is the history and physical examination report dictated by Dr. Kincaid after his examination and initial treatment of Mr. Clarke.

Questions about Medical Record 10.1

Write your answers in the spaces provided.

1. Below are medical terms used in this record you have not encountered in this text so far. Underline each where it appears in the record and define below.

   abrasion _____

   foci of atrophy _____

   ambulate _____

   cataract _____

2. In your own words, not using medical terminology, briefly describe Mr. Clarke's condition from the time he was found at home.

   _____

   Describe his condition after arriving at the ER.

   _____

3. Which of the following was *not* an emergency treatment provided for Mr. Clarke?

   a. administration of Valium

   b. assessment of respiratory rate

   c. CPR

   d. assistance with breathing

4. Define "postictal": _____

5. Mr. Clarke has a past medical history of several different illnesses. On the following list, check all health problems Mr. Clarke has experienced:

_____ skin bruising

_____ heart attacks

_____ excessive thyroid secretion

_____ COPD

_____ skin scrapes

_____ headaches

_____ nausea and vomiting

_____ atrial fibrillation

_____ pulmonary embolus

6. In your own words, describe the surgery Mr. Clarke had in the past:

_____

_____

_____

7. In lay language, what nervous system disorder did a family member experience?

_____

_____

_____

8. Dr. Kincaid's diagnosis identifies three possible conditions that may have led to Mr. Clarke's seizure. Put each in your own words:

a. _____

b. _____

c. _____

9. What three actions will now occur in the ICU?

a. _____

b. _____

c. _____

CENTRAL MEDICAL CENTER

211 Medical Center Drive • Central City, US 90000-1234 • PHONE: (012) 125-6784 • FAX: (012) 125-9999

HISTORY

DATE OF ADMISSION: August 1, 199x

REASON FOR ADMISSION: Seizure episode.

HISTORY OF PRESENT ILLNESS: The patient is a 76-year-old male brought to the emergency room following a seizure episode at home where he was found to be in mild tonic condition and was given intravenous Valium at which time his respiratory rate dropped, and he required some ventilatory assistance. He remained unresponsive postictal until an hour after emergency room arrival. He has a past history of a similar seizure in 1989 which was treated with Dilantin for a year and was then discontinued. No focal abnormality was noted at that time with the exception of an abnormality on CT showing small foci of atrophy possibly secondary to vascular disease. He has been evaluated by Dr. Levy, a neurologist. Please refer to Dr. Levy's consultation report.

PAST MEDICAL HISTORY: The patient has a past medical history of severe chronic obstructive airways disease; he is on multiple medications. He takes Slo-Bid 300 mg b.i.d., Medrol 5 mg q.o.d., and p.r.n. inhalation of Ventolin up to q.i.d. He has a long history of being steroid dependent and is daily symptomatic. He has a history of coronary artery disease with myocardial infarctions, questionable congestive heart failure, and chronic atrial fibrillation. He is being seen by Dr. Foley, a cardiologist. He is on Lanoxin 0.25 mg, Verelan 120 mg, Lasix 40 mg, and Micro-K 750 mg on a daily basis. He also has a history of hypothyroidism and takes Synthroid 0.1 mg. He has a history of steroid-dependent skin fragility with multiple ecchymoses; a recent fall resulted in a number of abrasions which were under treatment by Dr. Depmore, a family practitioner, with good healing.

PAST SURGICAL HISTORY: Septoplasty.

MEDICATIONS: As mentioned above.

ALLERGIES: The patient does not report any allergies to medications.

REVIEW OF SYSTEMS: The patient is not reported to have problems with headaches or dizzy spells. He does have exertional shortness of breath that he maintains control of with medications, and he is able to ambulate at least a mile a day. No abdominal or gastrointestinal symptoms are noted. There is no arthralgia.

(continued)

HISTORY AND PHYSICAL Page 1	PT. NAME:	CLARKE, ROBERT B.
	ID NO:	088676
	ROOM NO:	ICU
	ATT. PHYS.	G. KINCAID, M.D.

CENTRAL MEDICAL CENTER

211 Medical Center Drive • Central City, US 90000-1234 • PHONE: (012) 125-6784 • FAX: (012) 125-9999

HISTORY

FAMILY HISTORY: The patient's parents lived into their late 80s and died of old age. His brother died at age 70 of a cerebral vascular accident (CVA). There is no family history of diabetes, cardiac, pulmonary, renal, hepatic, or hematologic disorder; but his father did have cancer of the prostate.

PHYSICAL EXAMINATION

VITAL SIGNS: Blood Pressure: 173/78. Pulse: 90-100. Respirations: 12.

GENERAL APPEARANCE: The patient is able to respond to some degree to voice but poorly follows directions, this being due to the fact that he is still somewhat under the influence of Valium.

SKIN: Multiple ecchymoses of extremities. Only his back, abdomen, and head are free of signs of injury. The skin is dry. There are active abrasions from his seizure episode on the right ankle and both forearms.

HEENT: Tympanic membranes, nose, and throat appear to be normal. His teeth are in good condition. Both eyes are reactive to light. The right fundus is normal; however, the left fundus is not visualized secondary to cataract.

NECK: There is no cervical adenopathy or thyroid enlargement.

CHEST:
LUNGS: The patient's lungs are clear to percussion and auscultation. There are no rales, rhonchi, or wheezes.

HEART: Tones are regular without murmur.

ABDOMEN: The abdomen is flat, soft, and nontender without organ enlargement or masses. The bowel sounds are active.

RECTAL/GENITALIA: The rectal examination is normal. The patient has normal circumcised external genitalia.

(continued)

HISTORY AND PHYSICAL Page 2	PT. NAME: CLARKE, ROBERT B. ID NO: 088676 ROOM NO: ICU ATT. PHYS. G. KINCAID, M.D.

Medical Record 10.1. *Continued.*

CENTRAL MEDICAL CENTER

211 Medical Center Drive • Central City, US 90000-1234 • PHONE: (012) 125-6784 • FAX: (012) 125-9999

PHYSICAL EXAMINATION

EXTREMITIES: There are multiple ecchymoses. There are no deep tendon reflexes. Babinski's signs are negative. The patient is able to move all four extremities without any evidence of motor deficit. He is unable to report sensory activity.

IMPRESSION:
SEIZURE DISORDER, POSSIBLY SECONDARY TO CEREBRAL EMBOLI, HYPOXIA, OR UNKNOWN CAUSES, POSSIBLY DUE TO INTRACEREBRAL DISEASE.

PLAN: Recommend observation in Intensive Care Unit as workup proceeds and will ask for neurologic and pulmonary support from specialists R. Wilson, M.D., and E. Wong, M.D.

G. Kincaid, M.D.

G. Kincaid, M.D.

GK:wq

D: 8/2/9x
T: 8/5/9x

HISTORY AND PHYSICAL Page 3	PT. NAME: ID NO: ROOM NO: ATT. PHYS.	CLARKE, ROBERT B. 088676 ICU G.KINCAID, M.D.

Medical Record 10.1. *Continued.*

MEDICAL RECORD 10.2

Anne Cross has been fairly healthy until she had a stroke about two months ago. She was treated by Dr. Paul Jiang, her personal physician, at that time, and discharged from the hospital on medication. At the request of Ms. Cross, Dr. Jiang called for a consultation from a neurologist, Dr. Melvin Classen.

Directions

Read Medical Record 10.2 for Ms. Cross (pages 296–297) and answer the following questions. This record is a consultation report written by Dr. Classen as a letter back to Ms. Cross's physician, Dr. Jiang, after his consultation.

Questions about Medical Record 10.2

Write your answers in the spaces provided.

1. Below are medical terms used in this record you have not yet encountered. Underline each where it appears in the record and define below.

   homonymous hemianopsia _____

   finger-nose test _____

   apraxia _____

   clonus _____

2. In your own words, not using medical terminology, briefly describe Ms. Cross's symptoms in April before she was admitted to the hospital.

   _____

   _____

   _____

3. Write the missing parts in this table summarizing the diagnostic tests performed in April.

Test	Definition of Test	Findings
CT	_____	_____
_____	sound waves through heart	_____
carotid ultrasound	_____	_____

Test	Definition of Test	Findings
_____	_____	slowed electrical pulses on right side

4. What family member had a problem perhaps similar to Ms. Cross's?

_____

5. For each of the following medications given Ms. Cross, translate the dosage instructions:

Persantine _____

aspirin_____

Proventil_____

Procardia _____

6. Dr. Classen recommends two diagnostic studies. Describe both in your own words:

a. _____

b. _____

In one sentence, describe Dr. Classen's rationale for recommending the combination of these two tests:

_____

_____

7. Name the preventive surgical procedure Dr. Classen suggests that may be appropriate if changes are found in the carotid blood vessels.

_____

Describe that procedure in your own words:

_____

_____

CENTRAL MEDICAL GROUP, INC.

Department of Neurology

201 Medical Center Drive • Central City, US 90000-1234 • PHONE: (012) 125-8888 • FAX: (012) 125-3434

June 9, 199x

Paul Jiang, M.D.
1409 West Ninth Street
Central City, US 90000-1233

Dear Dr. Jiang:

RE: Anne Cross

I had the pleasure of meeting Mrs. Cross today. As you know, she is a 65-year-old right-handed female who began to have difficulties on or about April 17, 199x. She experienced dizziness that she described as occurring in the midday; there was also some associated slurring of speech. By the next morning, she seemed to have some disorientation with putting on her clothes, and she had some difficulties using the left side of her body. She had no headache or other problems. Prior to that time, she denied having any symptomatology. She was admitted to the hospital, as you are aware, and underwent a series of studies. A CT scan was reviewed and showed evidence of a right ischemic occipital infarct. In addition, she underwent an echocardiogram that was normal and an electroencephalogram that showed some right-sided slowing. A carotid ultrasound study suggested 60-70% stenosis of the bifurcation and/or internal carotids.

The patient was discharged on a combination of Persantine 50 mg t.i.d, enteric-coated aspirin 1 q d, Proventil 1 q 12 h p.r.n. for chronic obstructive pulmonary disease, and Procardia XL 1 q d for hypertension. The patient also has stopped smoking.

The patient reports that in the past, she has been essentially well except for some eye surgery. Additionally, after her discharge, she underwent visual field studies which confirmed the presence of an incomplete left-sided homonymous hemianopsia.

By way of family background, her brother died from complications of a stroke at age 78. Her mother died from liver cancer, and her father died from a myocardial infarction.

The patient has no specific allergy to drugs.

The patient's risk factors have been otherwise unremarkable.

On examination today, the patient is a slender female in no acute distress.

Blood pressure from the left arm in a sitting position is 130/95 and from the right arm in the sitting position is 145/95. Her pulse rate is 76 and regular.

No bruits are present over the carotid distributions. The temporal arteries are not enlarged or tender.

On examination of the eyes, the patient showed some mild arteriolar narrowing without hemorrhage or exudate. Gross visual confrontation suggests a neglect of left hemianopsia. The extraocular movements are full. The pupils are symmetrical. There is no ptosis. Facial movements are normal, and speech is normal.

Medical Record 10.2.

RE: Anne Cross
Page 2
June 9, 199x

There is no drift to the outstretched hands. Finger-to-nose test is performed symmetrically.

The patient does not have any asymmetrical topagnosis. She has no evidence of apraxia.

The patient's reflexes are physiologic: they are 2+ at the biceps, triceps, and brachioradialis. The knee and ankle jerks are 2+. No clonus is elicited.

Gait and stance are normal.

OVERALL ASSESSMENT:

Without prior warning, this woman had a new onset of a cerebral infarct. By her description, it is likely that she had a posterior circulatory infarct in the area of the occipital lobe. There may have been an association zone in the parietal area as well. Since that time, she has had some residual hemianopsia as described.

PLAN:

At this time, it is suggested that the most prudent approach would be to do an MRA and an MRI. This should include the great vessels of the neck and the vertebrobasilar system. The MRI would allow us to see the nature of residuals of the stroke, the distribution of the stroke, and would allow us to determine if there are any asymptomatic lesions, including microvascular infarcts which would not be seen on the CAT scan. The MRA would allow us to determine the overall anatomy of the vasculature--including the neck, the bifurcations, and the posterior circulation--in a noninvasive way. Depending on the results of both of these studies, we would have to consider if she needs a full angiogram done with selective views. If, in fact, she has had an infarct of the posterior occipital lobe, then the current treatment with aspirin and Persantine would be adequate. If, by the nature of the MRA, it is determined that there are significant changes or irregularity of the contour of the intima of the vessels at the bifurcations, then there may be an indication for prophylaxis for an endarterectomy despite not having a stroke in that distribution of the vessels. This, of course, would all be determined by the results of this study. The advantage of the MRA-MRI combined would allow us to visualize adequately the vessels combined with the detailed evaluation of her brain.

I think this would be the patient's best and most prudent approach to the patient's health and would help to prevent recurrence of this problem.

Please do not hesitate to call me if there are any questions regarding this patient's evaluation.

Sincerely,

Melvin Classen, M.D.
Department of Neurology
(012) 125-6899

MC:mar
DOT:6/10/9x

cc: Mrs. Anne Cross

Medical Record 10.2. *Continued.*

Endocrine System

OBJECTIVES

After completion of this chapter you will be able to

1. Define common combining forms used in relation to the endocrine system

2. Define the basic anatomical terms referring to the endocrine system

3. Define common symptomatic, diagnostic, operative, and therapeutic terms referring to the endocrine system

4. List the common diagnostic tests and procedures related to the endocrine system

5. Explain the terms and abbreviations used in documenting medical records involving the endocrine system

Combining Forms

Combining Form	Meaning	Example
aden/o	gland	adenoma ad-ĕ-nō'mă
adren/o	adrenal gland	adrenotrophic ă-drē-nō-trō'fik
andr/o	male	androgenous an-droj'ĕ-nŭs
crin/o	to secrete	endocrine en'dō-krin
dips/o	thirst	polydipsia pol-ē-dip'sē-ă
gluc/o	sugar	glucogenic glū-kō-jen'ik
glyc/o		hyperglycemia hī'per-glī-sē'mē-ă
glycos/o		glycosuria glī-kō-sū'rē-ă
hormon/o	hormone (an urging on)	hormonal hōr-mōn'ăl
ket/o	ketone bodies	ketogenic kē-tō-jen'ik
keton/o		ketonuria kē-tō-nū'rē-ă
pancreat/o	pancreas	pancreatitis pan'krē-ă-tī'tis
thym/o	thymus gland	thymoma thī-mō'mă
thyr/o	thyroid gland (shield)	thyroiditis thī-roy-dī'tis

Endocrine System Overview

The endocrine system is a network of ductless glands and other structures that affect the function of targeted organs by the secreting *hormones*. Figure 11.1 shows the locations of the endocrine glands. The hormones secreted by these glands and their functions are described under "Anatomical Terms" (also see Color Atlas, plates 23–24)

Anatomical Terms

Gland or Hormone	Location or Function
adrenal glands ă-drē'năl **suprarenal glands** sū'pră-rē'năl	located next to each kidney, the adrenal cortex secretes steroid hormones and the adrenal medulla secretes epinephrine and norepinephrine

continued

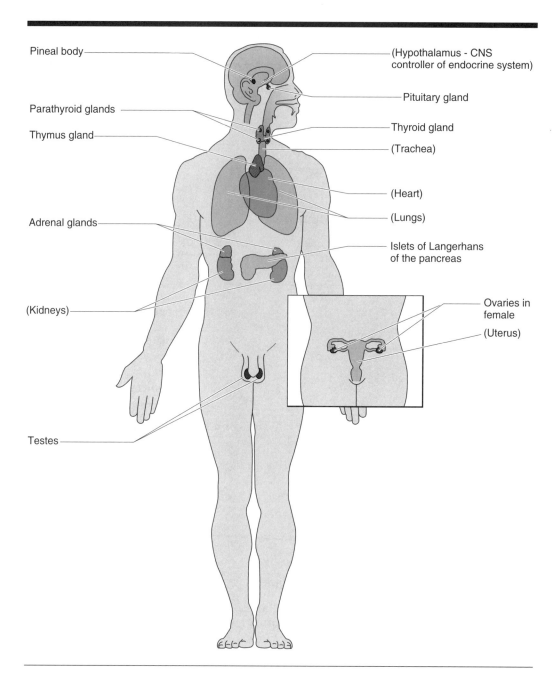

Figure 11.1. Endocrine system. Structures in parentheses are not part of endocrine system; they are shown for orientation only.

Gland or Hormone	Location or Function

steroid hormones
stĕr′oyd
    glucocorticoids
    glū-kō-kōr′ti-koydz
    mineral corticosteroids
    min′er-ăl kōr′ti-kō-stĕr′oydz
    androgens
    an′drō-jenz
	regulate carbohydrate metabolism and salt and water balance; some effect on sexual characteristics

continued

Gland or Hormone	Location or Function
epinephrine ep′i-nef′rin **norepinephrine** nōr′ep-i-nef′rin	affect sympathetic nervous system in stress response
ovaries ō′vă-rēz	located one on each side of the uterus in the female pelvis, functioning to secrete estrogen and progesterone
estrogen es′trō-jen **progesterone** prō-jes′ter-ōn	responsible for the development of female secondary sex characteristics and regulation of reproduction
pancreas (islets of Langerhans) pan′krē-as	located behind the stomach in front of the first and second lumbar vertebrae, functioning to secrete insulin and glucagon
insulin in′sŭ-lin **glucagon** glū′kă-gon	regulate carbohydrate/sugar metabolism
parathyroid glands par-ă-thī′royd	located on the posterior aspect of the thyroid gland in the neck, functioning to secrete parathyroid hormone (PTH)
parathyroid hormone (PTH)	regulates calcium and phosphorus metabolism
pineal gland pin′ē-ăl	located in the center of the brain, functioning to secrete melatonin and serotonin
melatonin mel-ă-tōn′in	exact function unknown, affects onset of puberty
serotonin	a neurotransmitter that serves as the precursor to melatonin
pituitary gland pi-tū′i-tār-ē **hypophysis** hī-pof′i-sis	located at the base of the brain, the anterior pituitary secretes thyroid-stimulating hormone, adrenocorticotrophic hormone, follicle-stimulating hormone, luteinizing hormone, melanocyte-stimulating hormone, growth hormone, and prolactin; the posterior pituitary releases antidiuretic hormone and oxytocin
anterior pituitary (adenohypophysis) ad′ĕ-nō-hī-pof′i-sis	
thyroid-stimulating hormone (TSH)	stimulates secretion from thyroid gland
adrenocorticotrophic hormone (ACTH) ă-drē′nō-kōr′ti-kō-trō′fik	stimulates secretion from adrenal cortex

continued

THYMUS. Derived from the Greek word for an offer or sacrifice, the thyme plant was burnt on altars because of its sweet smell. The term was applied to the thymus gland because of its likeness to a bunch of thyme.

THYROID. Thyroid is from a Greek word referring to a large oblong shield carried by soldiers. It had a deep notch at the top for the chin. The thyroid gland and the thyroid cartilage in the neck were named for this shield because of a similar appearance.

Gland or Hormone	Location or Function
follicle-stimulating hormone (FSH) fol'i-kl	initiates growth of ovarian follicle; stimulates secretion of estrogen in females and sperm production in males
luteinizing hormone (LH) lū'tē-ĭ-nīz-ing	causes ovulation; stimulates secretion of progesterone by corpus luteum; causes secretion of testosterone in testes
melanocyte-stimulating hormone (MSH) mel'ă-nō-sīt	affects skin pigmentation
growth hormone (GH)	influences growth
prolactin (lactogenic hormone) prō-lak'tin	stimulates breast development and milk production during pregnancy
posterior pituitary (neurohypophysis) nūr'ō-hī-pof'i-sis	
antidiuretic hormone (ADH) an'tē-dī-yū-ret'ik	influences the absorption of water by kidney tubules
oxytocin ok-sē-tō'sin	influences uterine contraction
testes tes'tēz	located one on each side within the scrotum in the male, functioning to secrete testosterone
testosterone tes-tos'tĕ-rōn	affects masculinization and reproduction
thymus gland thī'mŭs	located in the mediastinal cavity anterior to and above the heart, functioning to secrete thymosin
thymosin thī'mō-sin	regulates immune response
thyroid gland	located in front of the neck, functioning to secrete triiodothyronine (T_3), thyroxine (T_4), and calcitonin
triiodothyronine (T_3) trī-ī'ō-dō-thī'rō-nēn **thyroxine** (T_4) thī-rok'sēn	regulate metabolism
calcitonin kal-si-tō'nin	regulates calcium and phosphorus metabolism

Symptomatic and Diagnostic Terms

Term	Meaning
Symptomatic	
exophthalmos ek-sof-thal'mos **exophthalmus**	protrusion of one or both eyeballs, often because of thyroid dysfunction or a tumor behind the eyeball
glucosuria glū-kō-sū'rē-ă **glycosuria** glī-kō-sū'rē-ă	glucose (sugar) in the urine
hirsutism her'sū-tizm	shaggy; an excessive growth of hair especially in unusual places (e.g., a woman with a beard)
hypercalcemia hī'per-kal-sē'mē-ă	an abnormally high level of calcium in the blood
hypocalcemia hī'pō-kal-sē'mē-ă	an abnormally low level of calcium in the blood
hyperglycemia hī'per-glī-sē'mē-ă	high blood sugar
hypoglycemia hī'pō-glī-sē'mē-ă	low blood sugar
hyperkalemia hī'per-kă-lē'mē-ă	an abnormally high level of potassium in the blood (kalium = potassium)
hypokalemia hī'pō-ka-lē'mē-ă	deficient level of potassium in the blood
hypersecretion hī'per-se-krē'shŭn	abnormally increased secretion
hyposecretion hī'pō-se-krē'shŭn	decreased secretion
ketosis kē-tō'sis **acidosis** as-i-dō'sis **ketoacidosis** kē-tō-as-i-dō'sis	presence of an abnormal amount of ketone bodies (acetone, beta-hydroxybutyric acid, and acetoacetic acid) in the blood and urine indicating an abnormal utilization of carbohydrates as seen in uncontrolled diabetes and starvation (keto = alter)
metabolism mĕ-tab'ō-lizm	all chemical processes in the body that result in growth, generation of energy, elimination of waste, and other body functions
polydipsia pol-ē-dip'sē-ă	excessive thirst
polyuria pol-ē-yū'rē-ă	excessive urination
Diagnostic	
Adrenal Glands	
Cushing's syndrome	condition resulting from hypersecretion of the adrenal cortex; often caused by a tumor and characterized by obesity, hyperglycemia, and weakness

continued

Term	Meaning
adrenal virilism ă-drē′năl	excessive output of the adrenal secretion of androgen (male sex hormone) owing to tumor or hyperplasia in adult women evidenced by amenorrhea, acne, hirsutism, and deepening of the voice (virilis = masculine)
Pancreas pan′krē-as	
diabetes mellitus dī-ă-bē′tēz mel′i-tŭs	metabolic disorder caused by an abnormal utilization of insulin secreted by the pancreas evidenced by hyperglycemia and glycosuria (diabetes = passing through; mellitus = sugar)
insulin-dependent diabetes mellitus (IDDM) type I	patient is dependent on insulin for survival (Fig. 11.2)
non–insulin-dependent diabetes mellitus (NIDDM) type II	patient is not dependent on insulin for survival
hyperinsulinism hī′per-in′sū-lin-izm	condition resulting from an excessive amount of insulin in the blood that draws sugar out of the bloodstream, resulting in hypoglycemia, fainting, and convulsions; often caused by an overdose of insulin or by a tumor of the pancreas
pancreatitis pan′krē-ă-tī′tis	inflammation of the pancreas

continued

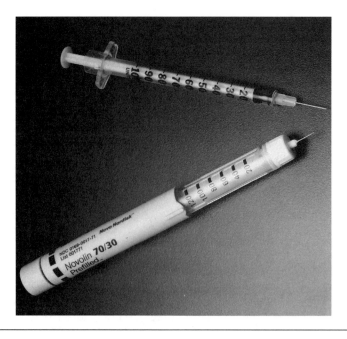

Figure 11.2. Insulin syringe prefilled with insulin.

Term	Meaning
Parathyroid Glands par-ă-thī′royd	
hyperparathyroidism hī′per-par-ă-thī′royd-izm	hypersecretion of the parathyroid glands, usually caused by a tumor
hypoparathyroidism hī′pō-par-ă-thī′royd-izm	hyposecretion of the parathyroid glands
Pituitary Gland (Hypophysis)	
acromegaly ak-rō-meg′ă-lē	disease characterized by enlarged features, especially face and hands, caused by hypersecretion of the pituitary hormone (Fig. 11.3)

continued

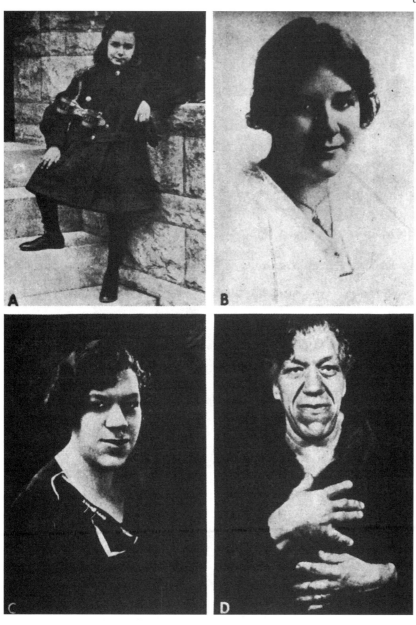

Figure 11.3. Progression of acromegaly. **A.** Normal, age 9 years. **B.** Age 16 years with possible early coarsening of features. **C.** Age 33 years, well-established acromegaly. **D.** age 52 years, end-stage acromegaly with gross disfigurement.

Term	Meaning
pituitary dwarfism dwōrf'izm	condition of congenital hyposecretion of growth hormone slowing growth and causing a short yet proportionate stature (not affecting intelligence)—often treated during childhood with growth hormone (Fig. 11.4) [note: there are many other forms of dwarfism, a condition of being markedly undersized; disproportionate types (short limb or short trunk) are most often caused by gene defects (Fig. 11.5)]
pituitary gigantism jī'gan-tizm	condition of hypersecretion of growth hormone before puberty that leads to an abnormal overgrowth of the bones, especially the long bones (Fig. 11.6)
Thyroid Gland	
goiter goy'ter	enlargement of the thyroid gland caused by thyroid dysfunction, tumor, lack of iodine in the diet, or inflammation (goiter = throat) (Fig. 11.7)
hyperthyroidism hī-per-thī'royd-izm **Graves' disease** grāvz di-zēz' **thyrotoxicosis** thī'rō-tok-si-kō'sis	condition of hypersecretion of the thyroid gland characterized by exophthalmia, tachycardia, goiter, and tumor (Fig. 11.8*A*)

continued

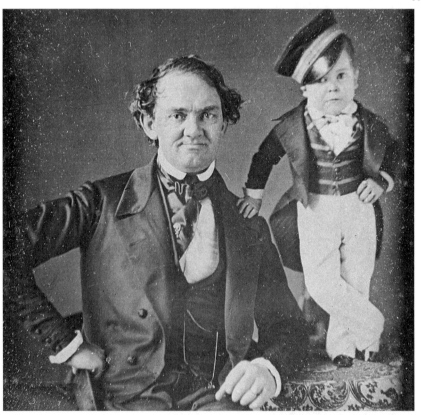

Figure 11.4. Tom Thumb, most famous proportionate dwarf and showman, poses with P. T. Barnum (left). Born January 4, 1838, weight 9 lb; at age 4, weight 15 lb, height 25 inches; died of a stroke at age 45, weight 70 lb, height 40 inches.

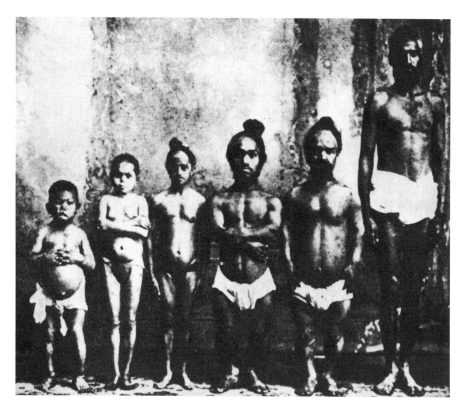

Figure 11.5. Normal male (extreme right) and three types of dwarfism. On the extreme left is a child who has failed to grow because of congenital absence of the thyroid gland (cretin). The next pair of dwarfs have entirely normal proportions but are half normal size. The next pair on the right show disproportionately short extremities but normal size trunk and head.

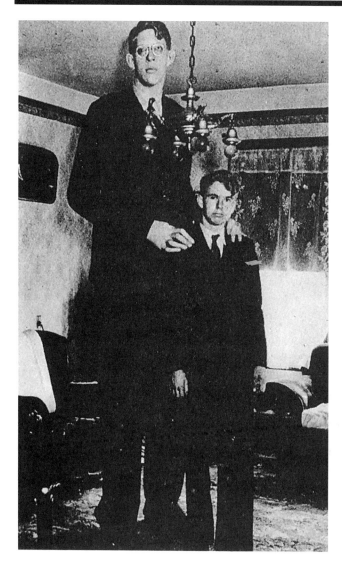

Figure 11.6. Robert Wadlow, famous giant, is shown with his brother. Born February 22, 1918, weight 8 lb. At age 8, weight 169 lb, height 6 feet; died at age 22, weight 491 lb, height 8 feet 11.1 inches. He died in 1940 after a long bout with a fever caused by a badly infected sore on his ankle (before availability of antibiotics).

Figure 11.7. Large masses in the neck in six of the seven persons in this photograph are typical of nontoxic goiter. The sixth (second from right) shows another abnormality characterized by the prominent exophthalmos and evidence of weight loss.

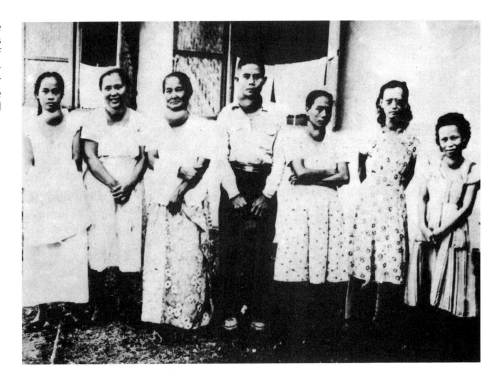

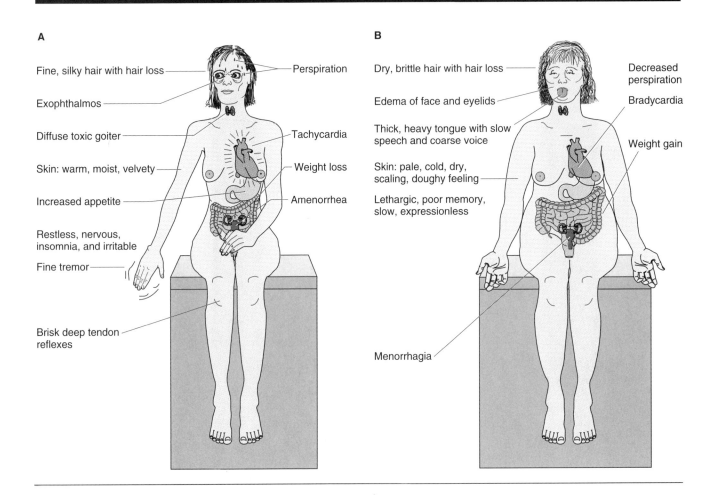

A

Fine, silky hair with hair loss

Exophthalmos

Diffuse toxic goiter

Skin: warm, moist, velvety

Increased appetite

Restless, nervous, insomnia, and irritable

Fine tremor

Brisk deep tendon reflexes

Perspiration

Tachycardia

Weight loss

Amenorrhea

B

Dry, brittle hair with hair loss

Edema of face and eyelids

Thick, heavy tongue with slow speech and coarse voice

Skin: pale, cold, dry, scaling, doughy feeling

Lethargic, poor memory, slow, expressionless

Menorrhagia

Decreased perspiration

Bradycardia

Weight gain

Figure 11.8. A. Hyperthyroidism. **B**. Hypothyroidism.

Term	Meaning
hypothyroidism hī′pō-thī′royd-izm	condition of hyposecretion of the thyroid gland causing low thyroid levels in the blood that result in sluggishness, slow pulse, and often obesity (Fig. 11.8B)
myxedema mik-se-dē′mă	advanced hypothyroidism in adults characterized by sluggishness, slow pulse, puffiness in hands and face, and dry skin (myx = mucous)
cretinism krē′tin-izm	condition of congenital hypothyroidism in children, that results in a lack of mental development and dwarfed physical stature (Fig. 11.5)

Diagnostic Tests and Procedures

Test or Procedure	Explanation
Laboratory Testing	
blood sugar (BS) **blood glucose**	measurement of the level of sugar (glucose) in the blood (Fig. 11.9)
fasting blood sugar (FBS)	measurement of blood sugar level after a fast of 12 hours
postprandial blood sugar (PPBS)	measurement of blood sugar level after a meal, commonly after two hours
glucose tolerance test (GTT)	measurement of the body's ability to metabolize carbohydrates by administering a prescribed amount of glucose after a fasting period, then measuring blood and urine for glucose levels every hour thereafter—usually for four to six hours
glycohemoglobin glī-kō-hē-mō-glō′bin	a molecule (fraction) in hemoglobin that rises in the blood as a result of an increased level of blood sugar; it is a common blood test used in diagnosing and treating diabetes

continued

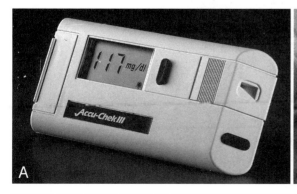
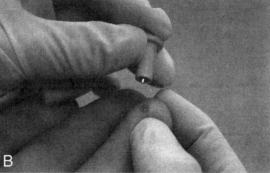

Figure 11.9. A. Blood glucose meter used to measure and monitor the level of sugar in blood obtained by capillary puncture. **B.** Skin puncture technique using a lancet.

Test or Procedure	Explanation
electrolytes ē-lek'tro-lītz	measurement of the level of specific ions (sodium, potassium, CO_2, and chloride) in the blood; electrolyte balance is essential for normal metabolism
thyroid function study	measurement of thyroid hormone levels in blood plasma to determine efficiency of glandular secretions including T_3, T_4, TSH
urine sugar and ketone studies kē'tōn	chemical tests to determine the presence of sugar or ketone bodies in urine; used as a screen for diabetes

Imaging Procedures

computed tomography (CT)	CT of the head is used to obtain a transverse view of the pituitary gland
magnetic resonance imaging (MRI)	nonionizing images of magnetic resonance are useful in identifying abnormalities of pituitary, pancreas, adrenal, and thyroid glands
sonography	sonographic images are used to identify endocrine pathology, such as with thyroid ultrasound
thyroid uptake and image	nuclear image involving scan of the thyroid to visualize the radioactive accumulation of previously injected isotopes to detect thyroid nodules or tumors (Fig. 11.10)

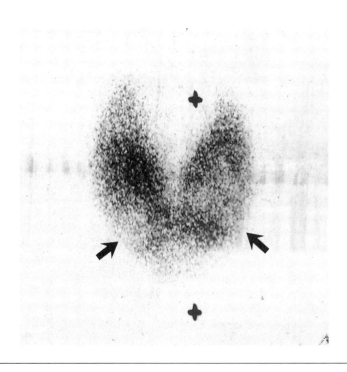

Figure 11.10. Thyroid uptake and image detecting presence of multiple nodules (*arrows*).

Operative Terms

Term	Meaning
adrenalectomy ă-drē-năl-ek′tō-mē	excision of adrenal gland
hypophysectomy hī′pof-i-sek′tō-mē	excision of pituitary gland
pancreatectomy pan′krē-ă-tek′tō-mē	excision of pancreas
parathyroidectomy pa′ră-thī-roy-dek′tō-mē	excision of parathyroid gland
thymectomy thī-mek′tō-mē	excision of thymus gland
thyroidectomy thī-roy-dek′tō-mē	excision of thyroid gland

Therapeutic Terms

Term	Meaning
radioiodine therapy rā′dē-ō-ī′ō-dīn	use of radioactive iodine to treat disease, such as to eradicate thyroid tumor cells

Common Therapeutic Drug Classifications

antihypoglycemic an′tē-hī′pō-glī-sē′mik	a drug that raises blood glucose
hormone replacement hōr′mōn	a drug that replaces a hormone deficiency (e.g., estrogen, testosterone, thyroid, etc.)
hypoglycemic antihyperglycemic hī′pō-glī-sē′mik an′tē-hī′per-glī-sē′mik	a drug that lowers blood glucose (e.g., insulin)

PRACTICE EXERCISES

For the following terms, draw a line or lines to separate prefixes, combining forms, and suffixes. Then define the term.

1. hypoparathyroidism _____

2. adenitis _____

3. hyperglycemia _____

4. thyrotoxicosis _____

5. polydipsia _____

6. hormonal _____

7. ketosis _____

8. polyuria _____

9. endocrine _____

10. thyroptosis _____

11. thymoma _____

12. acromegaly _____

13. android _____

14. adrenotrophic _____

15. pancreatogenic _____

Write the correct medical term for each of the following:

16. advanced hypothyroidism in adults _____

17. congenital hypothyroidism _____

18. another name for Graves' disease _____

19. condition resulting from hypersecretion of the adrenal cortex causing obesity, hyperglycemia, and weakness

_____

20. disease characterized by enlarged features caused by hypersecretion of the pituitary hormone

_____

21. enlargement of thyroid gland _____

22. protrusion of eyeball _____

23. condition of congenital hyposecretion of growth hormone _____

24. a deficient level of potassium in the blood _____

25. nuclear image of the thyroid _____

26. condition of congenital hypersecretion of the growth hormone _____

Match the following terms with their meanings:

27. congenital hypothyroidism   _____   a. gigantism

28. ketosis   _____   b. hirsutism

29. hyperthyroidism   _____   c. goiter

30. hypophysis   _____   d. IDDM

31. thyromegaly   _____   e. cretinism

32. adult hypothyroidism   _____   f. pituitary

33. adrenal virilism   _____   g. NIDDM

34. type II diabetes   _____   h. acidosis

35. pituitary hypersecretion   _____   i. myxedema

36. type I diabetes   _____   j. thyrotoxicosis

Complete the medical term by writing the missing part:

37. poly_____ ia = excessive thirst

38. _____ secretion = abnormally increased secretion

39. _____ glycemia = low blood sugar

40. glucos_____ = sugar in the urine

41. _____ secretion = decreased secretion

42. _____ glycemia = high blood sugar

43. _____ graphy = ultrasound imaging

Write the full medical term for the following abbreviations:

44. BS _____

45. IDDM _____

46. FBS _____

47. CT _____

48. PPBS _____

49. GTT _____

50. NIDDM _____

Medical Record Analyses

MEDICAL RECORD 11.1

Jane Dano, an 11-year-old girl, started experiencing a constant thirst accompanied by frequent urination. Gradually she lost weight. At the suggestion of Dr. Freeman, her family doctor, she was admitted to Central Medical Center for tests. Shortly after admission, her care was referred to Dr. Gallegos.

Directions

Read Medical Record 11.1 regarding Jane Dano (pages 318–320) and answer the following questions. These records represent the physician's orders from Dr. Gallegos, who assumed the care of Jane at the time of her admission, and his clinical summary dictated at the time of her discharge.

Questions about Medical Record 11.1

Write your answers in the spaces provided.

1. Below are medical terms used in this record you have not yet encountered in this text. Underline each where it appears in the records and define below.

   urinalysis _____

   nocturia _____

   dietician _____

   Kussmaul's respiration _____

2. In your own words, not using medical terminology, briefly describe Jane's condition as identified by the admitting and final diagnosis.

   _____

   _____

   _____

3. Dr. Gallegos requested that the unit nurses take Jane's blood pressure every ___ hours.

4. Explain in lay language Dr. Gallegos' instructions to the nurses for Jane's fluid intake.

   _____

   _____

5. By what route is Jane's regular insulin being administered?

   _____

6. Every nurse helping care for Jane needs to know to check her urine for acetone and sugar at what times?

_____

7. Part of Jane's care involves teaching her and others how to manage her diabetes when she returns home after discharge. The nurses and dietician provided this education to which of the following people (check all that apply):

_____ Jane's stepmother

_____ Jane's father

_____ Jane's teachers

_____ Jane's older brother

_____ a neighbor

_____ Dr. Gallegos

_____ the twins

8. Explain in lay language the two symptoms Jane had for 2 months before being admitted.

_____

What two additional symptoms occurred in the last 3 weeks?

_____

_____

9. At the time of discharge Jane weighed:

a. 40 pounds

b. 148 pounds

c. 89 pounds

d. 148 kg

10. Which of the following diagnostic tests will Jane and her family be performing at home?

    a. blood glucose monitoring

    b. vital signs

    c. body weight

    d. insulin injections

11. If you were Jane's parent, what guidance would you give about how active she can be at school? (Put in terms an 11-year-old can understand.)

    _____

    _____

    _____

CENTRAL MEDICAL CENTER

211 Medical Center Drive • Central City, US 90000-1234 • PHONE: (012) 125-6784 • FAX: (012) 125-9999

DOCTOR: PLEASE STATE PERTINENT CLINICAL INFORMATION WHEN ORDERING RADIOLOGY PROCEDURES

WRITE WITH BALLPOINT INK PEN; PRESS HARD

DATE	TIME	AUTHORIZATION IS GIVEN TO DISPENSE ANOTHER BRAND OF DRUG IDENTICAL IN FORM AND CONTENT UNLESS CHECKED
11-11-9x	1400	1. STAT Biochem Panel-18
		2. glyco hemoglobin
		3. anti-islet cell antibodies
		R Gallego M.D
		Noted 11/11/9x B.Hill, RN 1425
11-11-9x	1430	1. admit to 6 north
		2. Dx: IDDM new onset
		3. VS per routine BP q4° during day
		4. daily wt
		5. encourage p.o. fluids 1200 cc q8°
		6. a.m. insulin to be Novolin Regular and NPH Please have available on floor
		7. U.A
		8. accu check (blood sugar test) at 07-11-17-22-02
		9. Give 7 units of Regular insulin now
		10. Check urine for sugar, acetone and volume q void
		11. accucheck 1° p̄ above insulin given
		R Gallego M.D
		C. Wells 11-11-9x 1500
		Noted 11/11/9x B.Hill,RN 1600
11-11-9x	1530	1800 calorie ADA (American Diabetes Assoc) diet c̄ 3 meals and 2 snacks - no A.M. snack
		C. Wells 11-11-9x 1830 R Gallegos MD

PHYSICIAN'S ORDERS

PT. NAME: DANO, J.
ID NO: 4038315
SEX: F   AGE: 11   DOB: 02/13/9x
ATT. PHYS: R. GALLEGOS, M.D.

CENTRAL MEDICAL CENTER

211 Medical Center Drive • Central City, US 90000-1234 • PHONE: (012) 125-6784 • FAX: (012) 125-9999

DISCHARGE SUMMARY

ADMITTING DIAGNOSIS: New onset diabetes mellitus.

FINAL DIAGNOSIS: New onset diabetes mellitus.

HISTORY OF PRESENT ILLNESS: The patient is an 11-year-old white female who presented with a 3-week history of polyuria and polydipsia. She has also had nocturia for the past two months and associated weight loss. She was seen by E. Freeman, M.D., her private physician, on the day of admission. A urinalysis was positive for glucose. The patient was then referred to this examiner for further evaluation and management of new onset diabetes mellitus.

HOSPITAL COURSE: The patient was admitted to the third floor. She was initially treated with regular insulin and then progressed to a 2-shot regimen with regular insulin and NPH before breakfast and regular insulin and NPH before dinner. She also required some spot dosing at lunch time for hyperglycemia. Prior to discharge, her blood sugars had stabilized. She did not have any overnight hypoglycemia. She had spilled 10 gm of glucose in her urine but no ketones. Also, during the course of hospitalization, the parents, the patient, and a neighbor underwent extensive education with nursing and the dietician. The patient lives with her father and stepmother. Her stepmother is due to deliver twins in January, and her father travels quite a bit in his work; therefore, a neighbor was also trained to help in taking care of her diabetes. Prior to discharge, the patient and her parents have been able to give insulin injections and also do home blood glucose monitoring.

LABORATORY DATA: Initial laboratory studies showed the following: Sodium: 134. Potassium: 4.0. Chloride: 102. CO_2: 28. Blood urea nitrogen (BUN): 9. Creatinine: 0.7. Serum glucose: 517. Thyroid function was normal with: T_4: 6.5; free thyroxine index (FTI): 7.8; T_3: 1.02; TSH: 2.0. Total cholesterol was 146. Liver function tests were normal. Glycohemoglobin was 19.5. Anti-islet cell antibodies were sent out and are pending at the time of discharge. [islet cell antibodies commonly occur in newly diagnosed insulin dependent diabetics].

(continued)

DISCHARGE SUMMARY Page 1	PT. NAME: DANO, JANE V. ID NO: IP-403831 ROOM NO: 610 ADM. DATE: November 11, 199x DIS. DATE: November 18, 199x ATT. PHYS: R. GALLEGOS, M.D.

Medical Record 11.1. *Continued.*

CENTRAL MEDICAL CENTER

211 Medical Center Drive • Central City, US 90000-1234 • PHONE: (012) 125-6784 • FAX: (012) 125-9999

DISCHARGE SUMMARY

PHYSICAL EXAMINATION: Temperature: 36.9°C. Heart rate: 68. Respirations: 18. Discharge weight: 40.4 kg. Height: 148 cm. GENERAL: The patient is awake and alert and in no acute distress. Eyes reveal normal funduscopic examination. The neck is supple. The thyroid gland is nonpalpable. The chest is clear to percussion and auscultation. No Kussmaul's respirations were noted at discharge. CARDIOVASCULAR: Apical pulse is regular without murmur. ABDOMEN: The abdomen is soft and nontender. No enlargement or mass is noted. GENITOURINARY: Normal external female genitalia. EXTREMITIES: The patient did have significant improvement of the dryness on her hands and also around her mouth.

DISCHARGE PROGRAM: The patient is to be seen in the Diabetic Clinic in approximately two weeks. DIET: She is on a 1,950 calorie American Diabetes Association (ADA) diet with three meals and two snacks. Physical activity is ad lib. The patient may return to school at the end of the week. SPECIAL INSTRUCTIONS: The parents are to check blood sugar at 2 a.m. for the first two nights at home. They are also to call for insulin dose adjustments daily for the first week after discharge.

DISCHARGE MEDICATIONS: Novolin Human Insulin, 12 units of regular and 12 units of NPH, to be given 20 minutes before breakfast; 10 units of regular and 6 units of NPH to be given 20 minutes before dinner.

R. Gallegos, M.D.

RG:ti

D: 11/18/9x
T: 11/19/9x

DISCHARGE SUMMARY		
Page 2	PT. NAME:	DANO, JANE V.
	ID NO:	IP-403831
	ROOM NO:	610
	ADM. DATE:	November 11, 199x
	DIS. DATE:	November 18, 199x
	ATT. PHYS:	R. GALLEGOS, M.D.

Medical Record 11.1. *Continued.*

MEDICAL RECORD 11.2

Tara Nguyen had a long history of hyperthyroidism that was managed by pharmacological treatment for more than 5 years. She was often unhappy with how she felt, however, and decided on her own to stop taking the drug. Two months ago the symptoms of hyperthyroidism recurred, and she sought medical attention.

Directions

Read Medical Record 11.2 for Ms. Nguyen (page 322) and answer the following questions. This record is the report by Dr. Rincon, who analyzed Ms. Nguyen's thyroid uptake and imaging study.

Questions about Medical Record 11.2

Write your answers in the spaces provided.

1. Below are medical terms used in this record you have not yet encountered in this text. Underline each where it appears in the record and define below.

    propylthiouracil (PTU) _____

    uptake_____

    baseline (nonmedical term) _____

2. In your own words, not using medical terminology, briefly describe what seems to have been missing in Ms. Nguyen's past medical management.

    _____

    _____

3. In nonmedical terms, explain how the sodium iodide was administered.

    _____

4. In your own words, not using medical terminology, briefly describe Dr. Rincon's diagnosis.

    _____

    _____

    _____

5. What additional test did Dr. Rincon order on his own authority?

    a. thyroid function study

    b. fasting blood sugar

    c. thyroid MRI

    d. thyroid ultrasound

6. Which of the following tests is recommended to be peformed in 6 months?

    a. thyroid function study

    b. fasting blood sugar

    c. thyroid MRI

    d. thyroid ultrasound

CENTRAL MEDICAL CENTER

211 Medical Center Drive • Central City, US 90000-1234 • PHONE: (012) 125-6784 • FAX: (012) 125-9999

THYROID UPTAKE AND IMAGING STUDY

Date of Exam: 5/29/9x

CLINICAL HISTORY: The patient has more than a six year history of hyperthyroidism which was treated until approximately one year ago with propylthiouracil (PTU). The patient relates some instability in symptomatology during the treatment. She had no previous uptake and imaging study, and radioiodine therapy was never discussed with the patient. She spontaneously discontinued taking the PTU approximately one year ago and has had recurrent symptoms of hyperthyroidism in the last two months.

TECHNIQUE: The patient ingested a capsule containing 200 μCi^{123}I sodium iodide. Uptakes in the neck were measured at 6 and 24 hours. Images of the thyroid were obtained in multiple projections at 6 hours.

FINDINGS: Radioiodine uptake at 6 hours was 37% (normal: 0-15%), and at 24 hours, uptake was 57% (normal: 5-35%). Thyroid images reveal the gland to be diffusely modestly enlarged. Multiple areas of reduced function correlating with palpable nodules are present in both thyroid lobes with the largest nodule being present in the lower poles of both lobes but with the right lobe being somewhat more severely overall affected than the left lobe. No dominant functioning thyroid nodule is evident.

CONCLUSION:

TOXIC MULTINODULAR GOITER

NOTE: Because of the presence of the multiple nodules which are likely on a benign basis, I took the liberty of ordering a thyroid ultrasound as a baseline. This will be separately reported, and it is suggested that the thyroid ultrasound be repeated in six months to one year.

C. Rincon, M.D.

CR:se

D: 5/29/199x   T: 5/31/199x

THYROID UPTAKE AND IMAGING STUDY	PT. NAME: NGUYEN, TARA T. ID NO: NM-384023 Sex: F Age: 58 Y DOB: 02/18/9x ATT. PHYS. T. Hutton

Medical Record 11.2.

Eye

OBJECTIVES

After completion of this chapter you will be able to

1. Define the common combining forms used in relation to the eye

2. Locate and name the major structures of the eye

3. Define common symptomatic, diagnostic operative, and therapeutic terms referring to the eye

4. List the common diagnostic tests and procedures related to the eye

5. Explain the terms and abbreviations used in documenting medical records involving the eye

Combining Forms

Combining Form	Meaning	Example
aque/o	water	aqueous ak′we-ŭs
blephar/o	eyelid	blepharospasm blef′ă-ro-spazm
conjunctiv/o	conjunctiva (to join together)	conjunctival kon-jŭnk-tı′văl
corne/o	cornea	corneal kor′ne-ăl
ir/o irid/o	iris (colored circle)	iritis ı-rı′tis iridectomy ir′i-dek′to-me
kerat/o	hard or cornea	keratoplasty ker′ă-to-plas-te
lacrim/o dacry/o	tear	lacrimal lak′ri-măl dacryocyst dak′re-o-sist
ocul/o ophthalm/o opt/o	eye	ocular ok′yu-lăr ophthalmology of-thal-mol′o-je optometry op-tom′ĕ-tre
phac/o phak/o	lens (lentil)	phacolysis fă-kol′i-sis phakoma fa-ko′mă
phot/o	light	photophobia fo-to-fo′be-ă
presby/o	old age	presbyopia prez-be-o′pe-ă
scler/o	hard or sclera	scleritis sklĕ-rı′tis
vitre/o	glassy	vitreous vit′re-ŭs
-opia	condition of vision	hyperopia hı-per-ō′pē-ă

Eye Overview

The eye is the organ of sight that through pairing provides three-dimensional vision (Fig. 12.1). Each eye is located in a bony orbit (cavity) of the skull and is covered by the protective fold of the eyelid.

The *sclera*, the white of the eye, and the *cornea*, the transparent anterior coating, are part of the outer fibrous *tunic* (layer) that *refracts* (bends) light that enters the eye.

The *choroid*, a vascular layer located just beneath the sclera, contains blood vessels that nourish the outer portion of the retina. The *iris* contains blood vessels, pigment cells, and muscle fibers. Muscles of the iris regulate the amount of light that enters through the cen-

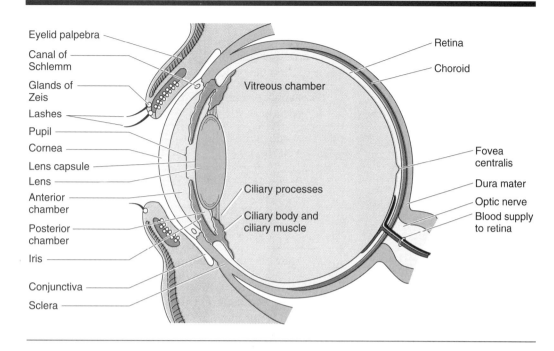

Figure 12.1. Anatomy of the eye (sagittal view).

tral opening known as the *pupil*. Melanin, the pigment present in the epithelial cells that cover the iris, gives color to the eyes. The *ciliary body* is a ring of muscle located behind the peripheral iris that controls the power of the lens. The elastic, transparent *lens*, located behind the pupil, focuses light rays on the *retina* in the inner, posterior part of the eye. *Aqueous humor*, produced by the surface epithelium of the ciliary body, provides nutrition to the avascular lens and cornea. *Vitreous* is the jelly-like material that occupies the space between the lens and retina.

The *retina* is the nerve tissue layer that contains cells for visual reception. The visual receptor neurons of the retina are the rods and cones. *Rods* are responsible for vision in dim light, and *cones* are responsible for vision in bright light. The *macula lutea* is the central region of the retina. It has a yellowish color caused by its pigment. At the center of the macula, a tiny, pinpoint depression known as the fovea centralis is the site of sharpest, central vision. The *optic disc* is the area in the retina where nerve fibers form the *optic nerve* for transmission to the optic tracts in the brain.

The *conjunctiva* provides a lining for the eye and eyelid. The *lacrimal gland*, located in the orbit above each eye, secretes tears that lubricate and protect the eye. Tears constantly flow across the eye and downward to the *lacrimal ducts*, to the *lacrimal sac*, and then into the *nasolacrimal duct* that drains into the nose. The *meibomian glands* are sebaceous glands located within the rim of the eyelid that secrete sebum to keep the lids from sticking together, and the *glands of Zeis* are sweat glands surrounding the hair follicles of the eyelashes.

Anatomical Terms

Term	Meaning
anterior chamber	fluid-filled space between cornea and iris
aqueous humor ak′wē-ŭs hyū′mer	watery liquid secreted at the ciliary body that fills the anterior and posterior chambers of the eye and provides nourishment for the cornea, iris, and lens (humor = fluid)

continued

Term	Meaning
canal of Schlemm	duct in anterior chamber that carries filtered aqueous humor to the veins and bloodstream
choroid kō'royd	vascular layer beneath the sclera that provides nourishment to outer portion of the retina
ciliary body sil'ē-ar-ē	ring of muscle behind the peripheral iris that controls the power of the lens
ciliary muscle	smooth muscle portion of the ciliary body, which contracts to assist in near vision capability
ciliary processes	epithelial tissue folds on the inner surface of the ciliary body that secrete aqueous humor
conjunctiva kon-jŭnk-tī'vă	joining together; mucous membrane that lines the eyelids and outer surface of the eyeball
cornea kōr'nē-ă	transparent, anterior part of the eyeball covering the iris, pupil, and anterior chamber that functions to refract (bend) light to focus a visual image
eyelid (palpebra) pal-pē'bră	movable protective fold that opens and closes, covering the eye
fovea centralis fō'vē-ă sen-trā'lis	pin point depression in the center of the macula lutea that is the site of sharpest vision (fovea = pit)
fundus (base) fŭn'dŭs	interior surface of the eyeball including the retina, optic disc, macula, and posterior pole (curvature at the back of the eye)
glands of Zeis	oil glands surrounding the eyelashes
meibomian glands mī-bō'mē-an	oil glands located along the rim of the eyelids
iris ī'ris	colored circle; colored part of the eye located behind the cornea that contracts and dilates to regulate light passing through the pupil
lacrimal gland lak'ri-măl	gland located in the upper outer region above the eyeball that secretes tears (Fig. 12.2)
lacrimal ducts	tubes that carry tears to the lacrimal sac
lacrimal sac	structure that collects tears before emptying into nasolacrimal duct
lens	transparent structure behind the pupil that bends and focuses light rays on the retina
lens capsule	capsule that encloses the lens
macula lutea (macula) mak'yū-lă	central region of the retina responsible for central vision; yellow pigment provides its color (lutea = yellow) (see Color Atlas, plate 25)
nasolacrimal duct nā-zō-lak'ri-măl	passageway for tears from the lacrimal sac into the nose

continued

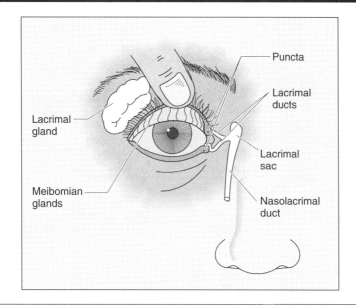

Figure 12.2. Lacrimal apparatus.

PUPIL. The Latin word, pupilla, the pupil of the eye, is derived from pupa, meaning a doll or little girl. The name is said to have been given to the pupil of the eye because a tiny image of the beholder may be seen reflected in it.

Term	Meaning
optic disc op'tik	exit site of retinal nerve fibers (see Color Atlas, plate 25)
optic nerve	nerve responsible for carrying impulses for the sense of sight from the retina to the brain
posterior chamber	space between the back of the iris and the front of the vitreous filled with aqueous fluid
pupil pyū'pĭl	black circular opening in the center of the iris through which light passes as it enters the eye
retina ret'i-nă	innermost layer that perceives and transmits light to the optic nerve (see Color Atlas, plate 25)
cones	cone-shaped cells within the retina that are color sensitive and respond to bright light
rods	rod-shaped cells within the retina that respond to dim light
sclera sklēr'ă	tough, fibrous, white outer coat extending from the cornea to the optic nerve
trabecular meshwork tră-bek'yū-lăr	mesh-like structure in the anterior chamber that filters the aqueous humor as it flows into the canal of Schlemm
vitreous vit'rē-ŭs	jelly-like mass filling the inner chamber between the lens and retina that gives bulk to the eye

Symptomatic and Diagnostic Terms

Term	Meaning
Symptomatic	
asthenopia as-thĕ-nō′pē-ă	eyestrain (asthenia = weak condition)
blepharospasm blef′ă-rō-spazm	involuntary contraction of the muscles surrounding the eye causing uncontrolled blinking and lid squeezing
diplopia di-plō′pē-ă	double vision
exophthalmos ek-sof-thal′mos **exophthalmus**	abnormal protrusion of one or both eyeballs
lacrimation lak-ri-mā′shŭn	secretion of tears
nystagmus nis-tag′mŭs	involuntary, rapid oscillating movement of the eyeball (nystagmos = a nodding)
photophobia fō-tō-fō′bē-ă	extreme sensitivity to, and discomfort from, light
scotoma skō-tō′mă	blind spot in vision (skotos = darkness)
Diagnostic	
refractive errors rē-frak′tiv	defects in the bending of light as it enters the eye, causing an improper focus on the retina
astigmatism ă-stig′mă-tizm	distorted vision caused by an oblong or cylindrical curvature of the lens or cornea that prevents light rays from coming to a single focus on the retina (stigma = point)
hyperopia hī-per-ō′pē-ă	farsightedness; difficulty seeing close objects when light rays extend beyond the proper focus on the retina (Fig. 12.3, *A* and *B*)
myopia mī-ō′pē-ă	nearsightedness; difficulty seeing distant objects when light rays fall short of the proper focus on the retina (Fig. 12.3, *A* and *C*)
presbyopia prez-bē-ō′pē-ă	impaired vision owing to old age loss of accommodation
accommodation ă-kom′ŏ-dā′shŭn	ability of the eye to adjust focus on near objects
aphakia ă-fā′kē-ă	absence of the lens, usually after cataract extraction
blepharitis blef′ă-rī′tis	inflammation of the eyelid

continued

Term	Meaning
blepharochalasis blef′ă-rō-kal′ă-sis **dermatochalasis** der′mă-tō-kal′ă-sis	baggy eyelid; overabundance and loss of elasticity of skin on the upper eyelid causing a fold of skin to hang down over the edge of the eyelid when the eyes are open (chalasis = a slackening)
blepharoptosis blef′ă-rop′tō-sis **ptosis**	drooping of the eyelid usually caused by paralysis
chalazion ka-lā′zē-on	chronic nodular inflammation of a meibomian gland, usually the result of a blocked duct (chalaza = hailstone) (Fig. 12.4)
cataract kat′ă-rakt	opaque clouding of the lens causing decreased vision (Fig. 12.5)
conjunctivitis kon-jŭnk-ti-vī′tis	pinkeye; inflammation of the conjunctiva

continued

CATARACT. This Greek word meaning waterfall, or something that rushes down to form an obstruction, like a portcullis, was probably related to the obstruction of vision that is symptomatic of a cataract. It was an ancient belief that the interference with vision occurred between the lens and the iris (like a veil).

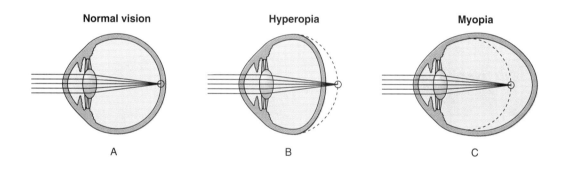

Figure 12.3. Proper focus of light rays on retina (**A**). Light rays extend beyond proper focus in hyperopia (**B**). Light rays fall short of proper focus in myopia (**C**).

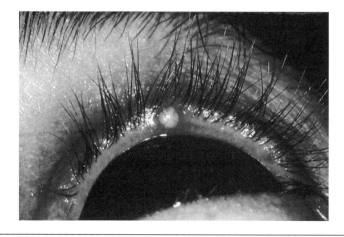

Figure 12.4. Upper lid chalazion.

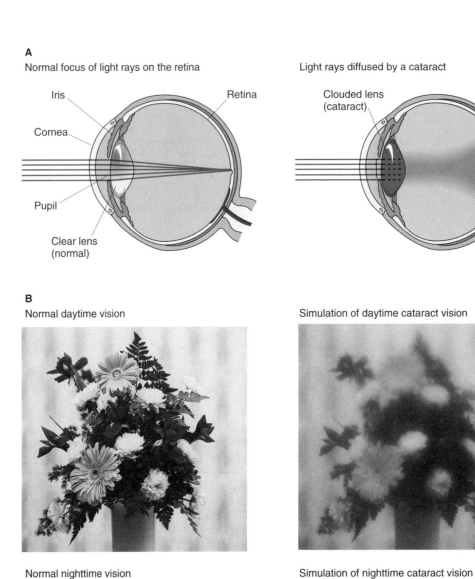

A

Normal focus of light rays on the retina

Light rays diffused by a cataract

B

Normal daytime vision

Simulation of daytime cataract vision

Normal nighttime vision

Simulation of nighttime cataract vision

Figure 12.5. Cataract. **A.** Normal light focus compared with light focus interference caused by cataract. **B.** Simulation of cataract vision.

Term	Meaning
dacryoadenitis dak're-o-ad-ĕ-nı'tis	inflammation of the lacrimal gland
dacryocystitis dak're-o'sis-tı'tis	inflammation of the tear sac (cyst/o = sac)
diabetic retinopathy dı-ă-bet'ik ret-i-nop'ă-the	disease of the retina in diabetics characterized by capillary leakage, bleeding, and new vessel formation (neovascularization) leading to scarring and loss of vision (see Color Atlas, plate 25)
ectropion ek-tro'pe-on	outward turning of the rim of the eyelid (tropo = turning) (Fig. 12.6*A*)
entropion en-tro'pe-on	inward turning of the rim of the eyelid (Fig. 12.6*B*)
epiphora e-pif'o-ră	abnormal overflow of tears caused by blockage of the lacrimal duct (epi = upon; phero = to bear)
glaucoma glaw-ko'mă	a group of diseases of the eye characterized by increased intraocular pressure that results in damage to the optic nerve, producing defects in vision
hordeolum hor-de'o-lŭm	a sty; an acute infection of a sebaceous gland of the eyelid (hordeum = barley)
iritis ı-rı'tis	inflammation of the iris
keratitis ker-ă-tı'tis	inflammation of the cornea
macular degeneration mak'yu-lăr de-jen-er-a'shŭn	breakdown or thinning of the tissues in the macula, resulting in partial or complete loss of central vision
pseudophakia su-do-fak'e-ă	an eye in which the natural lens is replaced with an artificial lens implant (pseudo = false)

continued

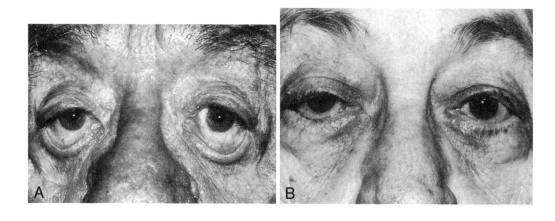

Figure 12.6. Eyelid abnormalities. **A.** Severe bilateral lower lid ectropion. **B.** Lower lid entropion causing lashes to rub on cornea.

STRABISMUS. Strabo, a geographer and prominent figure in Alexandria during the Roman period, suffered from a peculiar and noticeable squint. Any man with the same type of squint then was called Strabo, which led to the word strabismus.

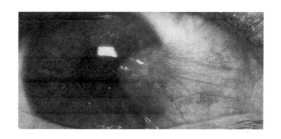

Figure 12.7. Pterygium caused by ultraviolet exposure and drying.

Esotropia 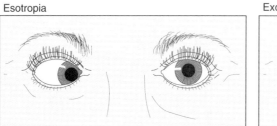   Exotropia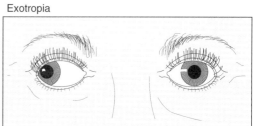

Figure 12.8. Strabismus.

Term	Meaning
pterygium tĕ-rij′ē-ŭm	a fibrous growth of conjunctival tissue that extends onto the cornea (Fig. 12.7)
retinal detachment ret-i-nal	separation of the retina from underlying epithelium, disrupting vision and resulting in blindness if not repaired surgically
retinitis ret-i-nī′tis	inflammation of the retina
strabismus stra-biz′mŭs **heterotropia** het′er-ō-trō′pē-ă	a condition of eye misalignment caused by intraocular muscle imbalance (strabismus = a squinting; hetero = other) (Fig. 12.8)
esotropia es-ō-trō′pē-ă	right or left eye deviates inward toward nose (eso = inward; tropo = turning)
exotropia ek-sō-trō′pē-ă	right or left eye deviates outward away from nose (exo = out; tropo = turning)
scleritis sklĕ-rī′tis	inflammation of the sclera
trichiasis trĭ-kī′ă-sis	misdirected eyelashes that rub on conjunctiva or cornea

Diagnostic Tests and Procedures

Test or Procedure	Explanation
distance visual acuity	a measure of the ability to see the details and shape of identifiable objects from a specified distance (usually 20 feet), typically using a Snellen Chart (Fig. 12.9)
fluorescein angiography flūr-es'ē-in an-jē-og'rǎ-fē	visualization and photography of retinal and choroidal vessels made as fluorescein dye, which is injected into a vein, circulates through the eye
ophthalmoscopy of-thal-mos'kō-pē	use of an ophthalmoscope to view the interior of the eye (see Color Atlas, plate 25)
slit lamp biomicroscopy bi'ō-mi-kros'kǒ-pē	use of a tabletop microscope used to examine the eye, especially the cornea, lens, fluids, and membranes (Fig. 12.10)
sonography sǒ-nog'rǎ-fē	use of high-frequency sound waves to detect pathology within the eye such as foreign bodies, detached retina, etc.
tonometry tō-nom'ě-trē	use of a tonometer to measure intraocular pressure—elevated in glaucoma (Fig. 12.11)

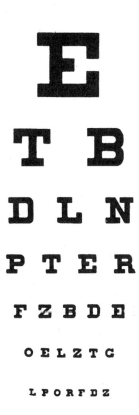

Figure 12.9. Snellen eye chart for testing distance visual acuity.

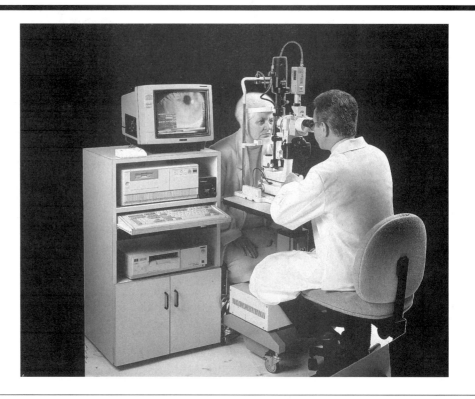

Figure 12.10. Slit lamp biomicroscope.

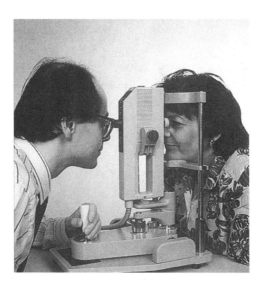

Figure 12.11. Tonometer.

Operative Terms

Term	Meaning
blepharoplasty blef'ă-ro-plast-tē	surgical repair of an eyelid
cataract extraction kat'ă-rakt ek-strak'shŭn	excision of a cloudy lens from the eye
cryoretinopexy krī-ō-ret'i-nō-pek-se **cryopexy**	use of intense cold to seal a hole or tear in the retina; used to treat retinal detachment
dacryocystectomy dak'rē-ō-sis-tek'tō-mē	excision of a lacrimal sac
enucleation ē-nū-klē-ā'shŭn	excision of an eyeball
iridectomy ir'i-dek'tō-mē	excision of a portion of iris tissue
iridotomy ir-i-dot'ō-mē	incision into the iris (usually with a laser) to allow for drainage of aqueous humor from the posterior to anterior chamber; used to treat a type of glaucoma
keratoplasty ker'ă-tō-plas-tē	corneal transplant
laser surgery	use of a laser to make incisions or destroy tissues (e.g., to create fluid passages, obliterate tumors, aneurysms, etc.) (Fig. 12.12)

continued

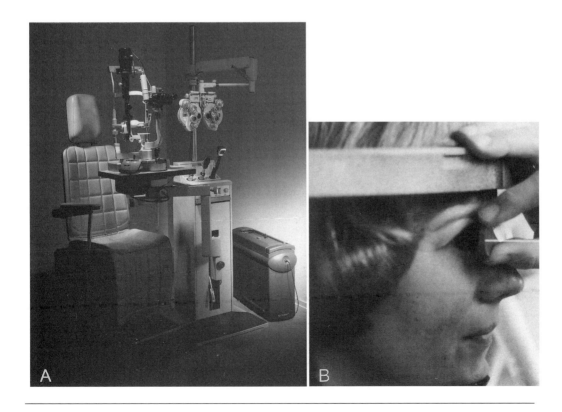

Figure 12.12. A. Ultima 2000 Argon Laser System. **B.** Placement of contact laser lens for laser treatment.

Term	Meaning
intraocular lens (IOL) implant in′tră-ok′yū-lăr	implantation of an artificial lens to replace a defective natural lens (e.g., after cataract extraction) (Fig. 12.13)
phacoemulsification fak′ō-ē-mŭl-si-fi-kā′shŭn	use of ultrasound to shatter and break up a cataract with aspiration and removal
radial keratotomy ker′ă-tot′ō-mē	technique designed to decrease myopia by making multiple symmetrical, spoke-like incisions in the cornea, allowing it to flatten centrally
trabeculectomy tră-bek′yū-lek′tō-mē	removal of a portion of the trabeculum to increase the flow of aqueous humor from the eye; used in treatment of glaucoma

Therapeutic Terms

Term	Meaning
contact lens	a small plastic curved disc with optical correction that fits over the cornea; used to correct refractive errors
eye instillation	introduction of a medicated solution in the eye
eye irrigation	washing of the eye with water or other fluid (e.g., saline)

continued

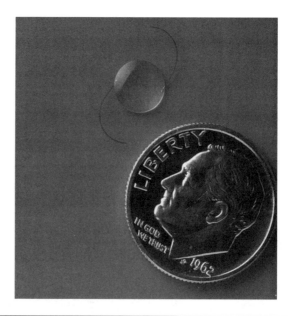

Figure 12.13. Intraocular lens and dime.

Term	Meaning

Common Therapeutic Drug Classifications

antibiotic ophthalmic solution an'tē-bī-ot'ik of-thal'mik	antimicrobial agent in solution, used to treat bacterial infections (e.g., conjunctivitis, corneal ulcers, etc.)
mydriatic (dilation of pupil) mi-drē-at'ik	an agent that causes dilation of the pupil (e.g., for certain eye examinations)
miotic mī-ot'ik	an agent that causes the pupil to contract (mio = less)

PRACTICE EXERCISES

For the following terms, draw a line or lines to separate prefixes, combining forms, and suffixes. Then define the term.

1. blepharoptosis _____

2. iridotomy _____

3. ophthalmology _____

4. vitrectomy _____

5. dacryocystitis _____

6. lacrimal _____

7. corneoscleral _____

8. keratotomy _____

9. blepharoplasty _____

10. dacryocystorhinostomy _____

11. photophobia _____

12. optical _____

13. scleromalacia _____

14. ocular _____

15. sclerostomy _____

Match the following terms for refractive disorders with their meanings:

16. myopia _____ a. old age loss of accommodation

17. strabismus _____ b. nearsightedness

18. presbyopia _____ c. farsightedness

19. astigmatism _____ d. crossed eyes

20. hyperopia _____ e. distorted vision

Complete the following medical term by writing the missing part:

21. _____ itis = inflammation of the cornea

22. _____ phobia = extreme sensitivity to light

23. dacryo _____ ectomy = excision of a tear sac

24. _____ ophthalmos = protrusion of the eyeball

25. _____ chalasis = baggy eyelids

Briefly define the following medical terms:

26. entropion _____

27. diplopia _____

28. tonometer _____

29. ectropion _____

30. scotoma _____

Write the correct medical term for each of the following:

31. pinkeye _____

32. inflammation of the eyelid _____

33. eyestrain _____

34. an agent that causes dilation of the pupil _____

35. absence of the lens of the eye _____

36. sty; acute infection of a sebaceous gland of the eyelid _____ _____

37. clouding of the lens causing decreased vision _____

38. breakdown or thinning of the tissues in the macula, resulting in partial or complete loss of central vision

_____

39. involuntary contraction of the muscles surrounding the eye

_____

40. an involuntary, rapid oscillating movement of the eyeball

_____

Medical Record Analysis

MEDICAL RECORD 12.1

Not long ago Cassandre Aquero had cataract surgery for her left eye and is now losing vision in her right eye because of another cataract. She is consulting an ophthalmologist, Dr. Oanh Tran, about surgery on the right eye.

Directions

Read Medical Record 12.1 for Ms. Aquero (pages 343–344) and answer the following questions. This record is the history and physical examination written by Dr. Tran in planning for her surgery.

Questions about Medical Record 12.1

Write your answers in the spaces provided.

1. Below are medical terms used in this record you have not yet encountered in this text. Underline each where it appears in the record and define below.

   appendectomy _____

   irides _____

2. In your own words, briefly describe Ms. Aquero's current complaint and diagnosis noted under "History of Present Illness."

   _____

   _____

   _____

3. Describe in lay language the two medical conditions Ms. Aquero has in addition to her current problem and past surgeries.

   _____

   _____

   _____

4. Which of the following findings on physical examination is related to her general medical condition in addition to her eye problems?

   a. rales on auscultation

   b. disoriented consciousness

   c. BP 180/100

   d. weight 135 lb

5. The planned operation involves several risks that the patient has accepted in the hopes of regaining good eyesight. Which of the following was *not* mentioned by Dr. Tran as a risk:

   a. hypertensive crisis

   b. retinal detachment

   c. edema of the macula

   d. bleeding

6. The preoperative nursing staff will ensure Ms. Aquero receives five medications before surgery. Translate the instructions for these:

   a. _____

   b. _____

   c. _____

   d. _____

   e. _____

7. In your own words, not using medical terminology, briefly describe what will occur in the surgery.

   _____

   _____

   _____

CENTRAL MEDICAL GROUP, INC.

Department of Ophthalmology

201 Medical Center Drive • Central City, US 90000-1234 • PHONE: (012) 125-8888 • FAX: (012) 125-3434

HISTORY

HISTORY OF PRESENT ILLNESS:

This 57-year-old female complains of progressive loss of vision in the right eye over the last two years which has been diagnosed as a cataract. The patient recently underwent cataract surgery in the left eye and is currently scheduled for surgery in the right eye due to her decreased vision.

PAST MEDICAL HISTORY:

The patient has had the normal childhood diseases and has essential hypertension and hypo-thyroidism.

SURGERIES: Appendectomy 40 years ago. Tonsillectomy and adenoidectomy as a child. Cataract surgery in the left eye with a posterior chamber lens implant in 199x.

ALLERGIES: None.

MEDICATIONS: Inderal 80 mg b.i.d. Hydrochlorothiazide 50 mg b.i.d. Clonidine, 0.1 mg, 2 tablets p.o. t.i.d. Synthroid 0.1 mg q.d. Slow-K 2 tablets p.o. q.d.

PHYSICAL EXAMINATION

VITAL SIGNS:

WEIGHT: 135 lb. BLOOD PRESSURE: 180/100.

HEENT:

HEAD, EARS, NOSE, THROAT: Normal.

EYES: Best corrected visual acuity in the right eye is counting fingers at two feet and 20/50 in the left eye. Pinhole vision in the left eye is 20/30. Slit lamp examination reveals normal lids, conjunctivae, and sclerae. Corneas are clear. Anterior chambers are clear and deep. Irides are within normal limits in the right eye. Evaluation of the lens reveals a 4+ posterior subcapsular plaquing with 3-4+ nuclear sclerosis, and in the left eye, there is a posterior chamber lens that is in place with posterior lens capsular plaquing. Intraocular pressure: OD: 18. OS: 17. Fundus examination in the right eye was severely hindered due to the dense cataract. However, evaluation of the posterior pole in the right eye was within normal limits.

(continued)

HISTORY AND PHYSICAL Page 1	PT. NAME: AQUERO,CASSANDRE D. ID NO: 008654 ATT PHYS: O. TRAN, M.D.

Medical Record 12.1.

CENTRAL MEDICAL GROUP, INC.

Department of Ophthalmology

201 Medical Center Drive • Central City, US 90000-1234 • PHONE: (012) 125-8888 • FAX: (012) 125-3434

PHYSICAL EXAMINATION

CHEST:
Clear to percussion and auscultation. The breasts were normal, and the lungs were clear.

PELVIC/RECTAL:
Within normal limits.

EXTREMITIES:
Within normal limits.

NEUROLOGICAL:
Within normal limits.

IMPRESSION:
1)   Cataract, right eye.
2)   Pseudophakia, left eye.
3)   Essential hypertension.
4)   Hypothyroidism.

RISKS/BENEFITS:
The patient is aware of the alternatives, risks, benefits, and possible complications of the procedure that include hemorrhage, infection, loss of vision, reoperation, retinal detachment, macular edema; and the patient still desires to undergo the procedure.

PLAN:
Extracapsular cataract extraction with posterior chamber lens implant under local anesthesia using a +21 diopter posterior chamber lens with the ultraviolet filter. Preoperative medication will consist of the patient's morning dose of Inderal, 80 mg; Hydrochlorothiazide, 50 mg; Clonidine, 0.2 mg; and Diamox, 250 mg with ¼ glass of water at approximately 10 a.m. on the day of surgery. The patient was also instructed to take Maxitrol, 1 gt OD, q 3 h starting 24 hours prior to the procedure, while awake.

O. Tran, M.D.

OT:mk
D: 10/19/9x   T: 10/20/9x

HISTORY AND PHYSICAL Page 2	PT. NAME: AQUERO, CASSANDRE D. ID NO: 008654 ATT PHYS: O. TRAN, M.D.

Medical Record 12.1. *Continued.*

Ear

OBJECTIVES

After completion of this chapter you will be able to

1. Define common combining forms used in relation to the ear

2. Locate and name the major structures of the ear

3. Define common symptomatic, diagnostic, operative, and therapeutic terms referring to the ear

4. List the common diagnostic tests and procedures related to the ear

5. Explain the terms and abbreviations used in documenting medical records involving the ear

Combining Forms

Combining Form	Meaning	Example
acous/o	hearing	**acoustic** ă-kūs′tik
audi/o		**audiometry** aw-dē-om′ĕ-trē
aer/o	air or gas	**aerotitis** ār-ō-tī′tis
aur/i	ear	**auricle** aw′ri-kl
ot/o		**otology** ō-tol′ŏ-jē
cerumin/o	wax	**ceruminosis** se-rū-mi-nō′sis
salping/o	eustachian tube or uterine tube	**salpingoscope** sal-ping′gō-skōp
tympan/o	eardrum	**tympanic** tim-pan′ik
myring/o		**myringotomy** mir-ing-got′ō-mē
-acusis (additional suffix)	hearing condition	**presbyacusis** prez′bē-ă-kū′sis

Overview of the Ear

The sense of hearing occurs through the mechanical action of the ear and its three divisions: outer ear, middle ear, and inner ear (Fig. 13.1) (see Color Atlas, plate 26)

Sounds are gathered by the projections of the *external ear* called the *pinna*, or auricle, and then dispersed through the external auditory canal to the *tympanum*, or eardrum, of the middle ear. Glands located throughout the external canal secrete a protective, waxy substance called *cerumen*.

The tympanum transmits sound vibrations through the auditory ossicles—*incus, malleus,* and *stapes*—to the oval window. Vibrations are increased as they are distributed from the tympanum to the incus, malleus, and stapes. When the stapes, held by a ligament called the *oval window*, vibrates, it stimulates the motion of the auditory fluids in the inner ear.

Within the *middle ear*, the *eustachian tube* or *auditory tube* provides a passageway to the throat, allowing air to pass to and from the outside of the body. This process is important for maintaining equal air pressure.

Located within the temporal bone of the skull, the *inner ear* receives sound vibrations passed from the oval window to the *cochlea*, the outer structure of the inner ear, that is part of the intricate intercommunicating tubes and chambers known as the *labyrinth*. Vibrations are passed through *perilymph*, a fluid within an area of the cochlea called the *scala vestibuli*, to the cochlear duct, which is filled with a fluid called *endolymph*. Finally, the vibrations are passed through the *organ of Corti* where hairs along its lining stimulate surrounding nerve fibers, generating impulses that then travel to the brain for processing of hearing.

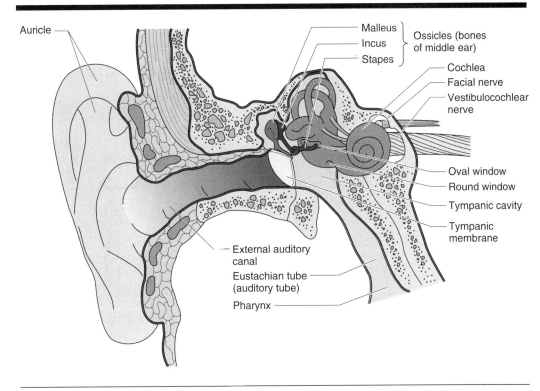

Figure 13.1. Anatomy of the ear.

TYMPANUM. Tympanum is the Latin word for tambourine or kettledrum, percussion instruments that are struck or beaten. Use of the term for eardrum was first introduced in 1255 and was adopted by the famous anatomist, Gabrielle Fallopius, because of the likeness of the eardrum to a tambourine.

In addition to hearing, the labyrinth is responsible for the equilibrium within the body. Within the labyrinth the *semicircular canals* are connected to the cochlea by a cavity called the *vestibule*. Within the vestibule are structures known as the *utricle* and *saccule*. Hair cells and surrounding nerve fibers within the canals that connect with the utricle respond to and are moved by endolymph to stimulate nerve conduction when changes in movement occur.

Anatomical Terms

Term	Meaning
external ear	
pinna pin′ă	auricle (little ear); projected part of the external ear (pinna = feather)
external auditory canal	external passage for sounds collected from the pinna to the tympanum
cerumen sĕ-rū′men	a waxy substance secreted by glands located throughout the external canal
middle ear	
tympanic membrane (TM) tim-pan′ik mem′brān	eardrum; drum-like structure that receives sound collected in the external auditory canal and amplifies it through the middle ear (see Color Atlas, plate 26)

continued

OSSICLE. Ossicle means a little bone; it is a diminutive of the Latin ossiculum meaning bone. Specifically ossicle means one of the small bones in the middle ear. The first authentic records indicate that the malleus and the incus were the first two to be discovered in 1514. The stapes was discovered around 1546.

Term	Meaning
malleus mal′ē-ŭs	hammer; first of the three auditory ossicles of the middle ear
incus ing′kŭs	anvil; middle of the three auditory ossicles of the middle ear
stapes stā′pēz	stirrup; last of the three auditory ossicles of the middle ear
eustachian tube yū-stā′shŭn **auditory tube**	tube connecting the middle ear to the pharynx (throat)
mastoid process mas′toyd	projection of the temporal bone (masto = breast)
oval window	membrane that covers the opening between the middle ear and inner ear
inner ear	structures and liquids that relay sound waves to the auditory nerve fibers on a path to the brain for interpretation of sound
labyrinth lab′i-rinth	maze; inner ear consisting of bony and membranous labyrinths
cochlea kok′lē-ă	coiled tubular structure of the inner ear that contains the organ of Corti (cochlea = snail)
perilymph per′i-limf	fluid that fills the bony labyrinth of the ear
endolymph en′dō-limf	fluid within the labyrinth of the ear
organ of Corti	organ located in the cochlea which contains receptors (hair cells) that receive vibrations and generate nerve impulses for hearing
vestibule ves′ti-būl	middle part of the inner ear in front of the semilunar canals and behind the cochlea that contains the utricle and the saccule
utricle ū′tri-kl	larger of two sacs within the membranous labyrinth of the vestibule in the inner ear (uter = leather bag)
saccule sak′yūl	smaller of two sacs within the membranous labyrinth of the vestibule in the inner ear (sacculus = small bag)
semicircular canals sem′ē-sir′kyū-lăr kă-nalz′	three canals within the inner ear that contain specialized receptor cells that generate nerve impulses with body movement

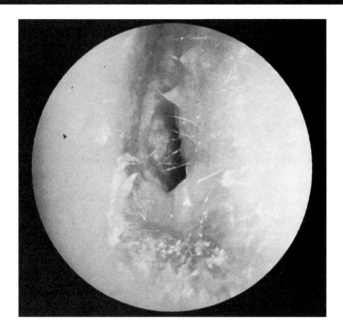

Figure 13.2. Otitis externa.

Symptomatic and Diagnostic Terms

Term	Meaning
Symptomatic	
anacusis an′ă-kū′sis	total hearing loss
otalgia ō-tal′jē-ă	earache
otorrhagia ō-tō-rā′jē-ă	bleeding from the ear
otorrhea ō-tō-rē′ă	purulent drainage from the ear
paracusis par′ă-kū′sis	impaired hearing
tinnitus ti-nī′tŭs	a jingling; ringing or buzzing in the ear
vertigo ver′ti-gō	a turning round; dizziness
Diagnostic	
otitis externa ō-tī′tis eks-ter′nă	inflammation of the external auditory canal (Fig. 13.2)
cerumen impaction sĕ-rū′men im-pak′shŭn	excessive buildup of wax in ear

continued

Term	Meaning
myringitis mir-in-jī′tis **tympanitis** tim-pă-nī′tis	inflammation of eardrum
otitis media ō-tī′tis mē′dē-ă	inflammation of the middle ear (see Color Atlas, plate 26)
aerotitis media ār-ō-tī′tis mē′dē-ă	inflammation of the middle ear from changes in atmospheric pressure; often occurs in frequent air travel
mastoiditis mas-toy-dī′tis	inflammation of the mastoid process
eustachian obstruction yū-stā′shŭn ob-strŭk′shŭn	blockage of the eustachian tube usually as a result of infection, as in otitis media
labyrinthitis lab′ĭ-rin-thī′tis	inflammation of the labyrinth
otosclerosis ō′tō-sklē-rō′sis	hardening of the bony tissue in the ear
deafness def′nes	general term for partial or complete hearing loss
conductive hearing loss kon-dŭk′tiv	hearing impairment caused by interference with sound or vibratory energy in the external canal, middle ear, or ossicles
sensorineural hearing loss sen′sōr-i-nū′răl	hearing impairment caused by lesions or dysfunction of the cochlea or auditory nerve
presbyacusis prez′bē-ă-kū′sis **presbycusis** prez-bē-kū′sis	hearing impairment in old age

Diagnostic Tests and Procedures

Test or Procedure	Explanation
audiometry aw-dē-om′ĕ-trē	process of measuring hearing (Fig. 13.3)
audiometer aw-dē-om′ĕ-ter	instrument to measure hearing
audiogram aw′dē-ō-gram	record of hearing measurement
audiologist aw-dē-ol′ō-jist	person who specializes in the study of hearing impairments
auditory acuity testing aw′di-tōr-ē ă-kyū′i-tē	physical assessment of hearing; useful in differentiating between conductive or sensorineural hearing loss (Fig. 13.4)
tuning fork	two-pronged, fork-like instrument that vibrates when struck: used to test for hearing, especially bone conduction

continued

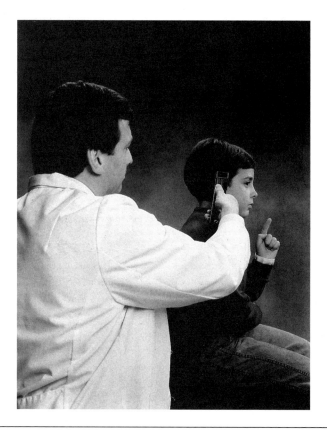

Figure 13.3. Audiometry: hearing screening.

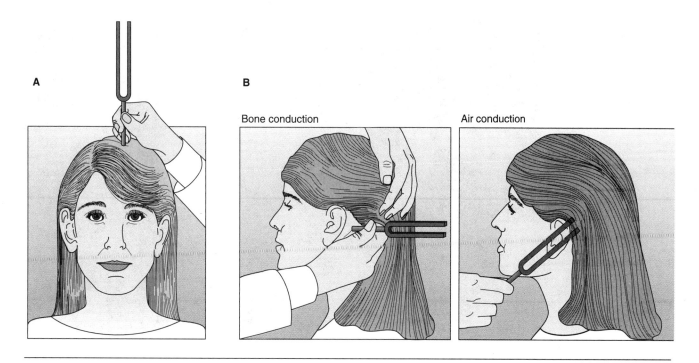

Figure 13.4. Tuning fork testing. **A.** Webber test. **B.** Rinne test.

Test or Procedure	Explanation
otoscopy ō-tos′kŏ-pē	use of an otoscope to examine the external auditory canal and tympanic membrane (Fig. 13.5) (see Color Atlas, plate 26)
tympanometry tim′pă-nom′ĕ-trē	measurement of the conductibility of the tympanic membrane and ossicles of the middle ear by monitoring the response after exposure to external airflow pressures

Operative Terms

Term	Meaning
microsurgery mī-krō-ser′jer-ē	surgery with the use of a microscope used in procedures involving delicate tissue such as the ear
myringotomy mir-ing-got′ŏ-mē	incision into the eardrum, most often for insertion of a small plastic tube made of polyethylene (PE) to keep the canal open, avoiding fluid buildup such as that which occurs as a result of otitis media (see Color Atlas, plate 26)
otoplasty ō′tō-plas-tē	surgical repair of the external ear

continued

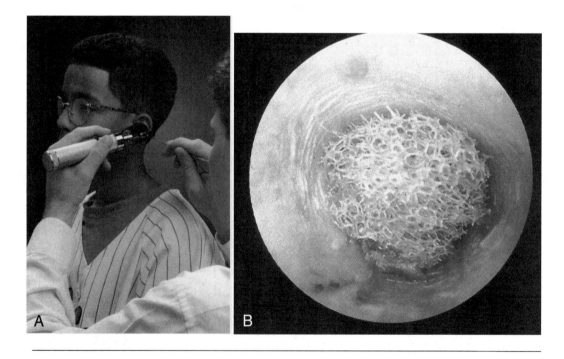

Figure 13.5. A. Otoscopic examination of external auditory canal. **B.** Otoscopic view of foreign body (sponge) in ear canal.

Term	Meaning
stapedectomy stā-pě-dek′tō-mē	excision of the stapes to correct otosclerosis
tympanoplasty tim′pă-nō-plas-tē	vein graft of a scarred tympanic membrane to improve sound conduction

Therapeutic Terms

Term	Meaning
ear lavage lă-vahzh′	irrigation of the external ear canal, commonly done to remove excessive buildup of cerumen
ear instillation in-sti-lā′shŭn	introduction of a medicated solution into the external canal

Common Therapeutic Drug Classifications

Term	Meaning
antibiotic an′tē-bī-ot′ik	drug that inhibits the growth of or destroys microorganisms; used to treat diseases caused by bacteria (e.g., otitis media)
antihistamine an-tē-his′tă-mēn	drug that blocks the effects of histamine
histamine his′tă-mēn	regulating body substance released in excess during allergic reactions causing swelling and inflammation of tissues; seen in hay fever, urticaria (hives), etc.
anti-inflammatory an′tē-in-flam′ă-tō-rē	a drug that reduces inflammation
decongestant dē-kon-jes′tant	a drug that reduces congestion and swelling of membranes, such as those of the nose and eustachian tube after infection

PRACTICE EXERCISES

For the following terms, draw a line or lines to separate prefixes, combining forms, and suffixes. Then define the term.

1. aerotitis _____

2. otosclerosis _____

3. myringoplasty _____

4. acoustic _____

5. tympanotomy _____

6. ceruminolysis _____

7. salpingoscope _____

8. otopyorrhea _____

9. audiometry _____

10. tympanocentesis _____

11. otodynia _____

12. audiogenic _____

13. myringectomy _____

14. ceruminal _____

15. tympanitis _____

Complete the medical term by writing the missing part:

16. oto_____osis = condition of hardening of the bony tissue of the ear

17. aero_____media = inflammation of the middle ear caused by changes in atmospheric pressure

18. _____logist = person who specializes in the study of hearing impairments

19. _____tomy = incision into the eardrum for the insertion of tubes

20. _____scope = instrument used to view the ear canal and tympanum

Write the correct medical term for each of the following:

21. inflammation of labyrinth _____

22. dizziness _____

23. bleeding from the ear _____

24. impaired hearing _____

25. hearing impairment of old age _____

26. ringing in the ear _____

27. excision of stapes to correct otosclerosis _____

28. excessive buildup of earwax _____

29. earache_____

30. the study of hearing _____

Medical Record Analysis

MEDICAL RECORD 13.1

Hank Ball, a preschooler, has had recurrent ear infections for one year that his doctor has not been able to treat successfully with antibiotics and other drugs. His preschool teacher also identified nasal speech patterns that his doctor later confirmed were related to his medical problems. After seeing several doctors who recommended surgery, Hank's parents have admitted him to Central Medical Center.

Directions

Read Medical Record 13.1 for Hank Ball (pages 359–361) and answer the following questions. These records are the history and physical examination before surgery and the subsequent operative report, both dictated by Dr. Baird, the surgeon.

Questions about Medical Record 13.1

Write your answers in the spaces provided.

1. Below are medical terms used in this record you have not yet encountered in this text. Underline each where it appears in the record and define below.

   hepatosplenomegaly _____

   turbinates _____

   extubation _____

2. In the left column, list the patient's medical problems noted in the HPI; in the right column write the diagnosis that pertains to each.

	Medical Problem	Diagnosis
a.	_____	
	_____	_____
b.	_____	
	_____	_____

3. In your own words explain how Hank's social history is related to his medical history.

   _____

   _____

   _____

4. Under the "Review of Systems" were any additional medical symptoms or problems identified? If so, list below.

   _____

   _____

5. What does it mean that at the time of the examination Hank was afebrile?

    _____

6. Carefully read the physical examination. Mark the body areas/systems in which Dr. Baird found any abnormalities.

    _____ general

    _____ HEENT

    _____ chest

    _____ back

    _____ rectal/genitalia

    _____ extremities

7. List the surgical procedures identified under "Plan" and briefly describe them in your own words, not using medical terminology.

    a. _____

    _____

    _____

    _____

    b. _____

    _____

    _____

    _____

    c. _____

    _____

    _____

    _____

8. In your own words, not using medical terminology, briefly describe oral intubation.

    _____

    _____

    _____

9. Put the following operative actions in correct order by numbering them 1 to 11:

_____ removal of adenoids

_____ incision in right eardrum

_____ PE tube placement in right tympanum

_____ repositioning in Rose's position

_____ incision in left eardrum

_____ aspiration of right middle ear

_____ extubation

_____ removal of wax in right ear

_____ nasopharynx examination

_____ polyethylene tube placement in left tympanum

_____ intubation

10. In your own words, not using medical terminology, briefly describe the condition of Hank's adenoids before adenoidectomy.

_____

_____

_____

CENTRAL MEDICAL CENTER

211 Medical Center Drive • Central City, US 90000-1234 • PHONE: (012) 125-6784 • FAX: (012) 125-9999

HISTORY

DATE OF ADMISSION: August 28, 199x

HISTORY OF PRESENT ILLNESS: The patient is a 4-year-old white male with recurrent ear infections and ear congestion nonresponsive to antibiotic and decongestant therapy over the past 12 months. The patient also has a history of nasal obstruction and nasal speech. The patient is being admitted for myringotomy, polyethylene tubes, and examination of the nasopharynx and adenoidectomy. The patient has also seen other doctors who have recommended surgery, including Dr. Feldman and Dr. Saunders.

PAST MEDICAL HISTORY: Medications: None. Allergies: None. Hospitalizations: None. Surgeries: None. Childhood Diseases: Normal.

FAMILY HISTORY: No cancer or diabetes, although the patient's grandparents have a history of adult-onset diabetes.

SOCIAL HISTORY: Normal development except for speech.

REVIEW OF SYSTEMS: CARDIOVASCULAR: No hypertension and no heart murmurs. PULMONARY: No croup or asthma. GASTROINTESTINAL: No hepatitis. RENAL: Negative. ENDOCRINE: No diabetes. MUSCULOSKELETAL: No joint disease. HEMATOLOGIC: `No anemia or bleeding tendencies.

(continued)

R. Baird, M.D.

RB:nn

D: 8/28/9x
T: 8/29/9x

HISTORY AND PHYSICAL Page 1	PT. NAME: BALL, HANK F. ID NO: OP-372201 ROOM: OPS ADM. DATE: August 28, 199x ATT. PHYS: R. BAIRD, M.D.

Medical Record 13.1.

CENTRAL MEDICAL CENTER

211 Medical Center Drive • Central City, US 90000-1234 • PHONE: (012) 125-6784 • FAX: (012) 125-9999

PHYSICAL EXAMINATION

GENERAL: The patient is alert and afebrile.

HEENT: TMs are dull and slightly retracted; there is decreased mobility. There is dull light reflex bilaterally. No sinus tenderness on percussion of the maxillary or frontal sinuses; there are swollen turbinates on nasal examination. The oropharynx shows hypertrophic tonsils, and there are hypertrophic adenoids on examination of the nasopharynx.

CHEST: LUNGS: Clear to percussion and auscultation. HEART: Pulse: 88 and regular. There are no murmurs, gallops, or rubs. ABDOMEN: There are no masses or tenderness. No hepatosplenomegaly was noted. There was no costovertebral angle (CVA) tenderness.

BACK: Supple. There are no masses or tenderness. There is mild anterior cervical adenopathy.

RECTAL/GENITALIA: Deferred.

EXTREMITIES: There was no peripheral edema, and there were no ecchymoses.

IMPRESSION: CHRONIC OTITIS MEDIA WITH EFFUSION, NASAL SPEECH, AND NASAL OBSTRUCTION SECONDARY TO ADENOID HYPERTROPHY.

PLAN: The patient is to be admitted as an outpatient for adenoidectomy, myringotomy, and polyethylene (PE) tubes as noted above. The surgery and potential risks and complications have been discussed with the grandfather and mother as well as the possible need for further repeat myringotomy and PE tubes.

R. Baird, M.D.

RB:nn

D: 8/28/9x
T: 8/29/9x

HISTORY AND PHYSICAL Page 2	PT. NAME:	BALL, HANK F.
	ID NO:	OP-372201
	ROOM NO:	OPS
	ADM. DATE:	August 28, 199x
	ATT. PHYS:	R. BAIRD, M.D.

Medical Record 13.1. *Continued.*

CENTRAL MEDICAL CENTER

211 Medical Center Drive • Central City, US 90000-1234 • PHONE: (012) 125-6784 • FAX: (012) 125-9999

OPERATIVE REPORT

DATE OF OPERATION: August 28, 199x

PREOPERATIVE DIAGNOSIS: Chronic otitis media with effusion bilaterally and nasal obstruction with chronic adenoiditis and adenoid hypertrophy.

POSTOPERATIVE DIAGNOSIS: Chronic otitis media with effusion bilaterally and adenoid hypertrophy and chronic adenoiditis.

OPERATION PERFORMED: Bilateral myringotomy and tubes with adenoidectomy.

SURGEON: R. Baird, M.D.

ANESTHESIOLOGIST: F. Kodama, M.D.

PROCEDURE AND FINDINGS: After general anesthesia induction and oral intubation, the patient's ears were prepped and draped in the usual manner for microscopic myringotomy surgery. A myringotomy in the right ear was carried out following debridement of cerumen. Incision of the circumferential inferior anterior quadrant was carried out. Mucoid material was aspirated from the middle ear. A Shepard polyethylene tube was placed in position without difficulty. Cotton dressing was applied to the ear. The left ear was examined. A similar dull, nonmobile TM was noted. An inferior anterior myringotomy was carried out again, and thick mucoid material was aspirated. A Shepard polyethylene tube was inserted again in the left ear. Cotton dressing was applied to the ear canal. The patient was repositioned in the Rose's position for examination of the nasopharynx which was carried out with a palate retractor, McIvor mouth gag, tongue retractor, and was stabilized with the Mayo stand. The marked adenoid hypertrophy was noted, and the adenoidectomy was carried out with curette technique. The patient tolerated the procedure well, and following extubation, he was sent back to the recovery room in satisfactory postoperative condition.

FINAL DIAGNOSIS: Chronic otitis media with effusion bilaterally, with chronic adenoiditis, adenoid hypertrophy, and nasal obstruction.

R. Baird, M.D.

RB:as
D: 8/28/9x   T: 8/29/9x

OPERATIVE REPORT
Page 1

PT. NAME: BALL, HANK F.
ID NO: OP-372201
ROOM NO: OPS
ATT. PHYS: R. BAIRD, M.D.

Medical Record 13.1. *Continued.*

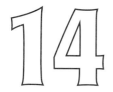

CHAPTER

Gastrointestinal System

OBJECTIVES

After completion of this chapter you will be able to

1. Define common combining forms used in relation to the gastrointestinal system

2. Define the basic anatomical terms referring to the gastrointestinal system

3. Name accessory organs of the gastrointestinal system

4. Identify clinical and anatomical divisions of the abdomen

5. Define common symptomatic, diagnostic, operative, and therapeutic terms referring to the gastrointestinal system

6. List common diagnostic tests and procedures related to the gastrointestinal system

7. Explain the terms and abbreviations used in documenting medical records involving the gastrointestinal system

Combining Forms

Combining Form	Meaning	Example
abdomin/o	abdomen	abdominocentesis ab-dom′i-nō-sen-tē′sis
celi/o		celiocentesis sē′lē-ō-sen-tē′sis
lapar/o		laparoscopy lap-ă-ros′kŏ-pē
an/o	anus	anal ā′năl
appendic/o	appendix	appendical ă-pen′di-kăl
bil/i	bile	biligenic bil-i-jen′ik
chol/e		cholelithiasis kō′lē-li-thī′ă-sis
bucc/o	cheek	buccal bŭk′ăl
cheil/o	lip	cheiloplasty kī′lō-plas-tē
choledoch/o	common bile duct	choledochotomy kō-led-ō-kot′ō-mē
col/o	colon	colitis kō-lī′tis
colon/o		colonoscopy kō-lon-os′kŏ-pē
dent/i	teeth	dental den′tăl
duoden/o	duodenum	duodenal dū′ō-dē′năl
enter/o	small intestine	enterocele en′ter-ō-sēl
esophag/o	esophagus	esophageal ē-sof′ă-jē′ăl
gastr/o	stomach	gastritis gas-trī′tis
gingiv/o	gum	gingivitis jin-ji-vī′tis
gloss/o	tongue	glossitis glo-sī′tis
lingu/o		lingual ling′gwăl

continued

Combining Form	Meaning	Example
hepat/o	liver	**hepatomegaly** hep′ă-tō-meg′ă-lē
hepatic/o		**hepaticotomy** he-pat-i-kot′ō-mē
herni/o	hernia	**herniorrhaphy** her′nē-ōr′ă-fē
ile/o	ileum	**ileostomy** il′ē-os′tō-mē
inguin/o	groin	**inguinal** ing′gwi-năl
jejun/o	jejunum (empty)	**jejunitis** je-jū-nī′tis
lith/o	stone	**lithiasis** li-thī′ă-sis
or/o	mouth	**oral** or′ăl
stomat/o		**stomatosis** stō-mă-tō′sis
pancreat/o	pancreas	**pancreatitis** pan′krē-ă-tī′tis
peritone/o	peritoneum	**peritoneoscopy** per′i-tō-nē-os′kŏ-pē
phag/o	eat or swallow	**aphagia** ă-fā′jē-ă
proct/o	rectum	**proctology** prok-tol′ō-jē
rect/o		**rectocele** rek′tō-sēl
pylor/o	pylorus (gatekeeper)	**pyloric** pī-lōr′ik
sial/o	saliva	**sialolithiasis** sī′ă-lō-li-thī′ă-sis
sigmoid/o	sigmoid colon (resembles s)	**sigmoidoscopy** sig′moy-dos′kŏ-pē
steat/o	fat	**steatolysis** stē-ă-tol′i-sis
-emesis (additional suffix)	vomiting	**hematemesis** hē-mă-tem′ĕ-sis

Gastrointestinal System Overview

The gastrointestinal (GI) system processes and transports nutrients and various wastes. The organs form a tube or tract, known as the *alimentary canal*, extending from the mouth to the anus. The alimentary canal is composed of the mouth, pharynx, esophagus, stomach and intestines (see Color Atlas, plate 27) (Fig. 14.1).

The gastrointestinal system has three functions: digestion, absorption, and excretion. *Digestion* is the process by which food is broken down by chewing and swallowing and is then mixed with digestive juices in the stomach to convert some of the food into absorbable molecules. *Absorption* is the passage of digested food molecules through the walls of the intestines into the bloodstream to be carried to the body cells. *Excretion* is the elimination of materials that are not absorbed (waste products) by transporting them to the outside of the body.

The accessory organs that aid in the digestion and absorption of food are the teeth, salivary glands, liver, gallbladder, and pancreas.

Anatomical Terms

Term	Meaning
oral cavity **mouth**	cavity that receives food for digestion
salivary glands sal'i-vār-ē	three pairs of exocrine glands in the mouth that secrete saliva: parotid, submandibular (submaxillary), and sublingual
cheeks	lateral walls of the mouth
lips	fleshy structures surrounding the mouth
palate pal'ăt	structure that forms the roof of the mouth; it is divided into the hard and soft palate
uvula yū'vyū-lă	small projection hanging from the back middle edge of the soft palate
tongue	muscular structure of the floor of the mouth covered by mucous membrane and held down by a band-like membrane known as the *frenulum*
gums	tissue covering the processes of the jaws
teeth	hard bony projections in the jaws that serve to masticate (chew) food
pharynx far'ingks	throat; passageway for food traveling to the esophagus and air traveling to the larynx
esophagus ē-sof'ă-gŭs	muscular tube that moves food from the pharynx to the stomach
stomach stŭm'ŭk	sac-like organ that chemically mixes and prepares food received from the esophagus
cardiac sphincter kar'dē-ak sfingk'ter	opening from esophagus to stomach (sphincter = band)

continued

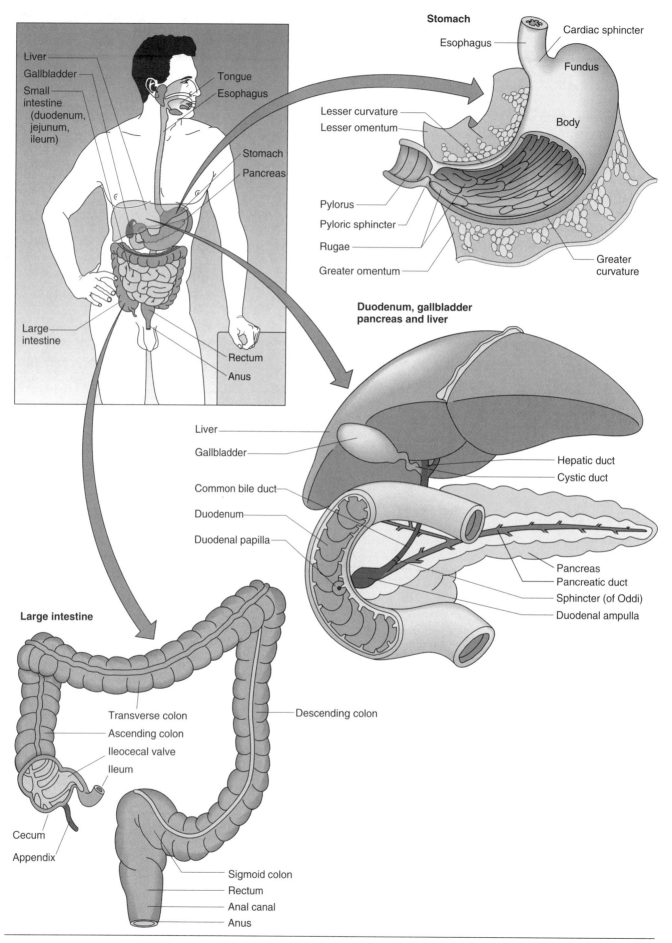

Figure 14.1. Gastrointestinal system.

Term	Meaning
pyloric sphincter pī-lōr'ik sfingk'ter	opening of the stomach into the duodenum
small intestine in-tes'tin	tubular structure that digests food received from the stomach
duodenum dū-ō-dē'nŭm	first portion of the small intestine
jejunum jĕ-jū'nŭm	second portion of the small intestine
ileum il'ē-ŭm	third portion of the small intestine
large intestine	larger tubular structure that receives the liquid waste products of digestion, reabsorbs water and minerals, and forms and stores feces for defecation
cecum se'kŭm	first part of the large intestine
vermiform appendix ver'mi-fōrm ă-pen'diks	worm-like projection of lymphatic tissue hanging off the cecum with no digestive function—may serve to resist infection (vermi = worm)
colon kō'lon	portions of the large intestine extending from the cecum to the rectum identified by direction or shape
ascending colon as-send'ing	portion that extends upward from the cecum
transverse colon trans-vers'	portion that extends across from the ascending cecum
descending colon dē-send'ing	portion that extends down from the transverse colon
sigmoid colon sig'moyd	portion (resembling an s) that terminates at the rectum
rectum rek'tŭm	distal (end) portion of the large intestine
rectal ampulla rek'tăl am-pūl'lă	dilated portion of the rectum just above the anal canal
anus ā'nŭs	opening of the rectum to the outside of the body
feces fē'sēz	refuse; solid waste formed in the large intestine
defecation def-ĕ-kā'shŭn	evacuation of feces from the rectum

DUODENUM. The Latin word for 12 is the origin of the name for the first part of the small intestine because the length of the structure was estimated to be 12 fingerbreadths.

JEJUNUM. The Latin word meaning empty or hungry was used for the portion of the small intestine that follows the duodenum because the ancients noted it was always empty after death.

continued

Term	Meaning
peritoneum per'i-tō-neŭm	membrane surrounding the entire abdominal cavity consisting of the parietal layer (lining the abdominal wall) and visceral layer (covering each organ in the abdomen)
peritoneal cavity per-i-tō-nē'ăl	space between the parietal and visceral peritoneum
omentum ō-men'tŭm	a covering; an extension of the peritoneum attached to the stomach and connecting it with other abdominal organs
liver	organ in the upper right quadrant that produces bile, which is secreted into the duodenum during digestion
gallbladder gawl'blad-er	receptacle that stores and concentrates the bile produced in the liver
pancreas pan'krē-as	gland that secretes pancreatic juice into the duodenum, where it mixes with bile to digest food
biliary ducts bil'ē-ār-ē	ducts that convey bile, including hepatic, cystic, and common bile ducts

HYPOCHONDRIAC. This Greek word meaning below the cartilage was used to refer to regions below the cartilages of the ribs. In these hypochondriac regions various sensations of a distressing nature were sometimes experienced without apparent organic disease. Persons with such complaints were called hypochondriacs. Today hypochondria refers to one who has an abnormal concern for one's health with the false belief that he or she is suffering from disease.

Anatomical and Clinical Divisions of the Abdomen

Anatomical and clinical divisions of the abdomen provide specific or general reference for descriptive purposes. There are nine specific anatomical divisions and four general clinical divisions (Figs. 14.2–14.4). All references are based on the *patient's* right or left.

Anatomical Divisions

Region	Location
hypochondriac regions hī-pō-kon'drē-ak	upper lateral regions beneath the ribs
epigastric region ep-i-gas'trik	upper middle region below the sternum
lumbar regions lŭm'bar	middle lateral regions
umbilical region ŭm-bil'i-kăl	region of the navel
inguinal regions ing'gwi-năl	lower lateral groin regions
hypogastric region hī-pō-gas'trik	region below the navel

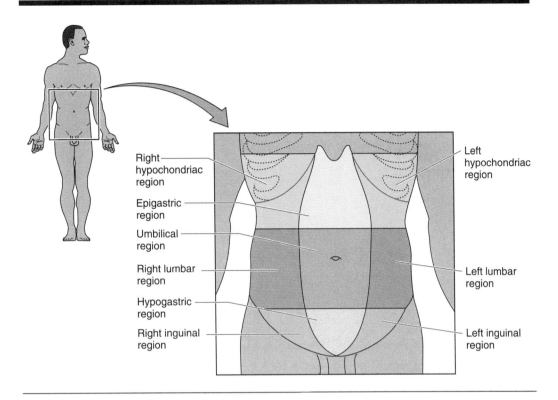

Figure 14.2. Anatomical divisions of abdomen.

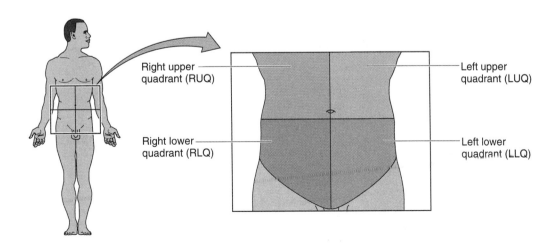

Figure 14.3. Clinical divisions of abdomen.

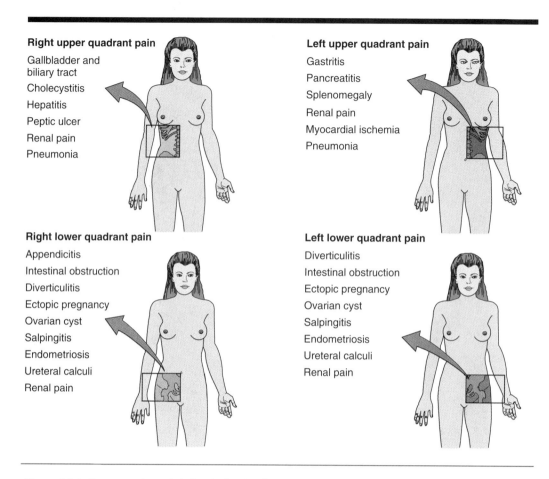

Right upper quadrant pain

Gallbladder and
biliary tract
Cholecystitis
Hepatitis
Peptic ulcer
Renal pain
Pneumonia

Left upper quadrant pain

Gastritis
Pancreatitis
Splenomegaly
Renal pain
Myocardial ischemia
Pneumonia

Right lower quadrant pain

Appendicitis
Intestinal obstruction
Diverticulitis
Ectopic pregnancy
Ovarian cyst
Salpingitis
Endometriosis
Ureteral calculi
Renal pain

Left lower quadrant pain

Diverticulitis
Intestinal obstruction
Ectopic pregnancy
Ovarian cyst
Salpingitis
Endometriosis
Ureteral calculi
Renal pain

Figure 14.4. Common sites of abdominal pain characteristic of various conditions.

Symptomatic and Diagnostic Terms

Term	Meaning
Symptomatic	
anorexia an-ō-rek′sē-ă	loss of appetite (orexis = appetite)
aphagia ă-fā′jē-ă	inability to swallow
ascites ă-sī′tēz	an accumulation of fluid in the peritoneal cavity (ascos = bag) (Fig. 14.5)
buccal bŭk′ăl	in the cheek
diarrhea dī-ă-rē′ă	frequent loose or liquid stools
dyspepsia dis-pep′sē-ă	indigestion (peptein = to digest)
dysphagia dis-fā′jē-ă	difficulty in swallowing

continued

Term	Meaning
eructation ē-rŭk-tā'shŭn	belch
flatulence flat'yū-lens	gas in the stomach or intestines (flatus = a blowing)
halitosis hal-i-tō'sis	bad breath (halitus = breath)
hematochezia hē'mă-tō-kē'zē-ă	red blood in stool (chezo = defecate)
hematemesis hē-mă-tem'ě-sis	vomiting blood
hepatomegaly hep'ă-tō-meg'ă-lē	enlargement of the liver
hyperbilirubinemia hī'per-bil'i-rū-bi-nē'mē-ă	excessive level of bilirubin (bile pigment) in the blood
icterus ik'ter-ŭs **jaundice** jawn'dis	yellow discoloration of the skin, sclera (white of the eye), and other tissues caused by excessive bilirubin in the blood (jaundice = yellow)

ASCITES. A Greek word for pouch or sac referring to the appearance of the abdomen with the collection of fluid in the peritoneal cavity.

continued

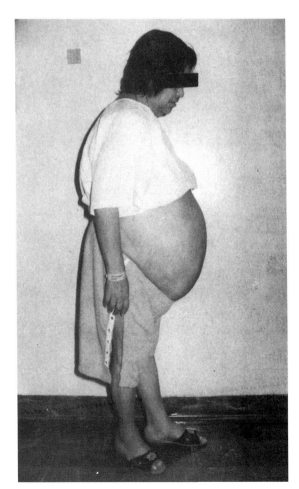

Figure 14.5. Side view of patient showing massive ascites and distention of abdomen.

ICTERUS. Icterus is a Greek word for jaundice meaning yellow bird. The yellow color associated with the condition was thought similar to the color of this bird. It was said that if a person suffering from jaundice looks at the bird, the bird dies and the patient recovers.

NAUSEA. Nausea is derived from a Greek word for ship referring to "ship sickness." Hippocrates used the term for seasickness; later it became generally applied to the sick and uneasy feeling that precedes vomiting.

Term	Meaning
melena me-le′nă	dark colored, tarry stool caused by old blood
nausea naw′ze-ă	sick in the stomach
steatorrhea ste′ă-to-re′ă	feces containing fat
sublingual sŭb-ling′gw ăl	under the tongue

Diagnostic

Term	Meaning
stomatitis sto-mă-tı′tis	inflammation of the mouth
sialoadenitis sı′ă-lo-ad-ĕ-nı′tis	inflammation of a salivary gland
parotitis (parotiditis) par-o-tı′tis	inflammation of the parotid gland; also called mumps
cheilitis kı-lı′tis	inflammation of the lip
glossitis glo-sı′tis	inflammation of the tongue
ankyloglossia ang′ki-lo-glos′e-ă	tongue-tie; a defect of the tongue characterized by a short, thick frenulum
gingivitis jin-ji-vı′tis	inflammation of the gums
esophageal varices e-sof′ă-je′ăl	swollen, twisted veins in the esophagus especially susceptible to ulceration and hemorrhage (see Color Atlas, plate 28)
esophagitis e-sof-ă-jı′tis	inflammation of the esophagus
gastritis gas-trı′tis	inflammation of the stomach (see Color Atlas, plate 28)
gastroesophageal reflux disease (GERD) gas′tro-e-sof′ă-je′ăl re′flŭks di-zez′	a backflow of contents of the stomach into the esophagus often as a result of abnormal function of the lower esophageal sphincter; causes burning pain in the esophagus
pyloric stenosis pı-lor′ik ste-no′sis	a narrowed condition of the pylorus
peptic ulcer pep′tik ŭl′ser	a sore on the mucous membrane of the stomach, duodenum, or any other part of the gastrointestinal system exposed to gastric juices (Fig. 14.6)
gastric ulcer gas′trik	ulcer located in the stomach

continued

Term	Meaning
duodenal ulcer dū'ō-dē'năl	ulcer located in the duodenum
gastroenteritis gas'trō-en-ter-ī'tis	inflammation of stomach and small intestine
enteritis en-ter-ī'tis	inflammation of small intestine
ileitis il-ē-ī'tis	inflammation of the lower portion of the small intestine
colitis kō-lī'tis	inflammation of the colon (large intestine)
ulcerative colitis ŭl'ser-ă-tiv	chronic inflammation of the colon along with ulcerations

continued

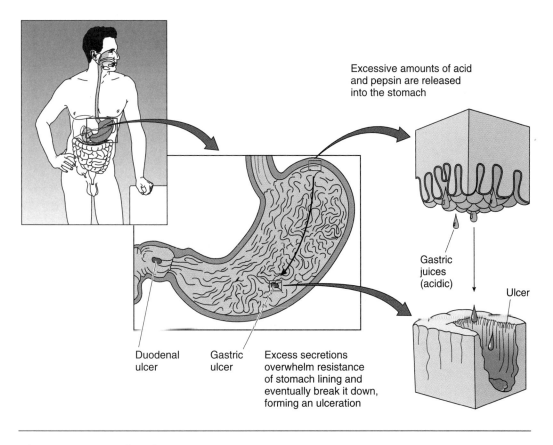

Duodenal ulcer

Gastric ulcer

Excess secretions overwhelm resistance of stomach lining and eventually break it down, forming an ulceration

Excessive amounts of acid and pepsin are released into the stomach

Gastric juices (acidic)

Ulcer

Figure 14.6. Peptic ulcer disease.

Term	Meaning
diverticulum dī-ver-tik′yū-lŭm	a by-way; an abnormal side pocket in the gastrointestinal tract usually related to lack of dietary fiber
diverticulosis dī′ver-tik-yū-lō′sis	presence of diverticula in the gastrointestinal tract, especially the bowel (Fig. 14.7) (see Color Atlas, plate 28)
diverticulitis dī′ver-tik-yū-lī′tis	inflammation of diverticula
dysentery dis′en-tār-ē	inflammation of the intestine characterized by frequent, bloody stools, most often caused by bacteria or protozoa (e.g., amebic dysentery)
appendicitis ă-pen-di-sī′tis	inflammation of the appendix
hernia her′nē-ă	protrusion of a part from its normal location
hiatal hernia hī-ā′tăl	protrusion of part of the stomach upward through the hiatal opening in the diaphragm (Fig. 14.8)
inguinal hernia ing′gwi-năl	protrusion of a loop of the intestine through layers of the abdominal wall in the inguinal region (Fig. 14.8)
incarcerated hernia in-kar′ser-ā-ted	hernia that is swollen and fixed within a sac, causing an obstruction
strangulated hernia strang′gyū-lā-ted	hernia that is constricted, cut off from circulation, and likely to become gangrenous
umbilical hernia ŭm-bil′i-kăl	protrusion of the intestine through a weakness in the abdominal wall around the umbilicus (navel)

continued

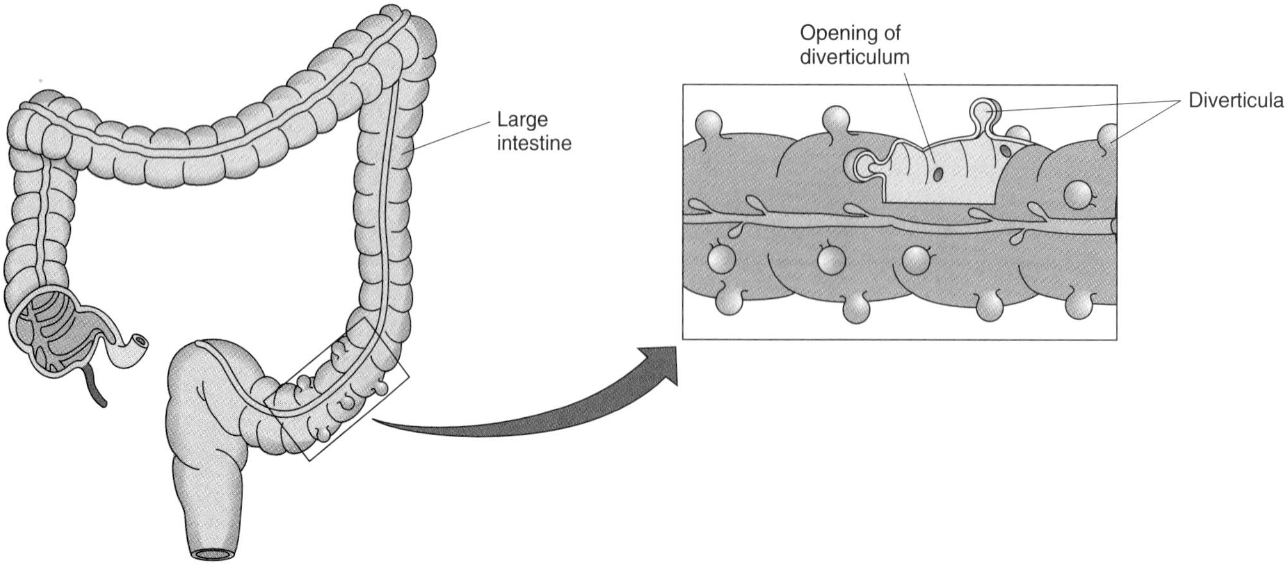

Figure 14.7. Diverticulosis.

Hiatal hernia

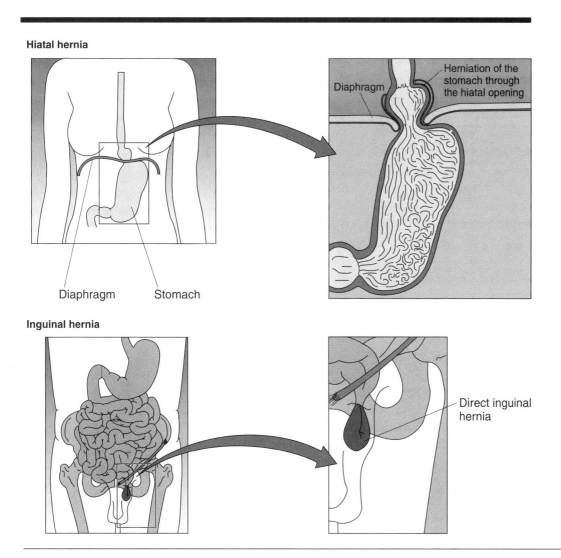

Inguinal hernia

Figure 14.8. Common hernias.

Term	Meaning
intussusception in′tŭs-sŭ-sep′shŭn	prolapse of one part of the intestine into the lumen of the adjoining part (intus = within; suscipiens = to take up) (Fig. 14.9)
volvulus vol′vū-lŭs	twisting of the bowel on itself, causing obstruction (volvo = to roll) (Fig. 14.10)
polyposis pol′i-pō′sis	multiple polyps in the intestine and rectum with a high malignancy potential (see Color Atlas, plate 28)
polyp pol′ip	tumor on a stalk
proctitis prok-tī′tis	inflammation of the rectum and anus
anal fistula ā′năl fis′tyū-lă	an abnormal tube-like passageway from the anus that may connect with the rectum (fistula = pipe) (Fig. 14.11)

continued

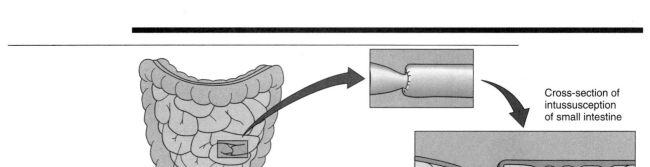

Figure 14.9. Intussusception.

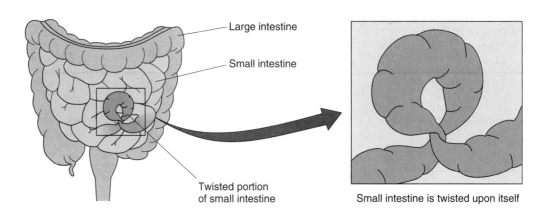

Figure 14.10. Volvulus.

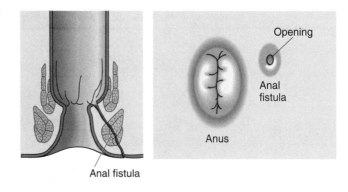

Figure 14.11. Anal fistula.

Term	Meaning
hemorrhoid hem′ŏ-royd	swollen, twisted vein (varicosity) in the anal region (haimorrhois = a vein likely to bleed)
peritonitis per′i-tō-nī′tis	inflammation of the peritoneum
hepatitis hep-ă-tī′tis	inflammation of the liver
hepatitis A	infectious inflammation of the liver caused by the hepatitis A virus, usually transmitted orally through fecal contamination of food or water
hepatitis B	hepatitis caused by the hepatitis B virus that is transmitted sexually or by exposure to contaminated blood or body fluids
cirrhosis sir-rō′sis	chronic disease characterized by degeneration of liver tissue most often caused by alcoholism or a nutritional deficiency (cirrho = yellow)
cholangitis kō-lan-jī′tis	inflammation of the bile ducts
cholecystitis kō′lē-sis-tī′tis	inflammation of the gallbladder
cholelithiasis kō′lē-li-thī′ă-sis	presence of stones in the gallbladder or bile ducts (Fig. 14.12)
choledocholithiasis kō-led′ō-kō-lith-ī′ă-sis	presence of stones in the common bile duct (Fig. 14.12) (see Color Atlas, plate 28)
pancreatitis pan′krē-ă-tī′tis	inflammation of the pancreas

CIRRHOSIS. A Greek word referring to a yellow condition, cirrhosis was first applied to the fibrosis of the liver in alcoholics because the granular deposits in the organ looked yellow.

continued

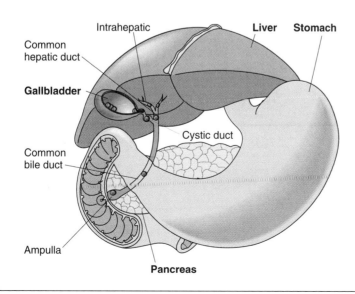

Figure 14.12. Sites of gallstones.

Diagnostic Tests and Procedures

Test or Procedure	Explanation
biopsy (Bx) bī′op-sē	removal and microscopic study of tissue
incisional Bx in-sizh′ŭn-ăl	removal of a portion of a lesion for pathological examination
excisional Bx ek-sizh′ŭn-ăl	removal of an entire lesion for pathological examination
endoscopy en-dos′kŏ-pē	examination within a body cavity with a flexible endoscope for diagnosis or treatment; used in the gastrointestinal tract to detect abnormalities and perform procedures such as biopsy, excision of lesions, dilations of narrowed areas, removal of swallowed objects, etc. (see Color Atlas, plate 28)
esophagoscopy ē-sof-ă-gos′kŏ-pē	examination of the esophagus with an esophagoscope
gastroscopy gas-tros′kŏ-pē	examination of the stomach with a gastroscope
upper gastrointestinal endoscopy gas′trō-in-tes′tin-ăl	examination of the lining of the esophagus, stomach, and duodenum with a flexible endoscope; also known as esophagogastroduodenoscopy (EGD) or panendoscopy (see Color Atlas, plate 28)
endoscopic retrograde cholangiopancreatography (ERCP) en-dos′kŏp′ik ret′rō-grād kō-lan′jē-ō-pan-krē-ă-tog′ră-fē	endoscopic procedure including x-ray fluoroscopy to examine the ducts of the liver, gallbladder, and pancreas (biliary ducts)
laparoscopy lap-ă-ros′kŏ-pē	examination of the abdominal cavity with a laparoscope—often including interventional surgical procedures (Fig. 14.13)

continued

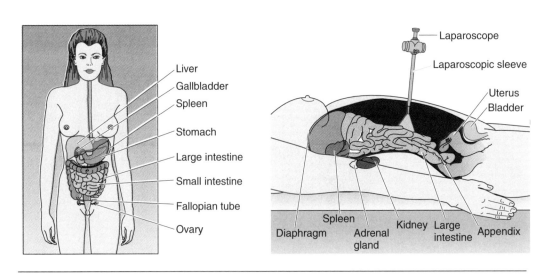

Figure 14.13. Laparoscopy.

Test or Procedure	Explanation
peritoneoscopy per′i-tō-nē-os′kŏ-pē	examination of the peritoneal cavity with a peritoneoscope; often performed to examine the liver and obtain a biopsy specimen
colonoscopy kō-lon-os′kŏ-pē	examination of the colon using a flexible colonoscope (see Color Atlas, plate 28)
sigmoidoscopy sig′moy-dos′kŏ-pē	examination of the sigmoid colon with a rigid or flexible sigmoidoscope
proctoscopy prok-tos′kŏ-pē	examination of the rectum and anus with a proctoscope
magnetic resonance imaging (MRI)	nonionizing imaging technique for visualizing the abdominal cavity to identify disease or deformity in the gastrointestinal tract
radiography rā′dē-og′ră-fē	x-ray imaging used to detect a condition or anomaly within the gastrointestinal tract (Fig. 14.14)
upper GI series	x-ray of the esophagus, stomach, and duodenum after the patient has swallowed a contrast medium (barium is most commonly used) (Fig. 14.15)
barium swallow ba′rē-ŭm	x-ray of the esophagus only; often used to locate swallowed objects

continued

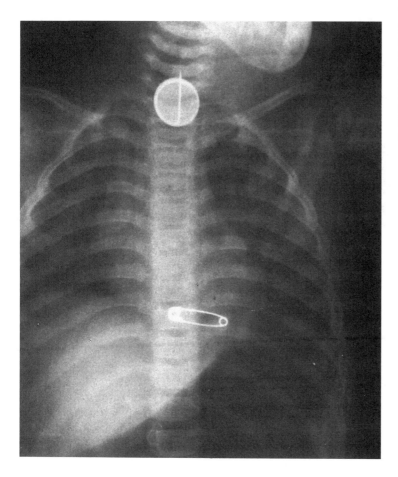

Figure 14.14. Radiograph showing two impacted foreign bodies in a child, aged two and one-half years. This child has ingested a safety pin and an ornamental pin. Endoscopic removal was required.

Test or Procedure	Explanation
fluoroscopy flŭr-os′kŏ-pe	x-ray using a fluorescent screen to visualize structures in motion (such as during a barium swallow)
lower GI series **barium enema** en′ĕ-mă	x-ray of the colon after administration of an enema containing a contrast medium (Fig. 14.16)
computed tomography **(CT) of abdomen** tō-mog′ră-fē	cross-sectional x-ray of the abdomen used to identify a condition or anomaly within the gastrointestinal tract (Fig. 14.17)
cholangiogram kō-lan′jē-ō-gram	x-ray of the bile ducts; often performed during surgery
cholecystogram kō-lē-sis′tō-gram	x-ray of the gallbladder taken after oral ingestion of iodine

continued

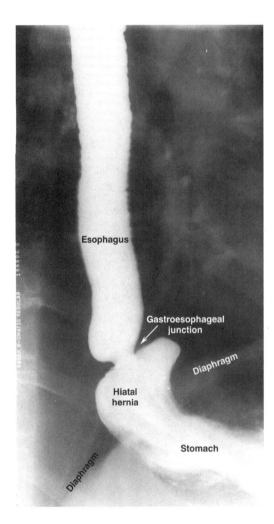

Figure 14.15. Upper gastrointestinal radiograph showing hiatal hernia.

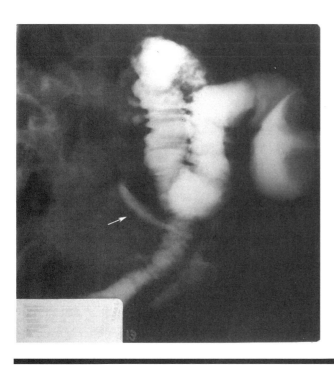

Figure 14.16. Barium enema radiograph of colon showing ruptured diverticulum. Its elongated appearance is similar to a deflated balloon.

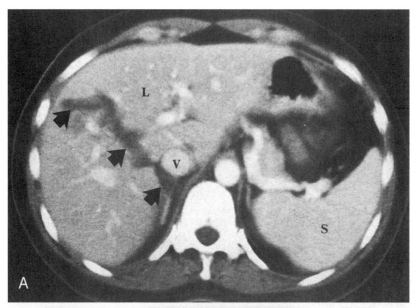

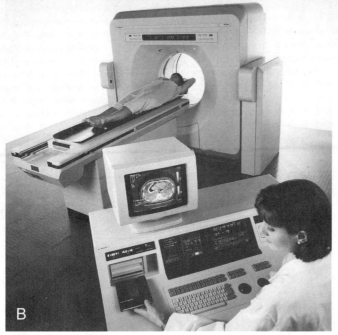

Figure 14.17. A. CT scan of a patient involved in a motor vehicle accident demonstrates a jagged laceration (*arrows*) extending from posterior to inferior vena cava (*V*) through right lobe of the liver (*L*). *S*, spleen. **B.** CT scanner.

Test or Procedure	Explanation
sonography sŏ-nog′ră-fē	ultrasound imaging
abdominal sonogram son′ō-gram	ultrasound image of the abdomen to detect disease or deformity in organs and vascular structures (e.g., liver, pancreas, gallbladder, spleen, aorta, etc.) (see Fig. 14.18)
endoscopic sonography	an endoscopic procedure using a sonographic transducer within an endoscope to examine a body cavity and make sonographic images of structures and tissues
stool culture and sensitivity	isolation of a stool specimen in a culture medium to identify disease-causing organisms; if present, the drugs to which they are sensitive are listed
stool occult blood study	a chemical test of a stool specimen to detect the presence of blood; positive findings indicate bleeding in the GI tract

Operative Terms

Term	Meaning
cheiloplasty kī′lō-plas-tē	repair of the lip

continued

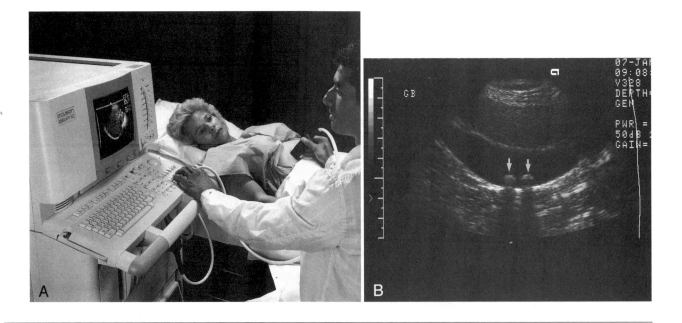

Figure 14.18. A. Abdominal sonography procedure **B.** Abdominal sonogram of two stones present in the gallbladder (*arrows*).

Term	Meaning
glossectomy glo-sek′tō-mē	excision of the tongue
glossorrhaphy glo-sōr′ă-fē	suture of the tongue
esophagoplasty ē-sof′ă-gō-plas-tē	repair of the esophagus
gastrectomy gas-trek′tō-mē	partial or complete removal of the stomach
gastric resection gas′trik rē-sek′shŭn	partial removal and repair of the stomach
gastroenterostomy gas′trō-en-ter-os′tō-mē	formation of an artificial opening between the stomach and small intestine; often performed at the time of a gastrectomy to route food from the remainder of the stomach to the intestine (also performed to repair a perforated duodenal ulcer)
abdominocentesis ab-dom′i-nō-sen-tē′sis **paracentesis** par′ă-sen-tē′sis	puncture of the abdomen for aspiration of fluid; e.g., fluid accumulated in ascites
laparotomy lap′ă-rot′ō-mē	incision into the abdomen
laparoscopic surgery lap′ă-rō-skō-pik	abdominal surgery using a laparoscope
herniorrhaphy her′nō-ōr′ă-fē **hernioplasty** her′nē-ō-plas-tē	repair of a hernia
colostomy kō-los′tō-mē	creation of an opening in the colon through the abdominal wall to create an abdominal anus; performed to treat a diseased colon such as that which occurs with ulcerative colitis, cancer, obstructions (Fig. 14.19)

continued

1. Ascending colostomy   2. Transverse colostomy   3. Descending colostomy

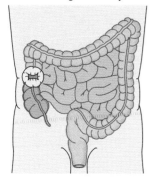 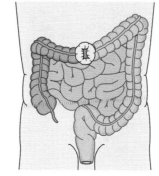 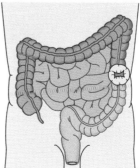

Figure 14.19. Common colostomy sites.

Term	Meaning
anastomosis ă-nas′tō-mō′sis	union of two hollow vessels; used in bowel surgery
ileostomy il′ē-os′tō-mē	surgical creation of an opening on the abdomen to which the end of the ileum is attached, providing a passageway for ileal discharges; performed after removal of the colon, which is done to treat chronic inflammatory bowel diseases such as ulcerative colitis, etc. (Fig. 14.20)
appendectomy ap-pen-dek′tō-mē	excision of a diseased appendix
incidental appendectomy	removal of the appendix during abdominal surgery for another procedure (e.g., a hysterectomy)
polypectomy pol-i-pek′tō-mē	excision of polyps
proctoplasty prok′tō-plas-tē	repair of the rectum
anal fistulectomy fis-tyū-lek′tō-mē	excision of an anal fistula
hemorrhoidectomy hem′ō-roy-dek′tō-mē	excision of hemorrhoids
hepatic lobectomy he-pat′ik lō-bek′tō-mē	excision of a lobe of the liver
cholecystectomy kō′lē-sis-tek′tō-mē	excision of the gallbladder

laparoscopic
   cholecystectomy
   lap′ă-rō-skŏp′ik
	excision of the gallbladder through a laparoscope

continued

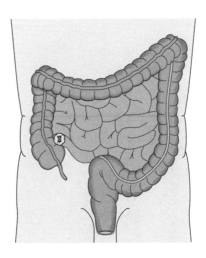

Figure 14.20. Ileostomy.

Term	Meaning
cholelithotomy kō'lē-li-thot'ō-mē	an incision for removal of gallstones
choledocholithotomy kō-led'ō-kō-li-thot'ō-mē	incision of the common bile duct for extraction of gallstones
cholelithotripsy kō-lē-lith'ō-trip-sē	crushing of gallstones
pancreatectomy pan'krē-ă-tek'tō-mē	excision of the pancreas

Therapeutic Terms

Term	Meaning
gastric lavage gas'trik lă-vahzh'	oral insertion of a tube into the stomach for examination and treatment; e.g., to remove blood clots from the stomach and monitor bleeding (lavage = to wash)
nasogastric (NG) **intubation** nā-zō-gas'trik in-tū-bā'shŭn	insertion of a tube through the nose into the stomach for various purposes, e.g., to obtain a gastric fluid specimen for analysis

Common Therapeutic Drug Classifications

antacid ant-as'id	drug that neutralizes stomach acid
antiemetic an'tē-ĕ-met'ik	drug that prevents or stops vomiting
antispasmodic an'tē-spaz-mod'ik	drug that decreases motility in gastrointestinal tract to arrest spasm or diarrhea
cathartic kă-thar'tik	drug that causes movement of the bowels; also called a laxative

PRACTICE EXERCISES

For the following terms, draw a line or lines to separate prefixes, combining forms, and suffixes. Then define the term.

1. gastrogenic _____

2. gingivoglossitis _____

3. stomatalgia _____

4. proctology _____

5. hematemesis _____

6. cheilostomatoplasty _____

7. enterocele _____

8. hyperemesis _____

9. cholecystectomy _____

10. gastroectasis _____

11. cheilophagia _____

12. glossospasm _____

13. gastroesophagitis _____

14. rectosigmoidal _____

15. choledochojejunostomy _____

16. dysphagia _____

17. laparoscopy _____

18. cholecystogram _____

19. glossopathy _____

20. orolingual _____

21. celiogastrotomy _____

22. pancreatoduodenostomy _____

23. coloenteritis _____

24. anoscope _____

25. sigmoidoscopy _____

26. hepatotoxic _____

27. buccal _____

28. sialorrhea _____

29. pylorectomy _____

30. hernioplasty _____

31. retroperitoneal _____

32. abdominocentesis _____

33. steatolysis _____

34. ileorrhaphy _____

35. dentalgia _____

Write the correct medical term for each of the following:

36. inflammation of the stomach _____

37. loss of appetite _____

38. inability to swallow _____

39. in the cheek _____

40. gas in the stomach or intestines _____

41. rupture or protrusion of a part from its normal location _____

42. black tarry stool _____

43. belch _____

44. instrument used to examine the rectum _____

45. inflammation of the large intestine _____

46. x-ray image of the esophagus only _____

47. accumulation of fluid in the peritoneal cavity _____

48. inflammation of the gallbladder _____

49. feces containing fat _____

50. presence of inflamed abnormal side pockets in gastrointestinal tract

    _____

51. peptic ulcer located in the stomach _____

52. enlargement of the liver _____

53. a tongue-tie condition _____

Complete the medical term by writing the missing part or word:

54. hemi_____ectomy = removal of half of the stomach

55. _____itis = inflammation of the appendix

56. _____rrhaphy = suture of the lip

57. cholelitho_____= crushing of gallstones

58. _____plasty = surgical repair of the mouth

59. chol_____gram = x-ray of bile ducts (vessels)

60. _____bilirubin_____ = excessive level of bilirubin
    in the blood

61. gastric _____ = partial removal and repair of the stomach

62. diverticulo_____ = the presence of diverticula

Name the anatomical divisions of the abdomen:

63. lower lateral groin regions _____

64. upper lateral regions beneath ribs _____

65. upper middle region below the sternum _____

66. region below the navel _____

67. middle lateral regions _____

68. region of the navel_____

Name the clinical divisions of the abdomen:

69. _____

70. _____

71. _____

72. _____

Match the following terms with the appropriate term on the right:

73. cathartic _____   a. cholelithotripsy

74. herniorrhaphy _____   b. barium swallow

75. appendicitis _____   c. oro

76. lower GI series _____   d. appendectomy

77. icterus _____   e. colostomy

78. chole _____   f. hernioplasty

79. abdominocentesis _____   g. bili

80. parotitis _____   h. barium enema

81. procto _____   i. mumps

82. upper GI series _____   j. paracentesis

83. ulcerative colitis _____   k. jaundice

84. cholelithiasis _____   l. recto

85. stomato _____   m. laxative

An endoscope is an instrument used to examine within the body. Name the specific type of endoscope used to examine the following body parts:

86. abdomen _____

87. anus _____

88. stomach _____

89. colon_____

90. peritoneal cavity _____

91. esophagus _____

92. Which type of hernia is swollen and fixed within a sac, causing obstruction?

_____

93. Which type of biopsy involves the removal an entire growth? _____

Write the full medical term for the following abbreviations:

94. NG tube_____

95. ERCP _____

96. GERD _____

97. LUQ _____

98. GI _____

99. MRI _____

100. EGD _____

Medical Record Analyses

MEDICAL RECORD 14.1

At age 65, Thomas Kingman had a routine screening test from Dr. Ford, his personal physician, that led to the discovery of colon cancer. After surgery to remove his tumor, it was discovered that the cancer had spread to his liver. Dr. Ford referred Mr. Kingman to Dr. Rafferty for consultation and further evaluation.

Directions

Read Medical Record 14.1 for Mr. Kingman (pages 395–398) and answer the following questions. This record is the consultation report dictated by Dr. Rafferty after his examination of Mr. Kingman.

Questions about Medical Record 14.1

Write your answers in the spaces provided.

1. Below are medical terms used in this record you have not yet encountered in this text. Underline each where it appears in the record and define below.

   clubbing _____

   palliative therapy _____

   sepsis _____

   central venous catheter _____

   carcinoembryonic antigen (CEA)_____

2. In your own words, briefly describe the scope of practice of an oncologist.

   _____

   _____

   _____

3. Mr. Kingman has undergone several diagnostic procedures with Drs. Ford, Glenn, and Rafferty. Put the following diagnostic procedures in the order they were used by numbering them 1 to 5:

   _____ CT scan

   _____ lower GI series

   _____ sigmoidoscopy

   _____ exploratory laparotomy

   _____ palpation

4. Describe Mr. Kingman's symptoms at the time of the screening by Dr. Ford:

_____

_____

_____

Describe Mr. Kingman's symptoms at the time of his consultation with Dr. Rafferty:

_____

_____

_____

5. In your own words, not using medical terminology, describe what was done in Mr. Kingman's surgery.

_____

_____

_____

6. Define Mr. Kingman's three medical problems stated under "Past Medical History":

a. _____

b. _____

c. _____

7. Which problem in the list below did Dr. Rafferty find in the "Review of Systems"?

a. arthritis

b. ill-fitting dentures

c. strangulated hernia

d. icterus

8. Translate Mr. Kingman's medication instructions for these drugs:

Vasotec _____

Calan SR _____

Tenoretic _____

Zyloprim _____

9. Translate Mr. Kingman's current medical condition as described in Dr. Rafferty's assessment:

_____

_____

_____

10. Dr. Rafferty's plan calls for several actions. Put the following in the correct order by numbering them 1 to 4:

_____ baseline evaluation with CEA and CA 19-9

_____ follow-up scans

_____ placement of central venous catheter

_____ administration of leucovorin and 5-FU

CENTRAL MEDICAL GROUP, INC.

Department of Oncology/Hematology

201 Medical Center Drive • Central City, US 90000-1234 • PHONE: (012) 125-8888 • FAX: (012) 125-3434

MEDICAL ONCOLOGY CONSULTATION

REASON FOR CONSULTATION: The patient is a 65-year-old gentleman seen post-operatively due to colon carcinoma for further advice and systemic treatment.

HISTORY OF PRESENT ILLNESS: The patient has been followed by Dr. Ford. He was feeling well and presented for routine physical examination during which a screening sigmoidoscopy was done in early March 199x. At that time, the patient was asymptomatic without change in bowel habits, blood in stool, etc.

A barium enema was performed on March 11, 199x, which showed a large tumor with minimal remaining lumen at approximately 20 cm.

At that time, laboratory data revealed a normal hemoglobin of 14.5, but the patient was microcytic with an MCV of 75.

The patient was seen by Dr. Glenn in surgical consultation. On March 17, 199x, he underwent exploratory laparotomy at which time a large tumor growing into the posterior wall of the pelvis in the curve of the sacrum was found. In addition, a large metastasis in the right lobe of the liver was palpated near the gallbladder. The patient had a postoperative CT scan to confirm this. The patient will be obtaining this scan for my review. A left hemicolectomy was performed with primary anastomosis.

The patient was discharged on March 22, 199x, and has been doing pretty well except for constipation alternating with diarrhea; he is currently using Metamucil to try to even this out.

PAST MEDICAL HISTORY: PREVIOUS SURGERIES: Unremarkable except as per History of Present Illness. PAST MEDICAL PROBLEMS: 1) Hypertension for many years, medically controlled. 2) Hyperuricemia. 3) Hypercholesterolemia.

(continued)

MEDICAL ONCOLOGY CONSULTATION Page 1 March 28, 199x	PT. NAME: KINGMAN, THOMAS C. ID NO: 009159 REF. PHYS: J. FORD, M.D. CONSULTANT: P. RAFFERTY, M.D.

CENTRAL MEDICAL GROUP, INC.

Department of Oncology/Hematology

201 Medical Center Drive • Central City, US 90000-1234 • PHONE: (012) 125-8888 • FAX: (012) 125-3434

MEDICAL ONCOLOGY CONSULTATION

REVIEW OF SYSTEMS: CHILDHOOD DISEASES: Usual. OTHER SIGNIFICANT INFECTIOUS DISEASES: None. SKIN: Negative. HEMATOLOGIC: Negative. HEAD/NECK: Negative. PULMONARY: History of smoking; otherwise negative. CARDIOVASCULAR: Hypertension. GASTROINTESTINAL: As per History of Present Illness; otherwise negative. GENITOURINARY: Negative. MUSCULOSKELETAL: Arthritis affecting peripheral joints and some chronic back pain, stable. NEUROLOGIC: Negative. ENDOCRINE: Negative. GENERAL: The patient has lost approximately 10 lb postoperatively. He has had some anorexia as well as some nondrenching night sweats.

ALLERGIES: No known history of drug allergy.

CURRENT MEDICATIONS: Vasotec 10 mg b.i.d. Calan SR 250 mg q a.m. Tenoretic 100/25 1 q a.m. Zyloprim 300 mg q a.m.

SOCIAL HISTORY: The patient is an ex-smoker; he quit many years ago. He consumes alcohol, but he did not specify the amount per day.

FAMILY HISTORY: Noncontributory, though three sisters died in the last two years. One sister died of sudden death of unclear etiology; one of cancer, possibly colon. Another sister died of an unknown type of cancer.

PHYSICAL EXAMINATION

GENERAL APPEARANCE: Reasonably well, somewhat frail-appearing gentleman appearing older than his stated age.

VITAL SIGNS: Height: 5 ft 6 in. Weight: 151 lb. Blood Pressure: 90/42. Pulse: 72. Respirations: 18. Temperature: 97.8°F.

HEENT: Normocephalic. Sclerae are nonicteric. Oropharynx: Upper and lower dentures; otherwise unremarkable.

NECK: Supple.

(continued)

MEDICAL ONCOLOGY CONSULTATION Page 2 March 28, 199x	PT. NAME: KINGMAN, THOMAS C. ID NO: 009159 REF. PHYS: J. FORD, M.D. CONSULTANT: P. RAFFERTY, M.D.

Medical Record 14.1. *Continued.*

CENTRAL MEDICAL GROUP, INC.

Department of Oncology/Hematology

201 Medical Center Drive • Central City, US 90000-1234 • PHONE: (012) 125-8888 • FAX: (012) 125-3434

MEDICAL ONCOLOGY CONSULTATION

LYMPH NODES: No pathologic peripheral lymphadenopathy appreciated.

BACK/SPINE: Nontender. No CVA tenderness.

HEART: Regular rhythm without murmurs, rubs, or gallops.

LUNGS: Clear to percussion and auscultation.

ABDOMEN: Soft, minimal tenderness, healing midline incision subxiphoid to supraumbilical.

EXTREMITIES: No cyanosis, clubbing, or edema.

GENITALIA//RECTAL: Not performed.

NEUROLOGIC: Grossly nonfocal.

LABORATORY DATA: No laboratory work was performed today since the patient has very poor peripheral veins.

PROBLEM LIST:
1. Colon carcinoma with probable persistent pelvic side wall tumor as well as a large hepatic metastasis.

2. Hypertension.

3. Hyperuricemia.

4. Hypercholesterolemia.

ASSESSMENT/PLAN: The patient has incurable metastatic colon carcinoma. This was discussed frankly with the patient and his wife. Palliative therapy is available. Though radiation therapy could be used, it is unlikely to offer significant benefit given his hepatic metastasis. Systemic chemotherapy utilizing leucovorin and 5-FU would be a reasonable alternative with approximately a 30-40% chance of response rate.

(continued)

MEDICAL ONCOLOGY CONSULTATION Page 3 March 28, 199x	PT. NAME: KINGMAN, THOMAS C. ID NO: 009159 REF. PHYS: J. FORD, M.D. CONSULTANT: P. RAFFERTY, M.D.

Medical Record 14.1. *Continued.*

CENTRAL MEDICAL GROUP, INC.

Department of Oncology/Hematology

201 Medical Center Drive • Central City, US 90000-1234 • PHONE: (012) 125-8888 • FAX: (012) 125-3434

MEDICAL ONCOLOGY CONSULTATION

In order to safely administer this treatment due to poor peripheral veins, Dr. Glenn will be placing a central venous catheter and Port-a-Cath access system subcutaneously in the right chest wall.

Side effects including diarrhea, sepsis, nausea, vomiting, minimal chance of hair loss, etc., were discussed.

Treatment will commence after placement of the Port-a-Cath catheter, and the patient will be evaluated at that time with a baseline carcinoembryonic antigen (CEA) and CA 19-9. If these are elevated, follow-up scans will be performed several months into treatment to verify whether or not the patient is responding.

I appreciate the opportunity of seeing Mr. Kingman in consultation and will be following him carefully with you.

P. Rafferty MD

P. Rafferty, M.D.

PR:jj

D: 3/28/9x
T: 3/29/9x

cc: J. Ford, M.D.

MEDICAL ONCOLOGY CONSULTATION Page 4 March 28, 199x	PT. NAME: KINGMAN, THOMAS C. ID NO: 009159 REF. PHYS: J. FORD, M.D. CONSULTANT: P. RAFFERTY, M.D.

Medical Record 14.1. *Continued.*

MEDICAL RECORD 14.2

At age 77 Kathleen Hillman has been in fairly good health. But one week ago she developed what she called "stomach problems" that led to frequent vomiting. She refused to seek medical help at first, until her daughter coaxed her into calling her family practitioner, Dr. Shigeda. Once she learned how serious Ms. Hillman's problem had become, Dr. Shigeda urged her to go to the emergency room immediately.

Directions

Read Medical Record 14.2 for Kathleen Hillman (pages 401–403) and answer the following questions on the next page. This record is the consultation report dictated by Dr. Flagstone after he examined her in the emergency room at Central Medical Center.

Questions about Medical Record 14.2

Write your answers in the spaces provided.
1. Below are medical terms used in this record you have not yet encountered in this text. Underline each where it appears in the record and define below.

   rebound tenderness _____

   abdominal guarding _____

   dehydration_____

   stasis dermatitis _____

   intractable _____

2. What was Ms. Hillman's complaint that led her to call Dr. Shigeda, who then sent her to the emergency room at Central Medical Center?

   _____

3. According to Dr. Flagstone's initial impression, which factor in Ms. Hillman's present history might be a cause of her gastrointestinal symptoms?

   a. her drinking

   b. stress from living with her daughter

   c. her allergies

   d. her arthritis medications

4. Describe the two previous operations Ms. Hillman has had involving the musculoskeletal system:

   _____

   _____

   _____

5. Using nonmedical language, explain what Ms. Hillman does not remember exactly about her gastrointestinal history two decades ago.

   _____

   _____

   _____

6. Check all of the findings below that Dr. Flagstone noted in the physical examination of Ms. Hillman:

_____ dehydration

_____ pulse 98

_____ icterus in the whites of eyes

_____ chronic stasis dermatitis

_____ varicose veins

_____ irregular heart rate

_____ vaginal infection

_____ possible atrial fibrillation

_____ parotitis

_____ yellowing of skin

_____ multiple ecchymoses

_____ clear lungs

7. Does Ms. Hillman have blood in her stool? Write the phrase from the medical record that indicates this.

_____

8. In your own words, explain the initial diagnoses, including the possibilities to eliminate:

a. _____

b. _____

c. _____

9. Dr. Flagstone's plan calls for administering medications, checking tests, and performing a procedure. Fill in the details below.

Administered to Ms. Hillman

a. _____

b. _____

c. _____

Check Ms. Hillman's

d. _____

e. _____

f. _____

Perform

g. _____

10. In your own words, describe stool culture and sensitivity.

_____

_____

_____

CENTRAL MEDICAL CENTER

211 Medical Center Drive • Central City, US 90000-1234 • PHONE: (012) 125-6784 • FAX: (012) 125-9999

CONSULTATION

REASON FOR CONSULTATION:
This 77-year-old female presented herself to the emergency room with a one week history of rather severe nausea and vomiting and also diarrhea and epigastric pain; she was sent by Dr. Shigeda, her family practitioner. The most troubling symptom for her is the vomiting and nausea because she vomits everything she drinks and eats. The epigastric pains are tolerable. The diarrhea also has somewhat improved. The patient's bowel movements usually are normal without history of black or bloody stools. Her appetite has been down markedly, and she has lost at least two to three pounds in the last several days. Her urination is normal. She does not drink or smoke. Her last admission was about a month ago after a fall.

MEDICATIONS: Prednisone, 10 mg, 1 q.i.d.; Naprosyn, 250 mg, 1 q noc; Voltaren 1 q d; penicillamine t.i.d.; and Mylanta and Tylenol p.r.n.

ALLERGIES: Demerol which gives her severe confusion lasting for days.

PAST MEDICAL HISTORY/REVIEW OF SYSTEMS:
The patient has reading glasses. There is no history of cephalalgia, diplopia, or tinnitus. There is no history of thyroid disease. CARDIOPULMONARY: There is no history of angina, dyspnea, hemoptysis, emphysema, hypertension, or heart murmurs. GASTROINTESTINAL: The patient had peptic ulcer disease about 20 years ago, nonbleeding, and does not remember whether it was gastric or duodenal. It was healed by diet and antacids. There has been no recurrence since. There is no history of gallbladder disease, hepatitis, pancreatitis, or colitis. However, years ago, she was told she had diverticulosis. GENITOURINARY: She is Gravida III Para III (3 pregnancies and 3 live births). Her last menstrual period was some 25 years ago. There is no history of dysuria, hematuria, or nephrolithiasis. MUSCULOSKELETAL: The patient has had severe rheumatoid arthritis for about 20 years and has been in treatment with Dr. Clemons. The disease is relatively well controlled with the above-mentioned medications. She had a right hip replacement in 199x and left knee arthroscopy. NEUROMUSCULAR: There is no history of loss of consciousness or seizure disorder. PSYCHIATRIC REVIEW: Negative.

FAMILY HISTORY:
All siblings and parents died of old age.

SOCIAL HISTORY:
The patient is a widow. She lives with her daughter.

(continued)

CONSULTATION
Page 1
October 19, 199x

PT. NAME: HILLMAN, KATHLEEN E.
ID NO: IP-990960
ROOM NO: 508
ATT. PHYS: R. FLAGSTONE, M.D.

Medical Record 14.2.

CENTRAL MEDICAL CENTER

211 Medical Center Drive • Central City, US 90000-1234 • PHONE: (012) 125-6784 • FAX: (012) 125-9999

CONSULTATION

PHYSICAL EXAMINATION:

GENERAL: The patient appeared to be in moderate to severe distress, appearing pale, chronically ill, with dehydration.

VITAL SIGNS: Blood pressure, lying: 100/70. Blood pressure, sitting: 90/65. Temperature: 98°F. Pulse: 80; went to 100 on sitting up. Respirations: 12.

HEENT: Head: Normocephalic. Eyes: Pupils equal, round, reactive to light and accommodation. No scleral icterus. Fundi benign. Ears, nose throat, and mouth were unremarkable.

NECK: Supple. No lymphadenopathy. No thyromegaly.

CHEST: Chest, costovertebral angle, and back were nontender.

LUNGS: Clear to percussion and auscultation.

HEART: There was an irregular rate, possibly atrial fibrillation, with a II/VI systolic ejection-type murmur mostly along the left sternal border.

ABDOMEN: Soft. There was moderate epigastric tenderness. There was no hepatospleno-megaly, no guarding, no rebound tenderness, no masses, no ascites, no abdominal bruits.

VAGINAL EXAMINATION: Refused.

RECTAL EXAMINATION: Good sphincter tone. Light brown, semiformed stool in the rectal ampulla which was occult blood negative.

EXTREMITIES: No edema. No varicose veins. Good peripheral pulses. No clubbing. No palmar erythema. There were, however, brownish changes of chronic stasis dermatitis.

SKIN: The skin showed 10-15% dehydration without jaundice. There were multiple ecchymoses secondary to the patient's prednisone.

(continued)

CONSULTATION Page 2 October 19, 199x	PT. NAME: HILLMAN, KATHLEEN E. ID NO: IP-990960 ROOM NO: 508 ATT. PHYS: R. FLAGSTONE, M.D.

Medical Record 14.2. *Continued.*

CENTRAL MEDICAL CENTER

211 Medical Center Drive • Central City, US 90000-1234 • PHONE: (012) 125-6784 • FAX: (012) 125-9999

CONSULTATION

INITIAL IMPRESSION:
1. SEVERE NAUSEA AND VOMITING, INTRACTABLE, WITH DEHYDRATION, PROBABLY SECONDARY TO MEDICATION-INDUCED GASTRITIS OR POSSIBLE RECURRENT PEPTIC ULCER DISEASE

2. R/O POSSIBLE PANCREATITIS SECONDARY TO PREDNISONE OR PENICILLAMINE.

3. R/O POSSIBLE VIRAL GASTROENTERITIS, THOUGH LESS LIKELY.

SECONDARY DIAGNOSES:
1. HISTORY OF LONGSTANDING, ADVANCED RHEUMATOID ARTHRITIS WITH LEFT KNEE SURGERY AND RIGHT HIP REPLACEMENT.

2. HISTORY OF DIVERTICULOSIS AND PREVIOUS PEPTIC ULCER DISEASE.

PLAN:
The patient will be admitted at least for a 23-hour hold and is then to be re-evaluated and will receive fluid volume replacement and potassium replacement; she will have her electrolytes checked, as well as her blood count, and will also be placed on Zantac intravenously. She will then have a gastroscopy in the morning. Her stools will also be checked, if they are still loose, for further occult blood, ova and parasites, and a possible culture and sensitivity.

R. Flagstone, M.D.

RF:ti

D: 10/19/9x
T: 10/20/9x

CONSULTATION	PT. NAME:	HILLMAN, KATHLEEN E.
Page 3	ID NO:	IP-990960
October 19, 199x	ROOM NO:	508
	ATT. PHYS:	R. FLAGSTONE, M.D.

Medical Record 14.2. *Continued.*

15

Urinary System

OBJECTIVES

After completion of this chapter you will be able to

1. Define common combining forms used in relation to the urinary system

2. Define the basic anatomical terms referring to the urinary system

3. Define common symptomatic, diagnostic, operative, and therapeutic terms referring to the urinary system

4. List the common diagnostic tests and procedures related to the urinary system

5. Explain terms and abbreviations used in documenting medical records involving the urinary system

Combining Forms

Combining Form	Meaning	Example
albumin/o	protein	**albuminoid** al-byū′min-oyd
bacteri/o	bacteria	**bacterium** bak-tēr′ē-ŭm
cyst/o	bladder or sac	**cystoscope** sis′tō-skōp
vesic/o		**vesicotomy** ves′i-kot′ō-mē
dips/o	thirst	**polydipsia** pol-ē-dip′sē-ă
glomerul/o	glomerulus (little ball)	**glomerular** glō-mār′yū-lăr
gluc/o	sugar	**glucose** glū′kōs
glyc/o		**glycogenesis** glī-kō-jen′ě-sis
glycos/o		**glycosuria** glī-kō-sū′rē-ă
ket/o	ketone bodies	**ketosis** kē-tō′sis
keton/o		**ketonuria** kē-tō-nū′rē-ă
lith/o	stone	**lithiasis** li-thī′ă-sis
meat/o	opening	**meatal** mē-ā′tăl
nephr/o	kidney	**nephrosis** ne-frō′sis
ren/o		**renal** rē′năl
pyel/o	basin	**pyelonephrosis** pī′ě-lō-ne-frō′sis
py/o	pus	**pyonephritis** pī′ě-lō-ne-frī′tis
ureter/o	ureter	**ureterolithiasis** yū-rē′ter-ō-li-thī′ă-sis
urethr/o	urethra	**urethrodynia** yū-rē-thrō-din′ē-ă
ur/o	urine	**urologist** yū-rol′ō-jist
urin/o		**urinary** yūr′i-nār-ē

Urinary System Overview

The urinary system includes the organs and structures involved in the secretion and elimination of urine: kidneys, ureters, urinary bladder, and urethra (Fig. 15.1). The principal organs of the urinary system, the *kidneys*, are located on each side of the lumbar region. They filter the blood and secrete water and nitrogenous wastes (urea, creatinine, etc.) in the form of *urine*.

The functional unit of the kidney is called the *nephron*. Each nephron consists of a *glomerulus*, the little ball-shaped cluster of capillaries at the top; *Bowman's capsule*, the top part that encloses the nephron; and a *renal tubule*, the stem portion of the nephron. Approximately one million nephrons make up the *cortex*, the outer part of each kidney. They gather waste substances by filtering the blood that enters the kidney through the *renal artery* at the *hilum*, the prominent indented portion. In the *medulla*, the inner portion of the kidney, the *calyces* collect urine from the tubules of the nephrons and drain their contents into the *renal pelvis*, the basin-like portion of the ureter within the kidney.

The *ureters*, usually one for each kidney, are tubes that carry the urine from the kidney to the *urinary bladder*, where it is held until being expelled during *urination* (micturition). The *urethra* is the single canal that carries urine from the bladder to the outside of the body. The *urethral meatus* is the opening in the urethra to the outside of the body (see Color Atlas, plate 29).

In addition to excreting waste products such as urea and creatinine, the kidney's play an essential life-sustaining role by regulating the levels of critical elements such as water, sodium, and potassium.

Anatomical Terms

Term	Meaning
kidneys kid'nēz	two structures located on each side of the lumbar region that filter blood and secrete impurities, forming urine (Fig. 15.2)

continued

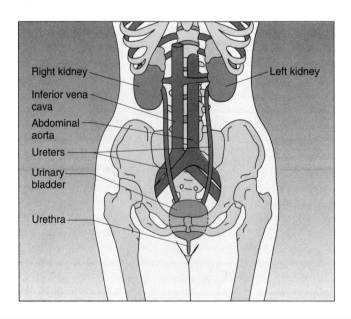

Right kidney

Inferior vena cava

Abdominal aorta

Ureters

Urinary bladder

Urethra

Left kidney

Figure 15.1. Urinary system.

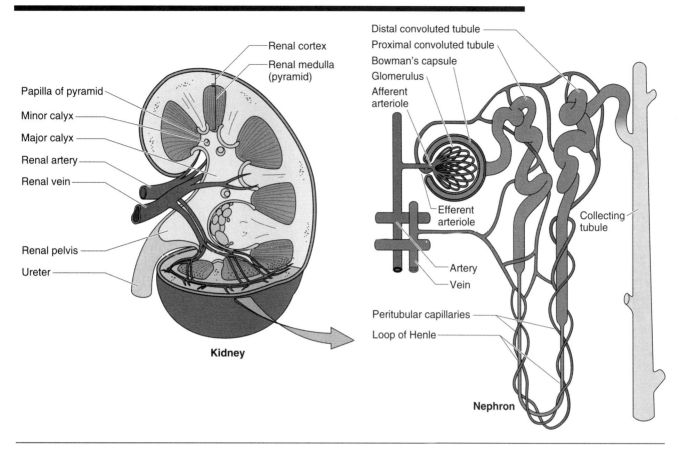

Figure 15.2. Kidney and nephron.

Term	Meaning
cortex kōr'teks	outer part of the kidney (cortex = bark)
hilum hī'lŭm	indented opening in the kidney where vessels enter and leave
medulla me-dūl'ă	inner part of the kidney
calyces kal'i-sēz	a system of ducts carrying urine from the nephrons to the renal pelvis (calyx = cup of a flower)
nephron nef'ron	microscopic functional units of the kidney, comprised of kidney cells and capillaries, each capable of forming urine
glomerulus glō-mār'yū-lŭs	little ball-shaped cluster of capillaries located at the top of each nephron
Bowman's capsule bō-mĕnz kap'sūl	top part of the nephron that encloses the glomerulus
renal tubule rē'năl tū'byūl	stem portion of the nephron

continued

INCONTINENCE. The Latin continent means to hold in, and the prefix in means not. In Shakespeare's time incontinently was used to mean immediately. Today incontinence specifically refers to the inability to prevent the discharge of excretions, especially urine or feces.

Term	Meaning
ureter ū-rē′ter	tube that carries urine from the kidney to the bladder
renal pelvis rē′năl pel′vis	basin-like portion of the ureter within the kidney
ureteropelvic junction yū′rē′ter-ō-pel′vik	point of connection between the renal pelvis and ureter
urinary bladder yūr′i-năr-ē	sac that holds the urine
urethra yū-rē′thră	single canal that carries urine to the outside of the body
urethral meatus mē-ā′tŭs	opening in the urethra to the outside of the body
urine yūr′in	fluid produced by the kidneys containing water and waste products
urea yū-rē′ă	waste product formed in the liver, filtered out of the blood by the kidneys, and excreted in urine
creatinine krē-at′i-nēn	waste product of muscle metabolism filtered out of the blood by the kidneys and excreted in urine

Symptomatic and Diagnostic Terms

Term	Meaning
Symptomatic	
albuminuria al-byū-mi-nū′rē-ă **proteinuria** prō-tē-nū′rē-ă	presence of albumin in the urine; occurs in renal disease or in normal urine after heavy exercise
anuresis an-yū-rē′sis **anuria** an-yū′rē-ă	no output of urine
bacteriuria bak-tēr-ē-ū′rē-ă	presence of bacteria in the urine
dysuria dis-yū′rē-ă	painful urination
enuresis en-yū-rē′sis	to void urine; involuntary discharge of urine, most often refers to a lack of bladder control
nocturnal enuresis nok-ter′năl	bed wetting during sleep
hematuria hē-mă-tū′rē-ă	presence of blood in the urine (Fig. 15.3)

continued

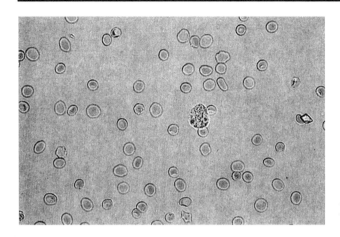

Figure 15.3. Hematuria. Microscopic urine showing a large number of red blood cells. One lone white blood cell is present in the center of the field.

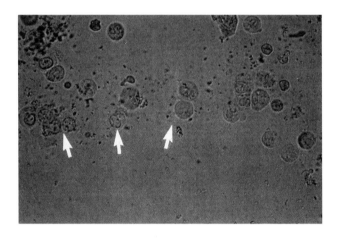

Figure 15.4. Pyuria. Microscopic urine showing the presence of white blood cells (*arrows*).

Term	Meaning
incontinence in-kon'ti-nens	involuntary discharge of urine, feces, or semen
stress incontinence	involuntary discharge of urine at the time of cough, sneeze, and/or strained exercise
ketonuria ke-to-nu're-ă	presence of ketone bodies in the urine

ketone bodies
   ke'ton
   ketone compounds
	acetone, beta-hydroxybutyric acid, and acetoacetic acid are products of metabolism that appear in the urine as a result of an abnormal utilization of carbohydrates; seen in uncontrolled diabetes and starvation

nocturia nok-tu're-ă	urination at night
oliguria ol-i-gu're-ă	scanty production of urine
pyuria pi-yu're-ă	presence of white cells in the urine, usually indicating infection (Fig. 15.4)

continued

Term	Meaning
urinary retention yūr′i-nār-ē rē-ten′shŭn	retention of urine owing to the inability to void (urinate) naturally because of spasm, obstruction, etc.

Diagnostic

Term	Meaning
glomerulonephritis glō-mār′yū-lō-nef-rī′tis	form of nephritis involving the glomerulus
hydronephrosis hī′drō-ne-frō′sis	dilation and pooling of urine in the renal pelvis and calyces of one or both kidneys caused by an obstruction in the outflow of urine (Fig. 15.5)
nephritis ne-frī′tis	inflammation of the kidney
pyelonephritis pī′ĕ-lō-ne-frī′tis	inflammation of the renal pelvis
nephrosis ne-frō′sis	degenerative disease of the renal tubules
nephrolithiasis nef′rō-li-thī′ă-sis	presence of a renal stone or stones (Fig. 15.6)
cystitis sis-tī′tis	inflammation of the bladder
urethritis yū-rē-thrī′tis	inflammation of the urethra
urethrocystitis yū-rē′thrō-sis-tī′tis	inflammation of the urethra and bladder
urethral stenosis yū-rē′thrăl ste-nō′sis	narrowed condition of the urethra
urinary tract infection (UTI)	invasion of pathogenic organisms (commonly bacteria) in the structures of the urinary tract, especially the urethra and bladder; symptoms include dysuria, urinary frequency, malaise

continued

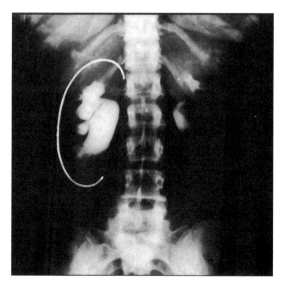

Figure 15.5. Collection of contrast media in the kidney displays an extraordinary amount of material, which indicates right-sided hydronephrosis caused by obstruction in the ureter.

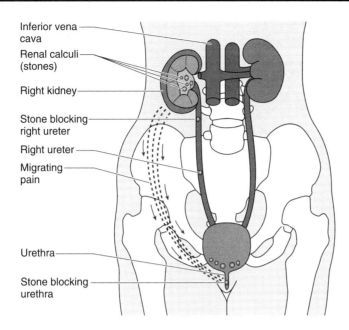

Figure 15.6. Kidney stone formation.

Term	Meaning
uremia yū-rē'mē-ă **azotemia** az-ō-tē'mē-ă	excess of urea and other nitrogenous waste in the blood as a result of kidney failure

Diagnostic Tests and Procedures

Test or Procedure	Explanation
cystoscopy sis-tos'kŏ-pē	examination of the bladder using a rigid or flexible cystoscope (Fig. 15.7)
kidney biopsy (Bx) **renal biopsy**	removal of kidney tissue for pathological examination
radiography rā'dē-og'ră-fē	x-ray studies commonly used in urology
intravenous pyelogram (IVP) in'tră-vē'nŭs pī'el-ō-gram **intravenous urogram**	x-rays of the urinary tract taken after iodine is injected into the bloodstream and as the contrast passes through the kidney, revealing obstruction, evidence of trauma, etc. (Fig. 15.5)
kidney, ureter, bladder (KUB)	abdominal x-ray of kidney, ureter, and bladder typically used as a scout film before doing an IVP (Fig. 15.8)
scout film	plain x-ray taken to detect any obvious pathology before further imaging (e.g., a KUB before an IVP)

continued

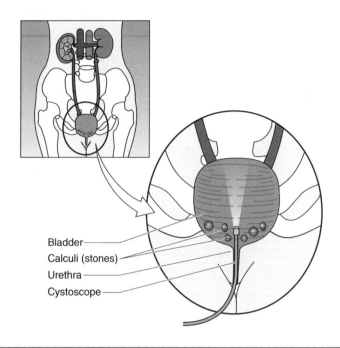

Bladder
Calculi (stones)
Urethra
Cystoscope

Figure 15.7. Cystoscopy.

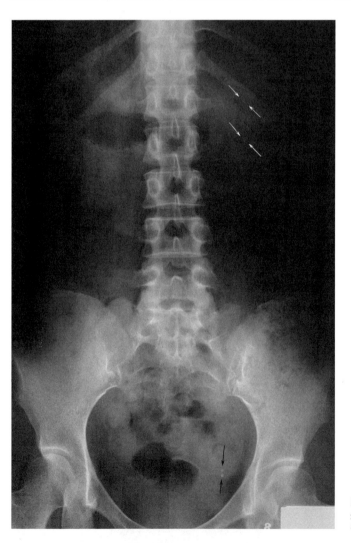

Figure 15.8. KUB showing kidney stones in ureters and bladder (arrows).

Test or Procedure	Explanation
renal angiogram an'jē-ō-gram	x-ray of the renal artery made after injecting contrast material into a catheter in the artery
retrograde pyelogram (RP) ret'rō-grād	x-ray of the ureters, bladder, and kidney taken after contrast medium is sent up through a small catheter passed through a cystoscope to detect the presence of stones, obstruction, etc.
voiding (urinating) cystourethrogram (VCU or VCUG) sis-tō-yū-rēth'rō-gram	x-ray of the bladder and urethra taken during urination
abdominal sonogram son'ō-gram	visualization of the urinary tract including the kidney, ureters, and bladder

Laboratory Testing

urinalysis (UA) yū-ri-nal'i-sis	physical, chemical, and microscopic examination of urine (Fig. 15.9)
specific gravity (SpGr)	measure of the kidney's ability to concentrate or dilute urine
pH	measure of the acidity or alkalinity of urine
glucose (sugar) glū'kōs	chemical test used to detect sugar in the urine, used most often to screen for diabetes
albumin (alb) al-byū'min **protein**	chemical test used to detect the presence of albumin in the urine
ketones **acid**	chemical test used to detect the presence of ketone bodies in the urine; if positive, fats are being utilized by the body instead of carbohydrates, which occurs in starvation or an unstable diabetic state
occult blood, urine	test for the presence of old blood in the urine
bilirubin bil-i-rū'bin	chemical test used to detect bilirubin in the urine
urobilinogen yūr-ō-bī-lin'ō-jen	chemical test used to detect bile pigment in the urine
microscopic findings mī-krō-skop'ik	microscopic identification of abnormal constituents present in the urine (e.g., red blood cells, white blood cells, casts, etc.) as reported per high or low power field (hpf or lpf) (Figs. 15.3 and 15.4)
urine culture and sensitivity	isolation of a urine specimen in a culture medium that propagates the growth of microorganisms; organisms that grow in the culture are identified and drugs to which they are sensitive are listed

continued

CENTRAL MEDICAL CENTER

211 Medical Center Drive • Central City, US 90000-1234 • PHONE: (012) 125-6784 • FAX: (012) 125-9999

11//02/9x
13:49

NAME : TEST, PATIENT   LOC: TEST   DOB: 2/2/XX   AGE: 38Y
MR#   :   TEST-221   SEX: M
ACCT # :   H111111111

M63560 COLL: 11/2/9x 13:24   REC: 11/2/9x 13:25

URINE BASIC
Color	STRAW		
Appearance	CLEAR		
Specific Gravity	1.010	[1.003 - 1.035]	
pH	5.5	[5.0 - 9.0]	
Protein	NEG	[0 - 10]	MG/DL
Glucose	NEG	[NEG]	
Ketones	NEG	[NEG]	
Bilirubin	NEG	[NEG]	
Urine Occult Blood	NEG	[NEG]	
Nitrites	NEG		

URINE MICROSCOPIC
Epithelial Cells	3 to 4	/HPF
WBCs	0 to 1	/HPF
RBCs	0	/HPF
Bacteria	0	
Mucous Threads	0	

TEST, PATIENT   TEST-221   END OF REPORT   PAGE 1
11/02/9x 13:49   INTERIM REPORT
INTERIM REPORT COMPLETED

Figure 15.9. Sample urinalysis report.

Test or Procedure	Explanation
blood urea nitrogen (BUN) yū-rē′ă nī′trō-jen	blood test to determine the level of urea in the blood—a high BUN indicates the kidney's inability to excrete urea
creatinine, serum krē-at′i-nen sēr′ŭm	test to determine the level of creatinine in the blood—useful in assessing kidney function
creatinine, urine	test to determine the level of creatinine in the urine
creatinine clearance testing	measurements of the level of creatinine in the blood and a 24-hour urine specimen to determine the rate that creatinine is "cleared" from the blood by the kidneys

Operative Terms

Term	Meaning
urologic endoscopic surgery yū-rō-loj′ik	use of specialized endoscopes (e.g., resectoscope) within the urinary tract to perform various surgical procedures such as resection of a tumor, repair of an obstruction, stone retrieval, placement of a stent, etc. (Fig. 15.10)
resectoscope rē-sek′tō-skōp	urologic endoscope sent through the urethra to resect (cut and remove) lesions of the bladder, urethra, and prostate
intracorporeal electrohydraulic lithotripsy in′tră-kōr-pō′rē-ăl ē-lek′trō-hī-dro′lik lith′ō-trip-sē	method of destroying stones within the urinary tract using high electrical energy discharges transmitted to a probe within a flexible endoscope—most commonly used to pulverize bladder stones (Fig. 15.11)
nephrotomy ne-frot′ō-mē	incision into the kidney
nephrorrhaphy nef-rōr′ă-fē	suture of an injured kidney

continued

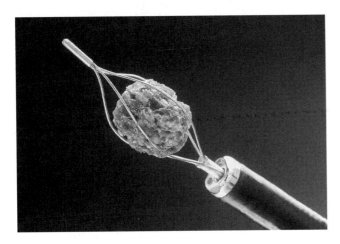

Figure 15.10. Stone basket used in kidney stone retrieval.

Term	Meaning
nephrolithotomy nef′rō-li-thot′ō-mē	incision into the kidney for the removal of stones
nephrectomy ne-frek′tō-mē	excision of a kidney
pyeloplasty pī′e-lō-plas-tē	surgical reconstruction of the renal pelvis
stent placement	use of a device to hold open vessels or tubes (e.g., an obstructed ureter) (Fig. 15.12)

continued

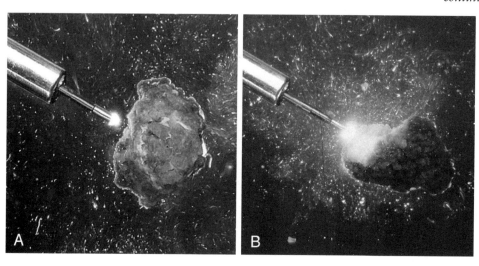

Figure 15.11. Simulation of the pulverizing of stones performed by intracorporeal electrohydraulic lithotripsy.

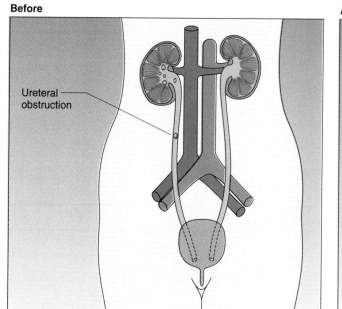
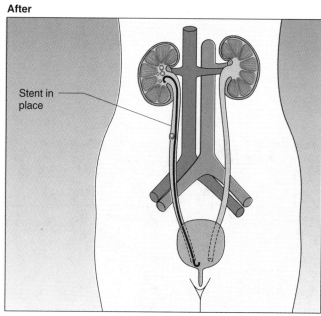

Figure 15.12. Placement of a double-J stent to relieve ureteral obstruction.

Term	Meaning
kidney transplantation **renal transplantation**	transfer of a kidney from the body of one person (donor) to another (Fig. 15.13)
urostomy yur-os′to-me	methods of temporary or permanent diversion of the urinary tract providing a new passage through which urine exits the body, most often by the creation of a stoma (opening) on the abdomen, done as a result of bladder disease or defect
ileal conduit il′e-ăl kon′du-it	removal of a portion of the ileum to use as a conduit to which the ureters are attached at one end; the other end is brought through an opening created in the abdomen (Fig. 15.14)

continued

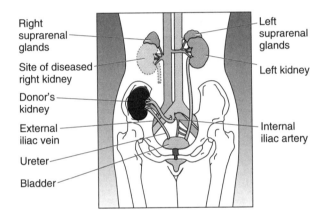

Right suprarenal glands

Left suprarenal glands

Site of diseased right kidney

Left kidney

Donor's kidney

External iliac vein

Internal iliac artery

Ureter

Bladder

Figure 15.13. Common site for donor kidney transplantation.

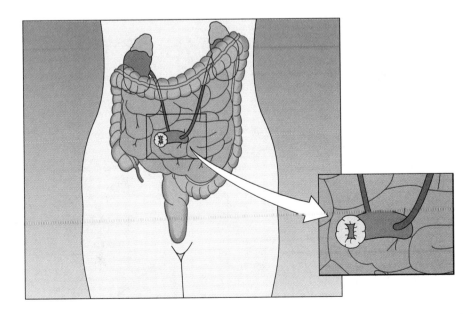

Figure 15.14. Urostomy: ileal conduit.

Therapeutic Terms

Term	Meaning
extracorporeal shock wave lithotripsy (ESWL) eks'tră-kōr-pō'rē-ăl lith'ō-trip-sē	procedure using shock waves to penetrate the body from outside and bombard and disintegrate a stone within—most commonly used to treat urinary stones above the bladder (Fig. 15.15)
kidney dialysis dī-al'i-sis	methods of filtering impurities from the blood to replace the function of one or both kidneys due to renal failure
hemodialysis hē-mō-dī-al'i-sis	method to remove impurities by pumping the patient's blood through a dialyzer, the specialized filter of the artificial kidney machine (hemodialyzer)
peritoneal dialysis per-i-tō-nē'ăl	method of removing impurities using the peritoneum as the filter; catheter insertion in the peritoneal cavity is required to deliver cleansing fluid (dialysate) that is washed in and out in cycles

Common Therapeutic Drug Classifications

analgesic an-ăl-jē'zik	drug that relieves pain
antibiotic an'tē-bī-ot'ik	drug that kills or inhibits the growth of microorganisms
antispasmodic an'tē-spaz-mod'ik	drug that relieves spasm
diuretic dī-yū-ret'ik	drug that increases the secretion of urine

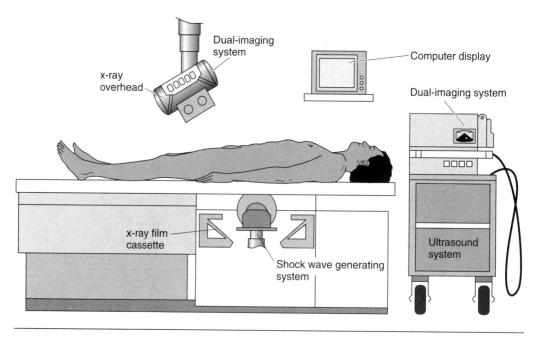

Figure 15.15. Shock wave therapy system for kidney stones.

PRACTICE EXERCISES

For the following terms, draw a line or lines to separate prefixes, combining forms, and suffixes. Then define the term.

1. pyuria _____

2. cystitis _____

3. nephromegaly _____

4. vesicostomy _____

5. urethrocystitis _____

6. nephroptosis _____

7. polydipsia _____

8. glomerulosclerosis _____

9. pyonephritis _____

10. dysuria _____

11. vesicotomy _____

12. glycosuria _____

13. meatal _____

14. pyelonephrosis _____

15. cystectomy _____

16. urologist _____

17. renogram _____

18. urethrostenosis _____

19. urostomy _____

20. urethropexy _____

21. nephrohypertrophy _____

22. transurethral _____

23. ureterolithotomy _____

24. ketosis _____

25. meatorrhaphy _____

26. bacteroid _____

27. renopathy _____

28. hydronephrosis _____

Identify the medical term for the following:

29. inflammation of the bladder _____

30. urinating at night _____

31. involuntary discharge of urine _____

32. suture of a torn kidney _____

33. degenerative disease of the kidney without inflammation_____

34. protein in urine_____

35. narrowed condition of the urethra _____

36. incision into the kidney _____

37. cytology study of kidney tissue_____

38. physical, chemical, and microscopic study of urine _____

Complete the following:

39. _____scopy = examination of the bladder

40. urethral _____osis = a narrowed condition of the urethra

41. extracorporeal shock wave _____ = procedure for disintegration of stones

42. _____scope = endoscope used to cut and remove lesions of the bladder, urethra and prostate

43. _____uria = scanty urination

44. _____uria = painful or difficult urination

45. _____uria = presence of infection in urine

46. _____uria = blood in the urine

47. _____uresis = no output of urine

48. _____uresis = involuntary discharge of urine

49. _____ incontinence = involuntary discharge of urine when coughing or sneezing

50. _____blood = old blood

Give the appropriate abbreviation for the following:

51. _____ kidney x-ray taken after contrast medium is sent "back-ward" through a cystoscope

52. _____ cytology study of kidney tissue

53. _____ physical, chemical, and microscopic study of urine

Match the following:

54. sugar   _____   a. cysto

55. proteinuria   _____   b. acid

56. uremia   _____   c. renal Bx

57. reno   _____   d. albuminuria

58. vesico   _____   e. nephro

59. ketones   _____   f. urination

60. diuretic   _____   g. azotemia

61. kidney biopsy _____   h. gluco

Define the following abbreviations:

62. C&S _____

63. VCU _____

64. alb _____

65. IVP _____

66. ESWL _____

67. KUB _____

68. SpGr _____

69. UTI _____

70. RP _____

Medical Record Analysis

MEDICAL RECORD 15.1

Charles Mercier had urination problems and abdominal pain when he saw his doctor, who referred him to Central Medical Center for a possible kidney infection. Dr. Zlatkin performed surgery, and Mr. Mercier was soon doing fine and was discharged. As planned, he later returned for surgical removal of a device that had been temporarily placed during the first surgery.

Directions

Read Medical Record 15.1 for Mr. Mercier (pages 425–426) and answer the following questions. The first record is the discharge summary from the first surgery, dictated by Dr. Zlatkin. The second record is the operative report for Mr. Mercier's return surgery 6 weeks later, also dictated by Dr. Zlatkin.

Questions about Medical Record 15.1

Write your answers in the spaces provided.

1. Below are medical terms used in this record you have not yet encountered in this text. Underline each where it appears in the record and define below.

   stent (double-J) _____

   drain (Jackson-Pratt) _____

   lithotomy position _____

   ureteral catheter _____

   patency _____

2. In your own words, not using medical terminology, briefly describe the history of Mr. Mercier's medical problems identified in the "Discharge Summary."

   _____

   _____

   _____

3. Put the following events reported in the "Discharge Summary" in chronological order by numbering them from 1 to 5:

   _____ removal of drain

   _____ reconstruction of renal pelvis

   _____ difficulty with micturition

   _____ urine test for microorganisms

   _____ insertion of stent

4. While at home after the operation, Mr. Mercier is instructed to do two things and *not* do three things. List them below:

   Mr. Mercier should _____

   _____

   Mr. Mercier should not _____

   _____

   _____

5. When Mr. Mercier returned 6 weeks later for follow-up surgery, describe in your own words the preoperative diagnosis:

   _____

   _____

   _____

6. During the second surgery, an endoscopic procedure and two different x-ray procedures were used to visualize internal structures. List and define each procedure and describe the findings:

Procedure	Definition	Finding
_____	_____	_____
_____	_____	_____
_____	_____	_____

7. The first surgery included insertion of a specialized device that was then removed in the second surgery. What was this device, and what function did it perform during the time between the two surgeries?

   _____

   _____

   _____

8. In the second surgery, did Mr. Mercier experience any complications? Write the sentence that supports your answer.

   _____

   _____

CENTRAL MEDICAL CENTER

211 Medical Center Drive • Central City, US 90000-1234 • PHONE: (012) 125-6784 • FAX: (012) 125-9999

DISCHARGE SUMMARY

DATE OF ADMISSION: 10/25/9x   DATE OF DISCHARGE: 10/29/9x

ADMITTING DIAGNOSIS:
Left ureteropelvic junction obstruction.

DISCHARGE DIAGNOSIS:
Left ureteropelvic junction obstruction.

PROCEDURE PERFORMED:
Left dismembered pyeloplasty and placement of stent.

BRIEF SUMMARY:
The patient is a 19-year-old male who was admitted to the hospital a month ago with left pyelonephritis. He was found to have a left ureteropelvic junction obstruction. The patient was brought to the hospital at this time for repair of the moderately to severely obstructed left kidney. A preoperative urine culture was sterile. The patient underwent the procedure without complication. A double-J stent was placed. The Jackson-Pratt drain was removed on the second postoperative day because of minimal drainage. The patient initially had urinary retention, but this resolved by the third postoperative day. He was doing fine at the time of discharge. His condition on discharge is good.

INSTRUCTIONS TO THE PATIENT:
1) Regular diet. 2) No heavy lifting, straining, or driving an automobile for six weeks from the day of surgery. He should also keep the incision relatively dry this week. 3) Follow up in my office in three weeks. 4) It is anticipated the stent will remain indwelling for six weeks and then will be removed cystoscopically at that time. 5) Discharge medication is Tylenol #3, 1-2 q 4 h p.r.n. pain.

L. Zlatkin, M.D.

LZ:mr

D: 10/29/9x
T: 10/30/9x

DISCHARGE SUMMARY	PT. NAME:	MERCIER, CHARLES F.
	ID NO:	IP-392689
	ROOM NO:	444
	ATT. PHYS:	L.ZLATKIN, M.D.

Medical Record 15.1.

CENTRAL MEDICAL CENTER

211 Medical Center Drive • Central City, US 90000-1234 • PHONE: (012) 125-6784 • FAX: (012) 125-9999

OPERATIVE REPORT

DATE: December 7, 199x

PREOPERATIVE DIAGNOSIS: Congenital left ureteropelvic junction obstruction status post pyeloplasty. Indwelling left ureteral stent.

POSTOPERATIVE DIAGNOSIS: Congenital left ureteropelvic junction obstruction status post pyeloplasty. Indwelling left ureteral stent, removed

OPERATION: Cystoscopy, removal of left ureteral stent, and left retrograde pyelogram.

PROCEDURE: The patient was identified, was placed on the operating table, and was administered a general anesthetic. He was placed in the lithotomy position, and a KUB was obtained. The genitalia were prepped and draped in a sterile fashion. After reviewing the KUB, it was noted at this time that the position of the stent was normal. Cystoscopy was performed with a #22 French cystoscope. The stent was identified coming from the left ureteral orifice, and the end was grasped with forceps and removed through the cystoscope. A #8 French cone-tipped ureteral catheter was then placed in the left ureteral orifice and passed to 10 cm. Then, 20 cm^3 of contrast was injected into a left collecting system. A film was exposed, and this showed patency without extravasation at the left ureteropelvic junction. There was some filling of calyces and partial filling of the dilated renal pelvis. A drainage film was subsequently obtained showing complete emptying of the pelvis and partial emptying of the mid and distal ureters. Dilated calyces were noted in the kidney. The patient was allowed to awaken and was returned to the recovery room in satisfactory condition. There were no intraoperative complications. He had no bleeding. The patient did receive 1 gm Ancef one-half hour prior to the onset of the procedure.

L. Zlatkin, M.D.

LZ:mr
D: 12/07/9x
T: 12/08/9x

OPERATIVE REPORT	PT. NAME:	MERCIER, CHARLES F.
	ID NO:	OP-912689
	ROOM NO:	ASC
	ATT. PHYS:	L.ZLATKIN, M.D.

Medical Record 15.1. *Continued.*

Male Reproductive System

16

OBJECTIVES

After completion of this chapter you will be able to

1. Define common combining forms used in relation to the male reproductive system

2. Define basic anatomical terms referring to the male reproductive system

3. Define common symptomatic, diagnostic, operative, and therapeutic terms referring to the male reproductive system

4. List the common diagnostic tests and procedures related to the male reproductive system

5. Explain terms and abbreviations used in documenting medical records involving the male reproductive system.

Combining Forms

Combining Form	Meaning	Example
balan/o	glans penis	**balanoplasty** bal'an-ō-plas-tē
epididym/o	epididymis	**epididymitis** ep-i-did-i-mī'tis
orch/o	testis or testicle	**orchitis** ōr-kī'tis
orchi/o		**orchiopexy** ōr'kē-ō-pek'sē
orchid/o		**orchidectomy** ōr-ki-dek'tō-me
test/o		**testicle** tes'tĭ-kl
perine/o	perineum	**perineal** per'i-nē'ăl
prostat/o	prostate	**prostatodynia** pros'tă-tō-din'ē-ă
sperm/o	sperm (seed)	**oligospermia** ol-i-gō-sper'mē-ă
spermat/o		**spermatic** sper-mat'ik
vas/o	vessel	**vasorrhaphy** vas-ōr'ă-fē

ORCHIO. Orchio is a Greek root for testicle, so named for the resemblance of the gland to the root of the orchid plant. At one time, orchid root was used to treat diseases of the testicle.

TESTICLE. Testicle is from the Latin testis, a word that also meant a witness or one who testifies. The presence of the testicles was evidence of virility, and it is said that under Roman law that no man could witness in court unless his testicles were present. An oath was taken with a hand on the testicles. The testicles are also associated with the swearing of oaths in the Old Testament.

Male Reproductive System Overview

The male reproductive system includes the *scrotum, testes, epididymides, vas deferens, seminal vesicles, prostate gland, bulbourethral glands, urethra,* and *penis* (Fig. 16.1). These parts produce and maintain *sperm,* the male reproductive cells, and introduce them into the female reproductive tract for the purpose of fertilizing the female ovum. The male reproductive organs also secrete certain hormones necessary for the maintenance of secondary sexual characteristics in the male (see Color Atlas, plate 30)

Anatomical Terms

Term	Meaning
scrotum skrō'tŭm	a bag; skin-covered pouch in the groin that is divided into two sacs, each containing a testis and an epididymis
testis (testicle) tes'tis	one of the two male reproductive glands, located in the scrotum, that produces sperm and the male hormone testosterone

continued

Term	Meaning
sperm **spermatozoon** sper'mă-tō-zō'on	male gamete or sex cell produced in the testes that unites with the ovum in the female to produce offspring
epididymis ep-i-did'i-mis	coiled duct on top and at the side of the testis that stores sperm before emission
penis pē'nis	erectile tissue covered with skin that contains the urethra for urination and ducts for the secretion of seminal fluid (semen)
glans penis glanz	bulging structure at the distal end of the penis (glans = acorn)
prepuce prē'pūs	foreskin; loose casing covering the glans penis—removed by circumcision
vas deferens vas def'er-ens	duct that carries sperm from the epididymis to the ejaculatory duct (vas = vessel; deferens = carrying away)
seminal vesicle sem'i-năl	one of two sac-like structures lying behind the bladder and connected to the vas deferens on each side—secretes an alkaline substance into the semen to enable the sperm to live longer
semen sē'men	a mixture of the secretions of the testes, seminal vesicles, prostate, and bulbourethral glands discharged from the male urethra during orgasm (semen = seed)

PENIS. Penis is a Latin word for tail. The name is also derived from pendere, to hang down. The Romans had a great many terms for the male organ, e.g., cauda (tail), clava (club), gladius (sword), radix (root), ramus (branch), and vomer (plough). Penis was adopted as the anatomical term, and it has been used in English since the 17th century.

continued

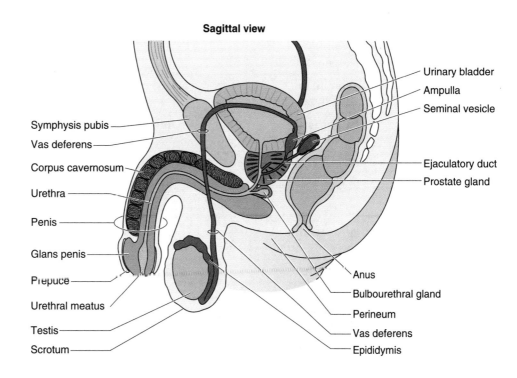

Frontal view

Sagittal view

Symphysis pubis
Vas deferens
Corpus cavernosum
Urethra
Penis
Glans penis
Prepuce
Urethral meatus
Testis
Scrotum

Urinary bladder
Ampulla
Seminal vesicle
Ejaculatory duct
Prostate gland
Anus
Bulbourethral gland
Perineum
Vas deferens
Epididymis

Figure 16.1. Male reproductive system.

Term	Meaning
ejaculatory duct ē-jak′yū-lă-tōr-ē	duct formed by the union of the vas deferens with the duct of the seminal vesicle; its fluid is carried into the urethra
prostate gland pros′tāt	trilobular gland that encircles the urethra just below the bladder—secretes an alkaline fluid into the semen
bulbourethral glands (Cowper's glands) bŭl′bō-yū-rē′thrăl	pair of glands below the prostate with ducts opening into the urethra—adds a viscid (sticky) fluid to the semen
perineum per′i-nē′ŭm	external region between the scrotum and anus in a male and between the vulva and anus in a female

Symptomatic and Diagnostic Terms

Term	Meaning
Symptomatic	
aspermia ā-sper′mē-ă	inability to secrete or ejaculate sperm
azoospermia ā-zō-ō-sper′mē-ă	semen without living spermatozoa, a sign of infertility in the male (zoo = life)
oligospermia ol-i-gō-sper′mē-ă	scanty production and expulsion of sperm
mucopurulent discharge myū-kō-pū′rū-lent	drainage of mucus and pus
Diagnostic	
anorchism an-ōr′kizm	absence of one or both testes
balanitis bal-ă-nī′tis	inflammation of glans penis
cryptorchism krip-tōr′kizm	undescended testicle; failure of a testis to descend into scrotal sac during fetal development; it most often remains lodged in the abdomen or inguinal canal requiring surgical repair (crypt = to hide) (Fig. 16.2)
epididymitis ep-i-did-i-mī′tis	inflammation of the epididymis
hydrocele hī′drō-sēl	hernia of fluid in the testis or tubes leading from the testis (Fig. 16.3)
hypospadias hī′pō-spā′dē-ăs	congenital opening of the male urethra on the undersurface of the penis (spadias = to draw away) (Fig. 16.4)
impotence im′pŏ-tens	failure to initiate or maintain an erection until ejaculation because of physical or psychological dysfunction (im = not; potis = able)

continued

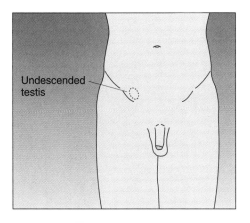

Figure 16.2. Cryptorchism.

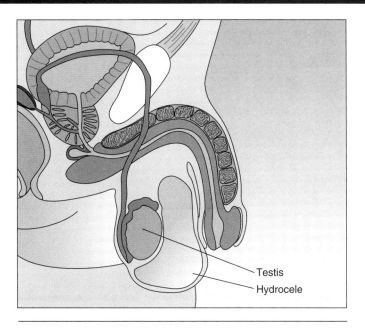

Figure 16.3. Hydrocele.

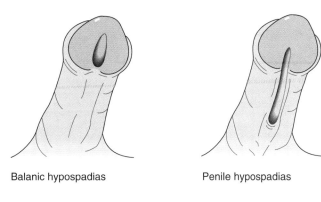

Balanic hypospadias   Penile hypospadias

Figure 16.4. Hypospadias

Term	Meaning
Peyronie's disease pā-rōn′ēz	disorder characterized by the induration (hardness) of the corpus cavernosum in the penis (Fig. 16.5)
benign prostatic hypertrophy/hyperplasia (BPH) bē-nīn′ pros-tat′ik hī-per′trō-fē	enlargement of the prostate gland; frequently seen in older men, causing urinary obstruction (Fig. 16.6)
prostate cancer	malignancy of the prostate gland
prostatitis pros-tă-tī′tis	inflammation of the prostate
seminoma sem-i-nō′mă	common type of malignant tumor of the testicle (testicular tumor)
varicocele var′i-kō-sēl	enlarged, swollen, herniated veins near the testis (varico = twisted vein)

continued

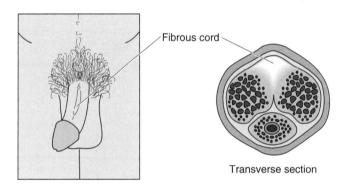

Fibrous cord

Transverse section

Figure 16.5. Peyronie's disease.

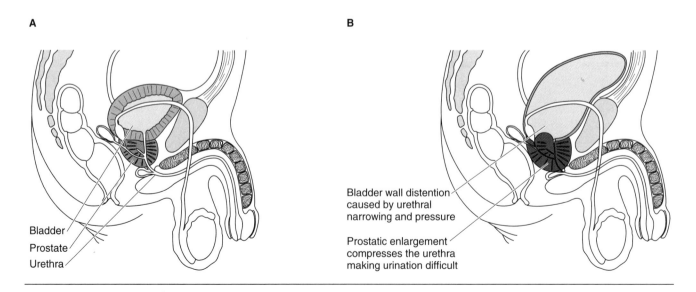

Bladder
Prostate
Urethra

Bladder wall distention caused by urethral narrowing and pressure

Prostatic enlargement compresses the urethra making urination difficult

Figure 16.6. A. Normal prostate. **B.** Hypertrophic prostate.

Term	Meaning
Sexually Transmitted Disease (STD)	
Major Bacterial STDs bak-tēr′ē-ăl	
chlamydia kla-mid′ē-ă	most common sexually transmitted bacterial infection in North America, often occurs with no symptoms and is treated only after it has spread
chancroid shang′kroyd	infection caused by a bacillus that erupts as a papule on the skin of the penis, urethra, or anus and ulcerates and spreads, causing enlarged lymph nodes in the groin (buboes) (chancre = ulcer; oid = resembling) (see Color Atlas, plate 4)
gonorrhea gon-ō-rē′ă	contagious inflammation of the genital mucous membranes caused by invasion of the gonococcus, *Neisseria gonorrhea* (gono = seed; rrhea = discharge)
syphilis sif′i-lis	infectious disease caused by a spirochete transmitted by direct intimate contact that may involve any organ or tissue over time, usually manifested first on the skin with the appearance of small, painless red papules that erode and form bloodless ulcers called chancres (see Color Atlas, plate 4)
Major Viral STDs vī′răl	
hepatitis B virus (HBV) hep-ă-tī′tis	virus that causes inflammation of the liver as a result of transmission through any body fluid, including vaginal secretions, semen, blood, etc.
herpes simplex virus Type II (HSV-2) her′pēz	virus that causes ulcer-like lesions of the genital and anorectal skin and mucosa; after initial infection the virus lies dormant in the nerve cell root and may recur at times of stress (see Color Atlas, plate 4)
human immunodeficiency virus (HIV) im′yū-nō-dē-fish′en-sē	virus that causes acquired immunodeficiency syndrome (AIDS), which permits various opportunistic infections, malignancies, and neurologic diseases; contracted through exposure to contaminated blood or body fluid (e.g., semen or vaginal secretions)
human papilloma virus (HPV) papi-lō′mă **condyloma acuminatum** kon-di-lō′mah ă-kyū′mĭ-nāt′ŭm **pl. condylomata acuminata** kon-di-lō′mah′t ă-kyū′mĭ-nah′t ă	virus transmitted by direct sexual contact that causes an infection that can occur on the skin or mucous membranes of the genitals; on the skin the lesions appear as cauliflower-like warts, and on mucous membranes they have a flat appearance (also known as venereal or genital warts) (see Color Atlas plate 4)

GONORRHEA. Derived from the Greek root gono meaning offspring or seed and suffix rrhea meaning flow or discharge, the word literally means flow of semen. It was once thought that the urethral discharge characteristic of the infection was a leakage of semen. Although the reasoning is wrong, attempts to change the term failed because its usage was too firmly established.

Diagnostic Tests and Procedures

Test or Procedure	Explanation
biopsy (Bx)	tissue sampling used to identify neoplasia
biopsy of the prostate	needle biopsy of the prostate often performed using ultrasound guidance

continued

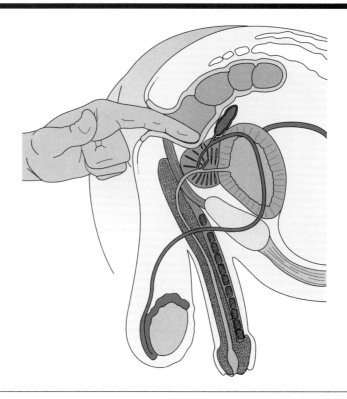

Figure 16.7. Digital rectal examination.

Test or Procedure	Explanation
testicular biopsy tes-tik′yū-lăr	a biopsy of a testicle
digital rectal exam (DRE)	insertion of a finger into the male rectum to palpate the rectum and prostate (Fig. 16.7)
prostate-specific antigen (PSA) **test** an′ti-jen	blood test used to screen for prostate cancer; an elevated level of the antigen indicates the possible presence of tumor
urethrogram yū-rē′thrō-gram	x-ray of urethra and prostate
semen analysis sē′men	study of semen including a sperm count with observation of form and motility; usually performed to rule out male infertility
endorectal (transrectal) **sonogram of the prostate** en′dō-rek′tăl trans-rek′tăl	scan of the prostate made after introducing an ultrasonic transducer into the rectum—also used to guide needle biopsy (Fig. 16.8)

Operative Terms

Term	Meaning
circumcision ser-kŭm-sizh′ŭn	removal of the foreskin (prepuce) exposing the glans penis

continued

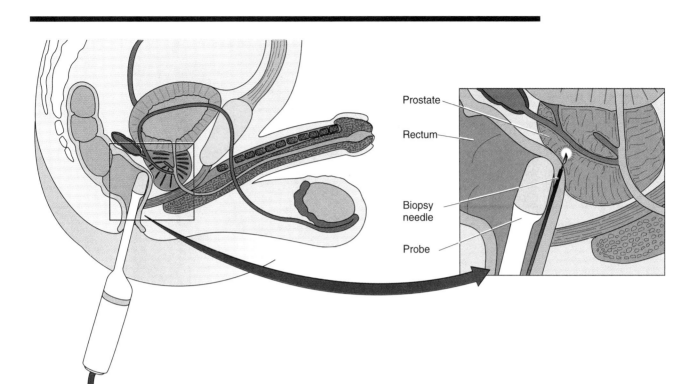

Figure 16.8. Ultrasound and biopsy (*inset*) of prostate.

Term	Meaning
epididymectomy ep'i-did-i-mek'tō-mē	removal of an epididymis
orchiectomy ōr-kē-ek'tō-mē **orchidectomy** ōr-ki-dek'tō-mē	removal of a testicle
orchioplasty ōr'kē-ō-plas-tē	repair of a testicle
orchiopexy ōr'kē-ō-pek'sē	fixation of an undescended testis in the scrotum
prostatectomy pros-tă-tek'tō-mē	excision of the prostate gland
transurethral resection of the prostate (TURP) trans-yū-rē'thrăl re-sek'shŭn	removal of prostatic gland tissue through the urethra using a resectoscope, a specialized urologic endoscope (Fig. 16.9)
vasectomy va-sek'tō-mē	removal of a segment of the vas deferens to produce sterility in the male (Fig. 16.10)
vasovasostomy vā'sō-vă-sos'tō-mē	restoration of the function of the vas deferens to regain fertility after vasectomy

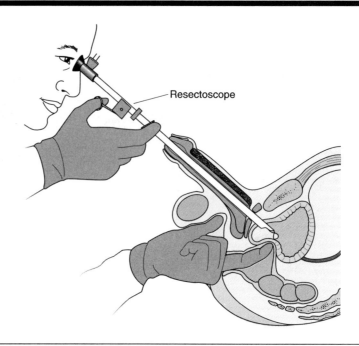

Figure 16.9. Transurethral resection of prostate (TURP).

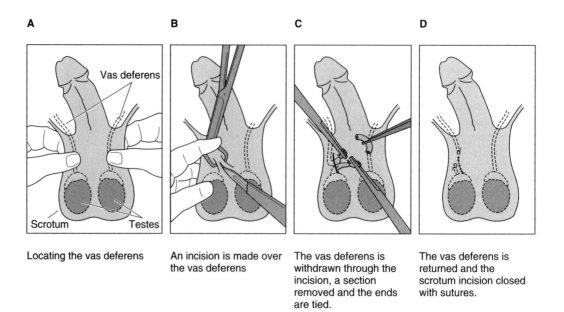

Figure 16.10. Vasectomy.

Therapeutic Terms

Term	Meaning
chemotherapy kem'ō-thār-ă-pē	treatment of malignancies, infections, and other diseases with chemical agents that destroy selected cells or impair their ability to reproduce
radiation therapy rā'dē-ā'shŭn	treatment of neoplastic disease by using radiation, usually from a cobalt source, to deter the proliferation of malignant cells
hormone replacement therapy (HRT)	use of a hormone to remedy a deficiency or regulate production (e.g., testosterone)
penile prosthesis pē'nĭl pros'thē-sis	implantation of a device designed to provide an erection of the penis—used to treat physical impotence

PRACTICE EXERCISES

For the following terms, draw a line or lines to separate prefixes, combining forms, and suffixes. Then define the term.

1. oligospermia _____

2. perineal _____

3. orchialgia _____

4. balanorrhagia _____

5. prostatodynia _____

6. orchidectomy _____

7. anorchism _____

8. vasectomy _____

9. aspermia _____

10. prostatitis _____

11. balanitis _____

12. orchioplasty _____

13. hydrocele _____

14. epididymectomy _____

15. vasovasostomy _____

Identify the medical term for the following:

16. absence of a testicle _____

17. inflammation of glans penis _____

18. failure to maintain an erection _____

19. enlarged, herniated veins near the testicle _____

20. testicular cancer tumor _____

21. semen without living sperm _____

22. scanty production of sperm _____

23. operative treatment for cryptorchism_____

24. specialized endoscope used to approach the prostate when performing a TURP

    _____

25. enlargement of prostate _____

26. fluid hernia in the testis _____

27. removal of a portion of the vas deferens to produce male sterility

    _____

28. disorder that causes induration of the corpora cavernosa in the penis

    _____

29. removal of foreskin to expose glans penis_____

Complete the following:

30. _____orchism = undescended testicle

31. _____ _____ exam = insertion of a finger into
    the male rectum to palpate rectum and prostate

32. _____ sonogram of prostate = ultrasound scan of prostate made
    after introduction of transducer into rectum

33. _____penis = bulging structure at the distal end of the penis

34. _____spermia = inability to secrete or ejaculate semen

Match the following:

35.	semen analysis	_____	a. orchiopexy
36.	testis	_____	b. foreskin
37.	testo	_____	c. sperm morphology
38.	BPH	_____	d. testes
39.	cryptorchism	_____	e. TURP
40.	prepuce	_____	f. orchido

Define the following abbreviations:

41. PSA_____

42. BPH _____

43. TURP _____

44. DRE _____

45. Bx _____

Medical Record Analyses

MEDICAL RECORD 16.1

Larry Phelps, age 31, has been happily married to his wife Nancy for almost five years. They have two children. The second child caused some health problems for Nancy, and her obstetrician recommended that they have no more children because of the risk to her health. After trying different forms of birth control, Nancy and Larry decided that he would have a vasectomy. His doctor referred him to Dr. Jerard Derrick in the urology department at Central Medical Group, Inc.

Directions

Read Medical Record 16.1 for Larry Phelps (pages 444–445) and answer the following questions. This record is a series of three chart notes written by Dr. Derrick after first meeting with Mr. Phelps to schedule surgery, after the surgery and discharge, and after seeing Mr. Phelps in a follow-up 10 days later.

Questions about Medical Record 16.1

Write your answers in the spaces provided.

1. Below are medical terms used in this record you have not yet encountered in this text. Underline each where it appears in the record and define below.

   sterility _____

   infiltrated _____

   resect _____

   ejaculation _____

   induration _____

2. The medical record suggests that Mr. Phelps signed which of these before surgery?

   a. last will and testament

   b. consent form

   c. application to sperm bank

   d. none of the above

3. In your own words, not using medical terminology, briefly summarize the procedure Dr. Derrick performed.

   _____

   _____

   _____

4. Complications of the surgery included the following:

    a. sterility

    b. fever

    c. nausea and vomiting

    d. bleeding

    e. all of the above

    f. none of the above

5. Translate the instruction for the immediate postoperative medication (how much, how often):

    _____

    _____

    _____

6. Mark any of the following that were symptoms Mr. Phelps reported to Dr. Derrick on his follow-up visit 10 days after surgery.

    a. fever

    b. bleeding

    c. pain in scrotum

    d. impotence

    e. suture loosening

7. Dr. Derrick carefully examined Mr. Phelps in the follow-up visit and noted the following objective findings (mark all that are appropriate):

    a. minor bruising in the scrotum

    b. small area of hard tissue at left vasectomy site

    c. bleeding at left vasectomy site

    d. pain at left vasectomy site

    e. very sore elevated mass at right vasectomy site

f. bleeding at right vasectomy site

g. pain at right vasectomy site

h. hard tissue areas along upper scrotum

i. black and blue penis

8. In your own words, define the diagnosis Dr. Derrick made in the follow-up visit:

_____

_____

_____

9. Translate Dr. Derrick's medication instructions after the follow-up visit:

Medication	Amount	How Often
_____	_____	_____
_____	_____	_____
_____	_____	_____
_____	_____	_____

CENTRAL MEDICAL GROUP, INC.

Department of Urology

201 Medical Center Drive • Central City, US 90000-1234 • PHONE: (012) 125-8888 • FAX: (012) 125-3434

PROGRESS NOTES

PHELPS, LAWRENCE

June 4, 199x

SUBJECTIVE: This 31-year-old male desires vasectomy for sterility. He and his wife have two children. He states that another pregnancy would put his wife at health risk.

OBJECTIVE: Normal genitalia with single vas bilaterally.

ASSESSMENT: The procedure, goals and risks were thoroughly discussed with the aid of pictures. The vasectomy booklet and consent form were provided to the patient.

PLAN: Schedule bilateral vasectomy.

DL:ti   T:6/7/9x

J. Derrick, M.D.
J. Derrick, M.D.

June 10, 199x

PROCEDURE: Bilateral vasectomy.

The patient was placed supine on the table; and the scrotum was shaved, prepped, and draped in the usual fashion. The right testicle was grasped, and the right vas was brought to the skin and was infiltrated with 1% Xylocaine. The vas was freed through a small incision. A segment was resected, and the ends were cauterized and tied with 3-0 silk suture. The skin was closed with 4-0 chromic suture. The same procedure was repeated on the left. There were no complications or bleeding.

PLAN: The patient is discharged to the care of his wife with an Rx for Darvocet-N, 100 mg, 1 q 4 h p.r.n. pain. He has been given a post-vasectomy instruction sheet. He is asked to call if there are any problems. He was also instructed to submit a semen specimen for analysis after 15-20 ejaculations.

DL:ti   T:6/12/9x

J. Derrick, M.D.
J. Derrick, M.D.

Medical Record 16.1.

CENTRAL MEDICAL GROUP, INC.

Department of Urology

201 Medical Center Drive • Central City, US 90000-1234 • PHONE: (012) 125-8888 • FAX: (012) 125-3434

PROGRESS NOTES

PHELPS, LAWRENCE

June 20, 199x

SUBJECTIVE: The patient has had pain in the right scrotum since surgery which became worse yesterday with pain in his right back. He states he has had no fevers, nausea, or vomiting.

OBJECTIVE:
1) Mild scrotal ecchymoses inferiorly. Normal testes and epididymides.
2) Small induration at left vasectomy site without tenderness.
3) Exquisitely tender 1.5 cm nodule at right vasectomy site; no induration in upper scrotum or cord.

ASSESSMENT: Probable small hematoma at right vasectomy site.

PLAN: Rx: Cipro 500 mg b.i.d. x 5 d
Darvocet-N 100 mg q 4 h p.r.n. pain
ibuprofen p.r.n.

RTO in one week.

DL:ti   T:6/22/9x

J. Derrick, M.D.

J. Derrick, M.D.

Medical Record 16.1. *Continued.*

MEDICAL RECORD 16.2

James Easley was having some difficulty urinating fully and was feeling gradually increasing pain in the perineal area. He went to see his personal physician, who after a digital rectal examination referred him to Dr. Lentz, a urologist at Central Medical Center.

Directions

Read Medical Record 16.2 for James Easley (page 447) and answer the following questions. This record is the ultrasound report dictated by Dr. Lentz after his session with Mr. Easley in the ultrasound suite at Central Medical Center.

Questions about Medical Record 16.2

Write your answers in the spaces provided:

1. Below are medical terms used in this record you have not yet encountered in this text. Underline each where it appears in the record and define below.

   needle biopsy _____

   MHz _____

   bifocal _____

2. In your own words, not using medical terminology, briefly describe the ultrasound procedure Mr. Easley underwent.

   _____

   _____

   _____

3. In your own words, describe the position Mr. Easley was put in for the ultrasound.

   _____

   _____

   _____

4. Mark any of the following that are abnormal findings in Dr. Lentz's report?
   a. enlarged prostate gland
   b. hemorrhage
   c. hypoechoic lesion
   d. obstructed urethra
   e. prostatic calculi
   f. multiplanar rectum

5. Because of the results of the ultrasound, Dr. Lentz decided to perform an additional diagnostic procedure while Mr. Easley was in the ultrasound suite. In your own words, describe that procedure.

   _____

   _____

6. Explain why Dr. Lentz's report does not include a plan or recommendations for further actions.

   _____

   _____

   _____

7. When and for how long should Mr. Easley take the Noroxin?

   _____

   _____

CENTRAL MEDICAL CENTER

211 Medical Center Drive • Central City, US 90000-1234 • PHONE: (012) 125-6784 • FAX: (012) 125-9999

PROSTATIC ULTRASOUND

EXAMINATION: Transrectal ultrasound of the prostate gland with biopsy.

DIGITAL RECTAL EXAMINATION: Grade I enlarged prostate gland, benign-feeling.

PSA: 5.7 ng%

PROCEDURE: An ultrasound unit with a 7.5 MHz bifocal multiplanar rectal transducer was used to scan the prostate gland. The patient was placed in the left lateral decubitus position. The prostate and seminal vesicles were thoroughly scanned in the transverse and sagittal modes.

The abnormal findings included a hypoechoic lesion at the right base of the prostate gland in the central zone. There were numerous prostatic calculi. The prostatic volume was 22 cc, and the PSA density was 0.25 (calculation based on PSA value and size of prostate). A prostatic needle biopsy was performed because of the increased PSA density and the hypoechoic lesion. This was accomplished without incident.

The patient tolerated the procedure well and had minimal bleeding and discomfort. The patient left the ultrasound suite in satisfactory condition. The patient was placed on Noroxin 400 mg b.i.d. x 3 days.

Further recommendations will be made following the biopsy report.

R. Lentz, M.D.

RL:kj

D: 9/11/9x
T: 9/14/9x

PROSTATIC ULTRASOUND	PT. NAME:	EASLEY, JAMES R.
	ID NO:	SI-350013
	ATT. PHYS:	R. LENTZ, M.D.

Medical Record 16.2.

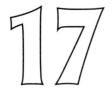

CHAPTER

Female Reproductive System

OBJECTIVES

After completion of this chapter you will be able to

1. **Define common combining forms used in relation to the female reproductive system**

2. **Define the basic anatomical terms referring to the female reproductive system**

3. **Define common symptomatic, diagnostic, operative, and therapeutic terms referring to the female reproductive system**

4. **List the common diagnostic tests and procedures related to the female reproductive system**

5. **Explain the terms used in documenting medical records involving the female reproductive system**

Combining Forms

Combining Form	Meaning	Example
cervic/o	neck or cervix	**cervical** ser′vĭ-kal
colp/o vagin/o	vagina (sheath)	**colposcope** kol′po-skop **vaginal** vaj′i-năl
episi/o vulv/o	vulva (covering)	**episiotomy** e-piz-e-ot′o-me **vulvar** vŭl′văr
gynec/o	woman	**gynecology** gı-nĕ-kol′o-je
hyster/o metr/o uter/o	uterus	**hysteroscopy** his-ter-os′kŏ-pe **metrorrhagia** me-tro-ra′je-ă **uterus** u′ter-ŭs
lact/o	milk	**lactogenic** lak-to-jen′ik
mast/o mamm/o	breast	**mastodynia** mas-to-din′e-ă **mammogram** mam′o-gram
men/o	menstruation	**menopause** men′o-pawz
oophor/o ovari/o	ovary	**oophoritis** o-of-or-ı′tis **ovarian** o-var′e-an
ov/i ov/o	egg	**ovigenesis** o-vi-jen′ĕ-sis **ovum** o′vŭm
salping/o	uterine (fallopian) tube (also eustachian tube)	**salpingitis** sal-pin-jı′tis
toc/o	labor or birth	**dystocia** dis-to′se-ă
-arche (additional suffix)	beginning	**menarche** me-nar′ke

Female Reproductive System Overview

The female reproductive system consists of the uterus, ovaries, uterine (fallopian) tubes, vagina, and vulva (Fig. 17.1). These structures are responsible for producing and maintaining female ova and providing a place for the implantation and nurturing of the fertilized ovum until birth. Treatment of the female reproductive system involves two medical specialties: gynecology and obstetrics (see Color Atlas, plates 31 and 32)

Anatomical Terms

Term	Meaning
uterus ū′ter-ŭs	womb; pear-shaped organ in the pelvic cavity in which the embryo develops
fundus fŭn′dŭs	upper portion of the uterus above the entry to the uterine tubes
endometrium en′dō-me′tre-ŭm	lining of the uterus that is shed approximately every 28–30 days in the nonpregnant female during *menstruation*

continued

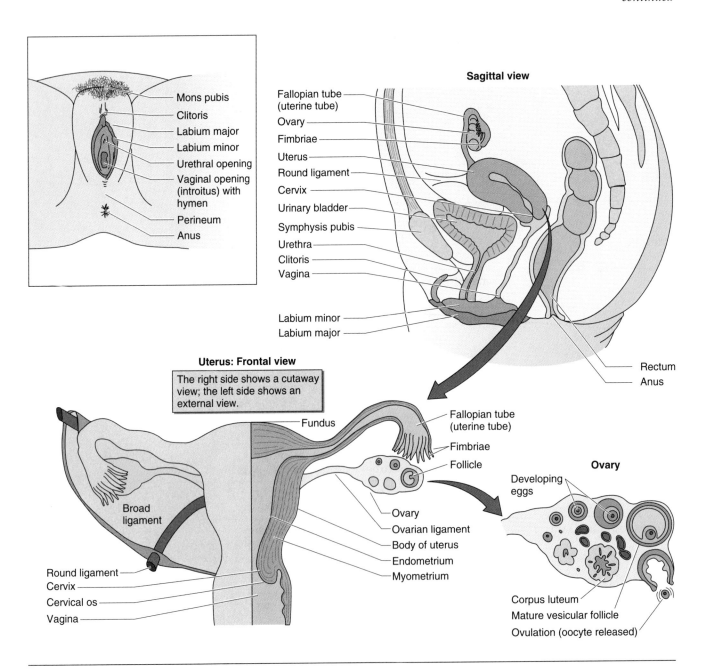

Figure 17.1. Female reproductive system.

Term	Meaning
myometrium mī′ō-mē′trē-ŭm	muscular wall of the uterus
uterine or fallopian tubes yū′ter-in fa-lō′pē-an	tubes extending from each side of the uterus toward the ovary that provide a passage for ova to the uterus
adnexa ad-nek′să	uterine tubes and ovaries (uterine appendages)
right uterine appendage	right tube and ovary
left uterine appendage	left tube and ovary
ovary ō′vă-rē	one of two glands located on each side of the pelvic cavity that produce ova and female sex hormones
cervix ser′viks	neck of the uterus
cervical os ser′vĭ-kăl os	opening of the cervix to the uterus
vagina vă-jī′nă	tubular passageway from the cervix to the outside of the body
vulva vŭl′vă	external genitalia of the female
labia lā′bē-ă	folds of tissue on either side of the vaginal opening known as the labia majora and labia minora
clitoris klit′ō-ris	female erectile tissue situated in the anterior portion of the vulva
hymen hī′men	a fold of mucous membrane that encircles the entrance to the vagina
introitus in-trō′i-tŭs	entrance to the vagina
Bartholin′s glands	two glands located on either side of the vaginal opening that secrete a lubricant during intercourse
perineum per′i-nē′ŭm	region between the vulva and anus
mammary glands mam′ă-rē	two glands of the female breasts capable of producing milk (see Color Atlas, plate 32)
mammary papilla pă-pil′ă	nipple
areola â-rē′ō-lă	dark pigmented area around the nipple
embryo em′brē-ō	developing organism from fertilization to the end of the eighth week (see Color Atlas, plate 32)

FALLOPIUS. Gabriele Fallopius, a 16th century Italian anatomist, made many important observations, especially concerning the female reproductive organs. His classical descriptions resulted in his name being associated with the uterine tubes. He compared the abdominal end of each tube to a trumpet.

MAMMA. Mamma is Latin for breast; the word is said to come from the cry of the infant for "ma-ma," which is a sound common to most languages and is the root for mother in many.

continued

Term	Meaning
fetus fē'tŭs	developing organism from the ninth week to birth (see Color Atlas, plate 32)
placenta plă-sen'tă	vascular organ that develops in the uterine wall during pregnancy that provides nourishment for the fetus (placenta = cake)
amniotic sac am-nē-ot'ik	membranes surrounding the embryo in the uterus filled with amniotic fluid
amniotic fluid	fluid within the amniotic sac that surrounds and protects the fetus
meconium mē-kō'nē-ŭm	intestinal discharges of the fetus that form the first stools in the newborn

Gynecological Symptomatic Terms
gī'nĕ-kō-loj'i-kăl

Term	Meaning
amenorrhea ă-men-ō-re'ă	absence of menstruation
anovulation an-ov-yū-lā'shŭn	absence of ovulation
dysmenorrhea dis-men-ōr-e'ă	painful menstruation
dyspareunia dis-pa-rū'nē-ă	painful intercourse (coitus) (dys = painful; para = alongside of; cunia = a lying)
leukorrhea lū-kō-re'ă	abnormal white or yellow vaginal discharge
menorrhagia men-ō-rā'jē-ă	excessive bleeding at the time of menstruation (menses)
metrorrhagia mē-trō-rā'jē-ă	bleeding from the uterus at any time other than normal menstruation
oligomenorrhea ol'i-gō-men-ō-re'ă	scanty menstrual period
oligo-ovulation ol'i-gō-ov'yū-lā'shŭn	irregular ovulation

Gynecological Diagnostic Terms

Term	Meaning
cervicitis ser-vi-sī'tis	inflammation of the cervix

continued

Term	Meaning
congenital anomalies (irregularities) kon-jen'i-tăl ă-nom'ă-lēz	birth defects causing the abnormal development of a female organ or structure (e.g., double uterus or absent vagina)
dermoid cyst der'moyd sist	congenital tumor composed of displaced embryonic tissue (teeth, bone, cartilage, and hair) more commonly found in an ovary; it is usually benign
displacements of uterus	displacement of the uterus from its normal position (Fig. 17.2)
anteflexion an-tē-flek'shŭn	abnormal forward bending of the uterus (ante = before; flexus = bend)
retroflexion re-trō-flek'shŭn	abnormal backward bending of the uterus
retroversion re-trō-ver'zhŭn	backward turn of the whole uterus—also called tipped uterus

continued

Anteflexion

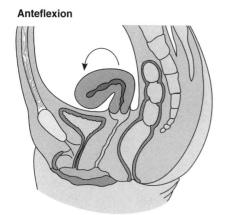

Retroflexion

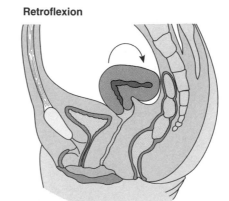

The three degrees of retroversion

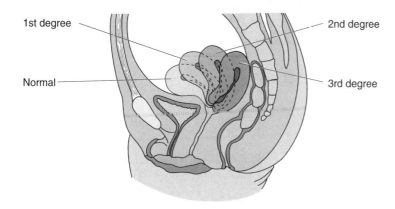

Figure 17.2. Displacements of the uterus.

Term	Meaning
endometriosis en'dō-mē-trē-ō'sis	condition characterized by migration of portions of endometrial tissue outside the uterine cavity
endometritis en'dō-mē-trī'tis	inflammation of the endometrium
fibroid fī'broyd **fibromyoma** fī'brō-mī-ō'mă **leiomyoma** lī'ō-mī-ō'mă	benign tumor in the uterus composed of smooth muscle and fibrous connective tissue (Fig. 17.3)
fistula fis'tyū-lă	abnormal passage such as from one hollow organ to another (fistula = pipe) (Fig. 17.4)
rectovaginal fistula rek-tō-vaj'i-năl	abnormal opening between the vagina and rectum
vesicovaginal fistula ves-i-kō-vaj'i-năl	abnormal opening between the bladder and vagina
cervical neoplasia	abnormal development of cervical tissue cells
cervical intraepithelial neoplasia (CIN) in'tră-ep-i-thē'lē-ăl nē-ō-plā'zē-ă **cervical dysplasia** dis-plā'zē-ă	potentially cancerous abnormality of epithelial tissue of the cervix, graded according to the extent of abnormal cell formation: CIN I mild dysplasia CIN II moderate dysplasia CIN III severe dysplasia (see Color Atlas, plate 31)

continued

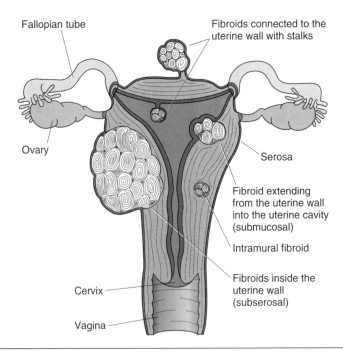

Figure 17.3. Fibroids.

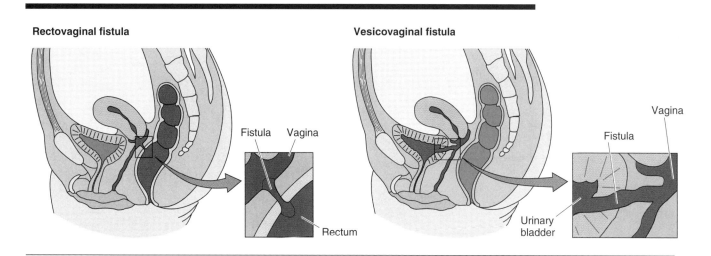

Figure 17.4. Fistulas.

Term	Meaning
carcinoma in situ (CIS) **of the cervix** kar-si-nō′mă in sī′tū	malignant cell changes of the cervix that are localized without any spread to adjacent structures
menopause men′ō-pawz	cessation of menstrual periods owing to lack of ovarian hormones
oophoritis ō-of-ōr-ī′tis	inflammation of one or both ovaries
parovarian cyst par-ō-var′ē-an	cyst of the fallopian tube
pelvic adhesions pel′vik ad-hē′zhŭnz	scarring of tissue within the pelvic cavity as a result of endometriosis, infection, or injury
pelvic inflammatory disease (PID)	inflammation of organs in the pelvic cavity usually including the fallopian tubes, ovaries, and endometrium—most often caused by bacteria
pelvic floor relaxation	relaxation of supportive ligaments of the pelvic organs (Fig. 17.5)
cystocele sis′tō-sēl	pouching of the bladder into the vagina
rectocele rek′tō-sēl	pouching of the rectum into the vagina
enterocele en′ter-ō-sēl	pouching sac of peritoneum between the vagina and rectum
urethrocele yū-rē′thrō-sēl	pouching of the urethra into the vagina
prolapse prō-laps′	descent of the uterus down the vaginal canal

continued

Term	Meaning
salpingitis sal-pin-jī′tis	inflammation of a fallopian tube

Sexually Transmitted Diseases (STDs) *(see Color Atlas, plate 4)*

Major Bacterial STDs

chlamydia kla-mid′ē-ă	most common sexually transmitted bacterial infection in North America that often occurs with no symptoms and is treated only after it has spread, such as to cause pelvic inflammatory disease
chancroid shang′kroyd	infection caused by a bacillus that erupts as a papule on the skin of the vulva or anus and ulcerates and spreads, causing enlarged lymph nodes in the groin (buboes) (chancre = ulcer; oid = resembling)
gonorrhea gon-ō-rē′ă	contagious inflammation of the genital mucous membranes caused by invasion of the gonococcus, *Neisseria gonorrhea* (gono = seed; rrhea = discharge)
syphilis sif′i-lis	infectious disease caused by a spirochete transmitted by direct intimate contact that may involve any organ or tissue over time, usually manifested first on the skin with the appearance of small, painless red papules that erode and form bloodless ulcers called *chancres*

continued

BUBO. Bubo is a Greek word for a swelling in the groin, especially a lymphatic gland. An herb called bulbonium was used by women who suffered from venereal swellings or buboes. It is unclear whether the plant or the swelling was first called bubo.

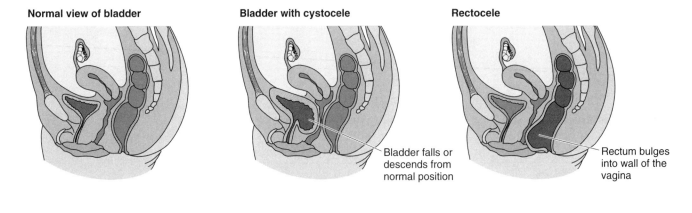

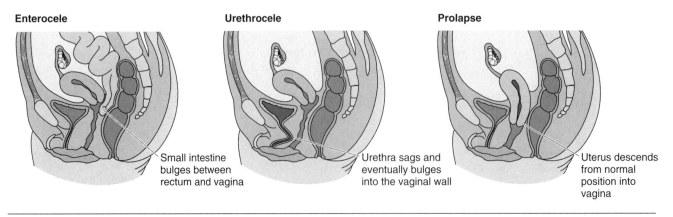

Figure 17.5. Pelvic floor relaxation.

Term	Meaning
Major Viral STDs	
hepatitis B virus (HBV) hep-ă-tī′tis	virus that causes an inflammation of the liver as a result of transmission through any body fluid, including vaginal secretions, semen, blood, etc.
herpes simplex virus Type II (HSV-2) her′pēz	virus that causes ulcer-like lesions of the genital and anorectal skin and mucosa; after initial infection the virus lies dormant in the nerve cell root and may recur at times of stress (see Color Atlas, plate 4)
human immunodeficiency virus (HIV) im′yū-nō-dē-fish′en-sē	virus that causes acquired immunodeficiency syndrome (AIDS), permitting various opportunistic infections, malignancies, and neurologic diseases—contracted through exposure to contaminated blood or body fluid (e.g., semen or vaginal secretions)
human papilloma virus (HPV) pap-i-lō′mă **condyloma acuminatum** kon-di-lō′mah ă-kyū′mĭ-nāt′ŭm **pl. condylomata acuminata** kon-di-lō′mah′t ă-kyū′mĭ-nah′t ă	virus that causes an infection that can occur on the skin or mucous membranes of the genitals transmitted by direct sexual contact—on the skin the lesions appear as cauliflower-like warts, and on mucous membranes they have a flat appearance (also known as venereal or genital warts) (see Color Atlas, plate 4)
vaginitis vaj-i-nī′tis	inflammation of the vagina with redness, swelling, and irritation—often caused by a specific organism, such as *Candida*, *Trichomonas*
atrophic vaginitis ă-trof′ik	thinning of the vagina and loss of moisture owing to depletion of estrogen, which causes inflammation of tissue
vaginosis vaj′i-nō-sis	infection of the vagina with little or no inflammation characterized by a milk-like discharge and an unpleasant odor—also known as nonspecific vaginitis
Breasts	
adenocarcinoma of the breast ad′ĕ-nō-kar-si-nō′mă	malignant tumor of glandular breast tissue
amastia ă-mas′tē-ă	absence of a breast
fibrocystic breasts fĭ-brō-sis′tik	benign condition of the breast consisting of fibrous and cystic changes that render the tissue more dense—patient feels painful lumps that fluctuate with menstrual periods
gynecomastia gī′nĕ-kō-mas′tē-ă	development of mammary glands in the male, caused by altered hormone levels
hypermastia hī-per-mas′tē-ă **macromastia** mak-rō-mas′tē-a	abnormally large breasts
hypomastia hī′po-mas′tē-ă **micromastia** mī′kro-mas′te-a	unusually small breasts

continued

Term	Meaning
mastitis mas-tī′tis	inflammation of breast—most common in women when breastfeeding
polymastia pol-ē-mas′tē-ă	presence of more than two breasts
polythelia pol-ē-thē′lē-ă **supernumerary nipples** sū-per-nū′mer-ār-ē	presence of more than one nipple on a breast

Gynecological Diagnostic Tests and Procedures

Test or Procedure	Explanation
biopsy (Bx)	removal of tissue for microscopic pathological examination (Fig. 17.6)
aspiration Bx as-pi-rā′shŭn	needle draw of tissue or fluid from a cavity for cytological examination—also called needle biopsy

continued

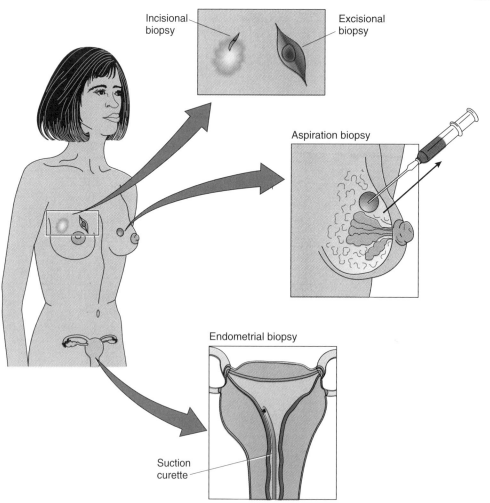

Incisional biopsy

Excisional biopsy

Aspiration biopsy

Endometrial biopsy

Suction curette

Figure 17.6. Biopsy.

Test or Procedure	Explanation
endoscopic Bx en'dō-skōp'ik	removal of a specimen for biopsy during an endoscopic procedure (e.g., colposcopy)
excisional Bx ek-sizh'ŭn-ăl	removal of an entire lesion for microscopic examination
incisional Bx in-sizh'ŭn-năl	removal of a piece of suspicious tissue for microscopic examination (e.g., cervical or endometrial biopsy)
needle biopsy	removal of a core specimen of tissue using a special hollow needle
stereotactic breast Bx ster'ē-ō-tak'tik	use of x-ray imaging, a specialized stereotactic frame, and a computer to calculate, precisely locate, and direct a needle into a breast lesion for the removal of a core specimen for biopsy
colposcopy kol-pos'kŏ-pē	examination of the vagina and cervix using a colposcope, a specialized microscope used to examine the vagina and cervix, often with a camera attachment for photographs—used to document findings and follow-up treatments (Fig. 17.7) (see Color Atlas, plate 31)

continued

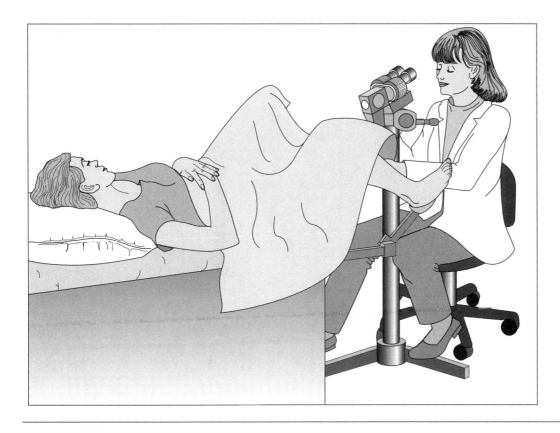

Figure 17.7. Colposcopy.

Test or Procedure	Explanation
hysteroscopy his-ter-os′kŏ-pē	use of a hysteroscope to examine the intrauterine cavity for assessment of abnormalities (e.g., polyps, fibroids, or anomalies) (Fig. 17.8)
magnetic resonance imaging (MRI) rez′ō-nans	use of nonionizing images to detect gynecological conditions (e.g., anomalies of the pelvis or soft tissues of the breast), stage tumors arising from the endometrium or cervix
Papanicolaou smear (Pap) pa-pĕ-nē′kĕ-low	study of cells collected from the cervix to screen for cancer and other abnormalities
radiography rā′dē-og′ră-fē	x-ray imaging
hysterosalpingogram his′ter-ō-sal-ping-ō-gram	x-ray of the fallopian tubes after injection of a contrast medium through the cervix—used to determine tubal patency
mammogram mam′ō-gram	low dose x-ray of breast tissue done to detect neoplasms (Fig. 17.9)
pelvic sonography sŏ-nog′ră-fē	ultrasound imaging of the female pelvis (Fig. 17.10)
endovaginal sonogram en′dō-vaj′i-năl **transvaginal sonogram** trans-vaj′i-năl son′ō-gram	ultrasound image of the uterus, tubes, and ovaries made after introduction of an ultrasonic transducer within the vagina to detect conditions such as ectopic pregnancy, missed abortion, etc.
transabdominal sonogram trans-ab-dom′i-năl	ultrasound image of the lower abdomen including the bladder, uterus, tubes, and ovaries to detect conditions such as cysts, tumors, etc.

continued

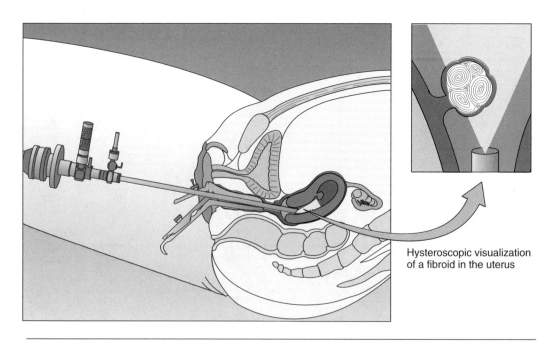

Hysteroscopic visualization of a fibroid in the uterus

Figure 17.8. Hysteroscopy.

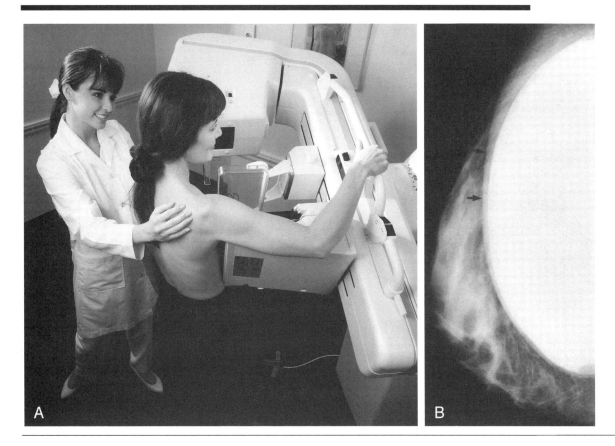

Figure 17.9. A. Mammography procedure. **B.** Mammogram of a patient with an implant. *Arrows,* pectoralis muscle anterior to implant.

Gynecological Operative Terms

Term	Meaning
adhesiolysis ad-hē′zē-ōl′i-sis **adhesiotomy** ad-hē-sē-ot′ō-mē	breaking down or severing of pelvic adhesions
cervical conization ser′vĭ-kal kō-nī-zā′shŭn	removal of a cone-shaped portion of the cervix
colporrhaphy kol-pōr′ă-fē	suture to repair the vagina
anterior repair	repair of a cystocele
posterior repair	repair of a rectocele
A&P repair	anterior and posterior repair of cystocele and rectocele
cryosurgery krī-ō-ser′jer-ē	method of destroying tissue by freezing—used for treating dysplasia and early cancers (Fig. 17.11)
culdocentesis kŭl-dō-sen-tē′sis	aspiration of fluid from the cul-de-sac (cavity that lies between the rectum and posterior wall of the uterus)—used for diagnosing ectopic pregnancy and pelvic inflammatory disease (Fig 17.12)

continued

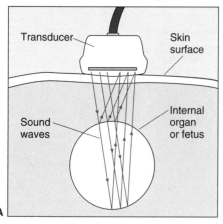

A

Energy in the form of sound waves is reflected off internal organs or, during pregnancy, the fetus and transformed into an image on a TV-type monitor

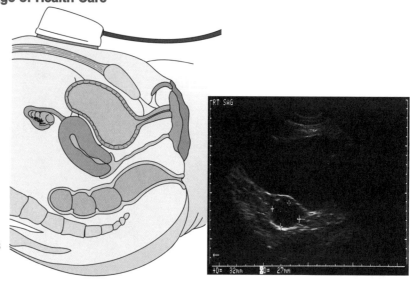

B

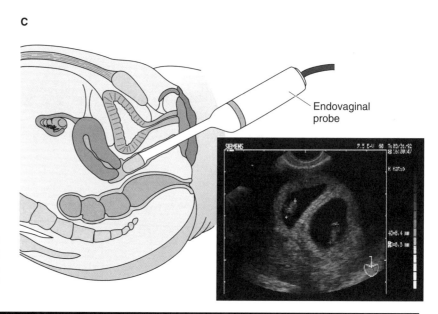

C

Figure 17.10. Pelvic sonography. **A.** Principles of sonography. **B.** Transabdominal imaging procedure. *Inset,* simple ovarian cyst. **C.** Transvaginal imaging procedure. *Inset,* twin pregnancies.

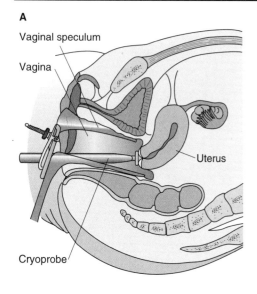

A

Vaginal speculum

Vagina

Uterus

Cryoprobe

Figure 17.11. Cryosurgical procedure.

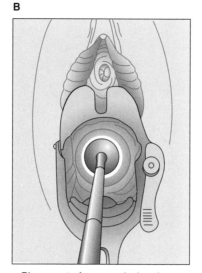

B

Placement of cryosurgical probe at treatment site

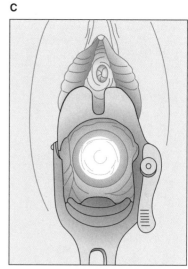

C

Ice crystals seen immediately after freezing treatment

Term	Meaning
dilation and curettage (D&C) dī-lā'shŭn kyū-rě-tahzh'	dilation of the cervix and scraping of the endometrium to control bleeding, obtain tissue for biopsy, or remove polyps or products of conception (Fig. 17.13)
hysterectomy his-ter-ek'tō-mē	removal of the uterus
abdominal hysterectomy	removal of the uterus through an incision in the abdomen
vaginal hysterectomy	removal of the uterus through the vagina

continued

HYSTERIA. Hysteria is a Greek word meaning a uterine condition. Ancient Greeks believed that nervous symptoms were due to the uterus and therefore were experienced by women only. Plato described the uterus as an animal endowed with spontaneous sensation and emotion that was lodged in a woman, ardently desiring to produce children. If the uterus remained sterile long after puberty, it became ill-tempered and caused a general disturbance in the body until it became pregnant. The common prescription for the hysterical female in those days was marriage and childbirth!

Speculum
Vagina
Forceps
Speculum
Uterus
Needle
Cul-de-sac

Figure 17.12. Culdocentesis.

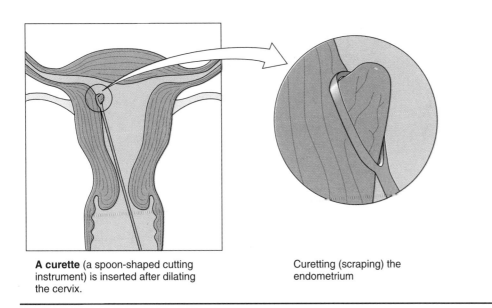

A curette (a spoon-shaped cutting instrument) is inserted after dilating the cervix.

Curetting (scraping) the endometrium

Figure 17.13. Dilation and curettage.

Term	Meaning
total hysterectomy	removal of the uterus and cervix
laparoscopy lap-ă-ros′kŏ-pē	inspection of the abdominal or pelvic cavity with a laparoscope, an endoscope used to examine the abdominal and pelvic regions
laparoscopic surgery	surgical procedures within the abdominal or pelvic region using a laparoscope
laser surgery lā′zer	use of a laser to destroy lesions or dissect or cut tissue—used frequently in gynecology
loop electrosurgical excision procedure (LEEP) **large loop excision of the transformation zone (LLETZ)**	use of electrosurgical or radio waves transformed through a loop-configured electrosurgical device to treat precancerous lesions by simultaneous excisional biopsy and treatment of affected tissue (e.g., cervical dysplasia or human papilloma virus lesions) (Fig. 17.14)
myomectomy mī-ō-mek′tō-mē	excision of fibroid tumors
oophorectomy ō-of-ōr-ek′tō-mē	excision of an ovary
ovarian cystectomy ō-var′ē-an sis-tek′tō-mē	excision of an ovarian cyst
salpingectomy sal-pin-jek′tō-mē	excision of a uterine tube
bilateral salpingo-oophorectomy bī-lat′er-ăl sal-ping′gō- ō-of-ō-rek′tō-mē	excision of both uterine tubes and ovaries

continued

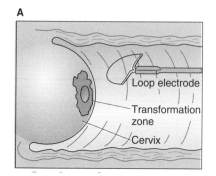 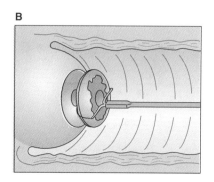 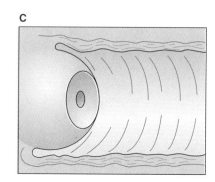

Figure 17.14. Loop electrosurgical excision procedure (LEEP) or large loop excision of the transformation zone (LLETZ). **A.** Electrode approach. **B.** Removal of transformation zone. **C.** Excision site (region between endocervix and ectocervix).

Term	Meaning
salpingotomy sal-pin-got′to-me	incision into a fallopian tube—often performed to remove an ectopic pregnancy (Fig. 17.15)
salpingostomy sal-ping-gos′to-me	creation of an opening in the fallopian tube to open a blockage
tubal ligation lı-ga′shŭn	sterilization of a woman by cutting and tying (ligating) the uterine tubes

Breasts

Term	Meaning
lumpectomy lŭm-pek′to-me	excision of a breast tumor without removing any other tissue or lymph nodes, most often followed by radiation and/or chemotherapy if cancerous
mastectomy mas-tek′to-me	removal of a breast (Fig. 17.16)
simple mastectomy	removal of an entire breast with underlying muscle and axillary lymph nodes left intact
radical mastectomy	removal of an entire breast, underlying chest muscles, and axillary lymph nodes
modified radical mastectomy	removal of an entire breast and lymph nodes of the axilla
mammoplasty mam′o-plas-te	surgical reconstruction of a breast
augmentation mammoplasty	reconstruction to enlarge the breast, often by insertion of an implant (Fig. 17.17)
reduction mammoplasty	reconstruction to remove excessive breast tissue (Fig. 17.18)
mastopexy mas′to-pek-se	elevation of pendulous breast tissue (Fig. 17.18*B*)

continued

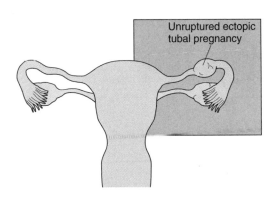
Unruptured ectopic tubal pregnancy

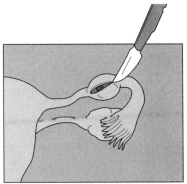
Surgical incision of uterine tube for removal of products of conception

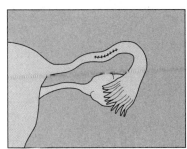
Suture of incision site

Figure 17.15. Salpingostomy.

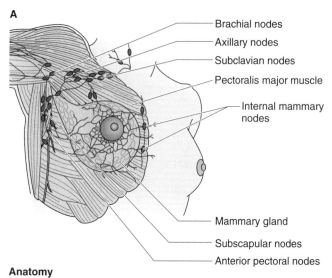

A

- Brachial nodes
- Axillary nodes
- Subclavian nodes
- Pectoralis major muscle
- Internal mammary nodes
- Mammary gland
- Subscapular nodes
- Anterior pectoral nodes

Anatomy
The breast, the underlying muscles, and the lymph nodes are the structures involved in breast cancer surgery. The lymph nodes, which act as barriers against bacteria or tumor cells, are useful in staging breast cancer.

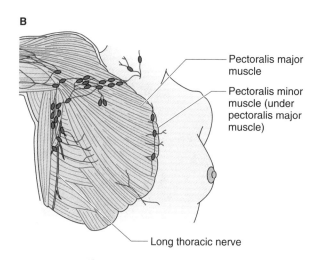

B

- Pectoralis major muscle
- Pectoralis minor muscle (under pectoralis major muscle)
- Long thoracic nerve

Simple Mastectomy
Only the breast is removed. The underlying muscle and associated lymph nodes are not removed.

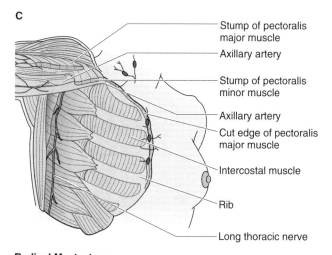

C

- Stump of pectoralis major muscle
- Axillary artery
- Stump of pectoralis minor muscle
- Axillary artery
- Cut edge of pectoralis major muscle
- Intercostal muscle
- Rib
- Long thoracic nerve

Radical Mastectomy
The breast, pectoralis muscles, and contents of the axilla (including lymph nodes and adipose tissue) are removed.

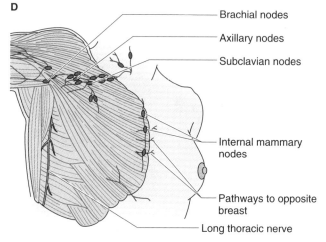

D

- Brachial nodes
- Axillary nodes
- Subclavian nodes
- Internal mammary nodes
- Pathways to opposite breast
- Long thoracic nerve

Modified Radical Mastectomy
The breast and lymph nodes of the axilla are removed. Occasionally the pectoralis minor muscle is transected or removed to approach the lymph nodes.

Figure 17.16. A. Anatomy of the breast. **B–D.** Mastectomy alternatives.

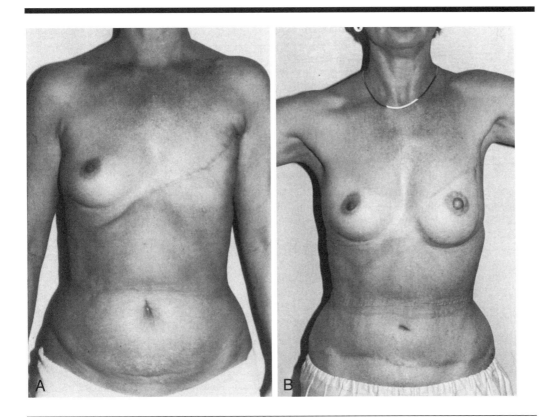

Figure 17.17. Augmentation mammoplasty. **A.** Left modified radical mastectomy in 53-year-old woman (three months postoperation). **B.** Same patient 10 months after augmentation mammoplasty.

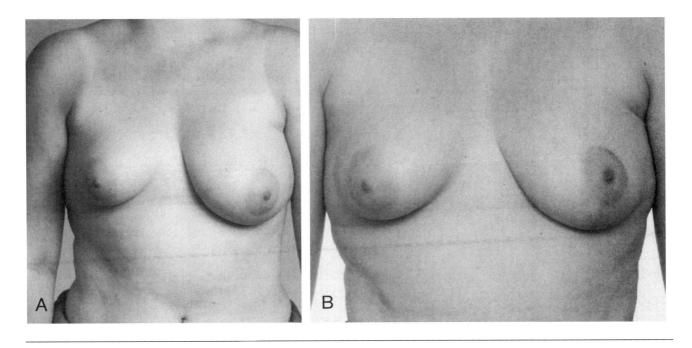

Figure 17.18. Mammoplasty and mastopexy. **A.** Micromastia of one breast and macromastia of opposite breast in 22-year-old patient. **B.** Same patient 15 months postreduction mammoplasty and mastopexy.

Therapeutic Terms

Term	Meaning
chemotherapy kem'ō-thār-ă-pē	treatment of malignancies, infections, and other diseases with chemical agents that destroy selected cells or impair their ability to reproduce
radiation therapy	treatment of neoplastic disease by using radiation, usually from a cobalt source, to deter the proliferation of malignant cells
hormone replacement therapy (HRT)	use of a hormone (e.g., estrogen or progesterone) to replace a deficiency or regulate production
hormonal contraceptives	hormones used to prevent conception by suppressing ovulation
oral contraceptive pill (OCP)	birth control pills
contraceptive injection	injection of the hormone into the body such as Depo-Provera
contraceptive implant	insertion of a contraceptive capsule under the skin providing a continual infusion over an extended time
barrier contraceptives	products that provide a physical barrier that prevents conception (e.g., condoms or diaphragms)
intrauterine device (IUD) in'tră-yū'ter-in	contraceptive device inserted into the uterus that prevents implantation of the fertilized egg
spermicidals sper-mi-sī'dălz	creams, jellies, lotions, or foams containing agents that kill sperm (cido = to kill)

Obstetrical (OB) Symptomatic and Diagnostic Terms
ob-stet'ri-kal

Term	Meaning
Symptomatic	
gravida grav'i-dă	a pregnant woman
nulligravida nŭl-i-grav'i-dă	having never been pregnant
primigravida prī-mi-grav'i-dă	first pregnancy

continued

Term	Meaning
para par′ă	to bear; a woman who has produced one or more viable (live outside the uterus) offspring
nullipara nŭl-i-par′ă	a woman who has not borne a child (nulli = none; para = to bear)
primipara pri-mip′ă-ră	first delivery (primi = first; para = to bear)
multipara mŭl-tip′ă-ră	a woman who has given birth to two or more children (multi = many; para = to bear)
cervical effacement ĕ-fās′ment	progressive obliteration of the endocervical canal during delivery
estimated date of confinement (EDC) kon-fīn′ment	expected date for delivery of the baby—normally 280 days or 40 weeks from conception
meconium staining mē-kō′nē-ŭm	presence of meconium in amniotic fluid
ruptured membranes rŭp′chūrd	rupture of the amniotic sac, usually at onset of labor
macrosomia mak-rō-sō′mē-ă	large bodied baby commonly seen in diabetic pregnancies (macro = large; soma = body)
polyhydramnios pol′ē-hī-dram′nē-os	excessive amniotic fluid

ECLAMPSIA. Eclampsia is a Greek word meaning to flash out or shine forth suddenly, first used in the 18th century for any sudden convulsion. Today it particularly refers to toxemia of pregnancy.

Diagnostic

Term	Meaning
abortion (AB) ă-bōr′shŭn	expulsion of the product of conception before the fetus can be viable (live outside the uterus)
spontaneous abortion spon-tā′nē-ŭs	miscarriage; expulsion of products of conception occurring naturally
habitual abortion	spontaneous abortion occurring in three or more consecutive pregnancies
incomplete abortion	incomplete expulsion of products of conception
missed abortion	death of a fetus or embryo within the uterus that is not naturally expelled after death (Fig. 17.10*B*)
threatened abortion	bleeding with threat of miscarriage
cephalopelvic disproportion (CPD) sef′ă-lō-pel′vik	conditions preventing normal delivery through the birth canal—either the baby's head is too large or the birth canal is too small
eclampsia ek-lamp′sē-ă	true toxemia of pregnancy characterized by high blood pressure, albuminuria, edema of the legs and feet, severe headaches, dizziness, convulsions, and coma

continued

Term	Meaning
preeclampsia **pregnancy-induced** **hypertension** (PIH) prē-ē-klamp′sē-ă	toxemia of pregnancy characterized by high blood pressure, albuminuria, edema of the legs and feet, and puffiness of the face, without convulsion or coma
ectopic pregnancy ek-top′ik	implantation of the fertilized egg outside the uterine cavity, often in the tube, ovary, or rarely the abdominal cavity (Fig. 17.19)
erythroblastosis fetalis ĕ-rith′rō-blas-tō′sis fē′tā′lis	disorder that results from the incompatibility of a fetus with an Rh positive blood factor and a mother who is Rh negative, causing red blood cell destruction in the fetus—necessitates a blood transfusion to save the fetus
Rh factor	presence, or lack, of antigens on the surface of red blood cells that may cause a reaction between the blood of the mother and fetus, resulting in fetal anemia (which causes erythroblastosis fetalis)
Rh positive	presence of antigens
Rh negative	absence of antigens
hyperemesis gravidarum hī-per-em′ĕ-sis grav-i-dā′rŭm	severe nausea and vomiting in pregnancy that can cause severe dehydration in the mother and fetus (emesis = vomit)
meconium aspiration mē-kō′nē-ŭm as-pi-rā′shŭn	fetal aspiration of amniotic fluid containing meconium

continued

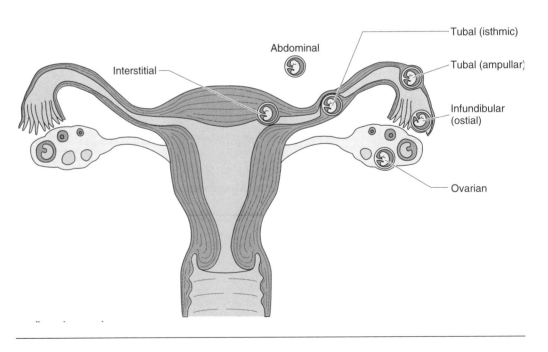

Figure 17.19. Ectopic pregnancy: sites of extrauterine implantation.

Term	Meaning
placenta previa plă-sen′tă prē′vēă	displaced attachment of the placenta in the lower region of the uterine cavity (Fig. 17.20)
abruptio placentae ab-rŭp′shē-ō pla-sen′tē	premature detachment of a normally situated placenta

Obstetrical Diagnostic Tests and Procedures

Test or Procedure	Explanation
chorionic villus sampling (CVS) kō-rē-on′ik vil′us	sampling of placental tissue for microscopic and chemical examination to detect fetal abnormalities (Fig. 17.21A)
amniocentesis am′nē-ō-sen-tē′sis	aspiration of a small amount of amniotic fluid for analysis of possible fetal abnormalities (Fig. 17.21B)
fetal monitoring	use of an electronic device for simultaneous recording of fetal heart rate and uterine contractions
pelvimetry pel-vim′ĕ-trē	obstetrical measurement of the pelvis to evaluate proper conditions for vaginal delivery
pregnancy test	test performed on urine or blood to detect the presence of human chorionic gonadotropin hormone (secreted by the placenta) that indicates pregnancy
endovaginal sonogram **transvaginal sonogram**	ultrasound image of the uterus, tubes, and ovaries made after introduction of an ultrasonic transducer within the vagina—useful in detecting pathology (e.g., ectopic pregnancy, missed abortion, etc.) (Fig. 17.11)
obstetrical sonogram	ultrasound image of the pregnant uterus to determine fetal development (Fig. 17.22)

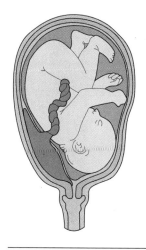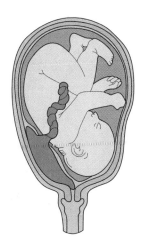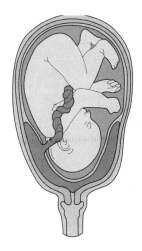

Figure 17.20. Placenta previa.

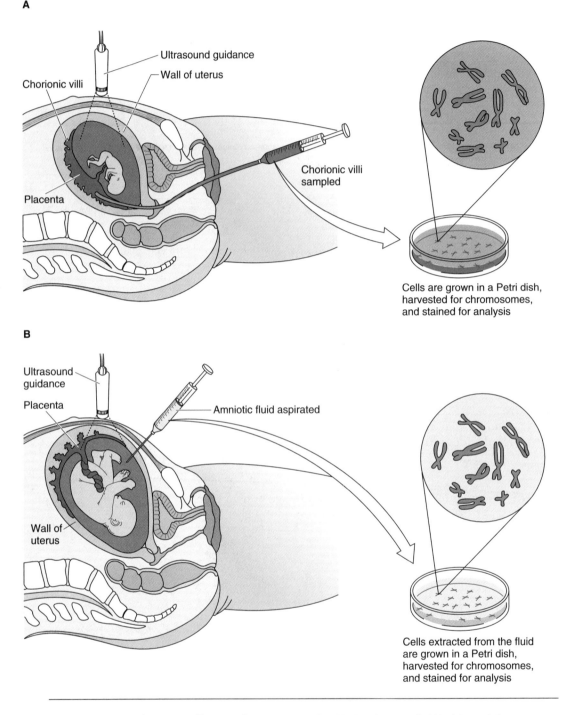

Figure 17.21. A. Chorionic villus sampling (9–11 weeks). **B.** Amniocentesis (15–18 weeks).

Chapter 17 • **Female Reproductive System** 473

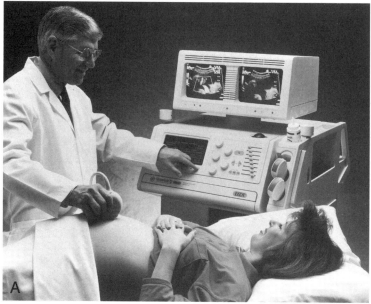
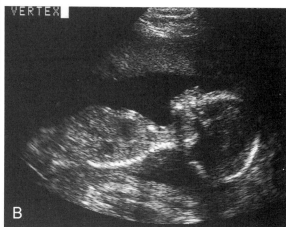

Figure 17.22. **A.** Obstetrical sonography. **B.** Sonographic image of fetus in breech position (vertex).

Obstetrical Operative and Therapeutic Terms

Term	Meaning
Operative	
cesarean section (C-section) se-zā′rē-ăn	surgical delivery of a baby by making an incision through the abdomen and into the uterus
episiotomy e-piz-ē-ot′ō-mē	incision of the perineum to facilitate delivery
Therapeutic	
amnioinfusion am′nē-ō-in-fyū′zhŭn	introduction of a solution into the amniotic sac—most commonly an isotonic solution used to relieve fetal distress
therapeutic abortion (TAB)	abortion induced by mechanical means or by drugs for medical consideration
version	manual method reversing the position of the fetus, usually done to facilitate delivery
external version	abdominal manipulation
internal version	intravaginal manipulation

Common Therapeutic Drug Classifications

abortifacient ă-bōr-ti-fā′shent	drug that causes abortion (e.g., RU-486)

CESAREAN SECTION. The fetus is removed from the uterus through an incision in the abdomen. The procedure was first used to save the baby when the mother had died. Julius Caesar is said to have been born in this manner.

Term	Meaning
oxytocin ok-sē-tō′sin	hormone secreted by the pituitary gland that causes myometrial contraction—used for induction of labor
Rh immune globulin glob′yū-lin	immunizing agent given to an Rh negative mother within 72 hours after delivering an Rh positive baby to suppress the Rh immune response
tocolytic agent tō-kō-lit′ik	drug used to stop labor contractions

PRACTICE EXERCISES

For the following words, draw a line or lines to separate prefixes, combining forms, and suffixes. Then define the term.

1. vulvitis _____

2. mastoptosis _____

3. vaginosis _____

4. tocolysis _____

5. salpingotomy _____

6. mammotrophic _____

7. episiorrhaphy _____

8. transvaginal _____

9. hysterorrhexis _____

10. gynecology _____

11. colposcopy _____

12. menostasis _____

13. hyperplasia _____

14. mammogram _____

15. metromalacia _____

16. ovariocentesis _____

17. menarche _____

18. polymastia _____

19. pyosalpingitis _____

20. oophorostomy _____

21. oligomenorrhea _____

22. vaginitis _____

23. mastotomy _____

24. dystocia _____

25. gynecologist _____

26. hysterectomy _____

27. colpocystitis _____

28. episiotomy _____

29. colporrhaphy _____

30. hysterospasm _____

31. ovariocele _____

32. vulvectomy _____

33. lactogenesis _____

34. endometritis _____

35. salpingolysis _____

36. mastectomy _____

37. pelvimeter _____

38. ovoid _____

39. adenocarcinoma _____

Define the following abbreviations:

40. IUD _____

41. HPV _____

42. CVS _____

43. D&C _____

44. HBV _____

45. EDC _____

46. HSV _____

47. STD_____

48. TAB_____

49. HRT _____

Match the following:

50. removal of a uterine tube _____   a. PID
    and an ovary

51. white vaginal discharge _____   b. chlamydia

52. condition when baby's _____   c. colporrhaphy
    head is too big for birth canal

53. presence of more than _____   d. LEEP
    one nipple on a breast

54. implantation of a fertilized _____   e. CPD
    egg outside the uterus

55. most common bacterial _____   f. leukorrhea
    STD in North America

56. excisional biopsy _____   g. polythelia

57. painful intercourse _____   h. ectopic

58. surgical repair of cystocele _____   i. salpingo-oophorectomy

59. inflammation of entire _____   j. dyspareunia
    female pelvic cavity

Give the medical term for the following:

60. condition of benign lumps in breast that fluctuate with menstrual cycle

    _____

61. abnormal opening between bladder and vagina _____

62. cutting and tying the uterine tubes_____

63. having more than two breasts _____

64. bacterial STD caused by a spirochete _____

65. x-ray of uterine tubes to determine patency _____

66. study of cervical cells to screen for cancer_____

67. condition of migration of endometrial tissue _____

68. abnormal opening between the rectum and vagina_____

69. surgical remedy for rectocele _____

Complete the following:

70. _____ pause = cessation of menstruation

71. _____ rrhea = painful menstruation

72. _____ rrhea = absence of menstruation

73. _____ rrhea = scanty menstruation

74. _____ rrhagia = excessive bleeding at time of menstruation

75. _____ rrhagia = bleeding from the uterus at any time other than the normal period

76. _____ mastia = development of mammary glands in male

77. _____ mastia = absence of a breast

78. _____ mastia = unusually small breasts—a common surgical remedy is _____mammoplasty

79. _____ mastia = unusually large breasts—a common surgical remedy is _____mammoplasty

80. masto_____ = surgical fixation of a pendulous breast

81. _____ ectomy = removal of a breast

82. _____ ectomy = removal of a breast lump

Identify terms related to abortion:

83. _____ a naturally occurring miscarriage

84. _____ a miscarriage occurring in three or more consecutive pregnancies

85. _____ fetal expulsion with parts of placenta remaining with bleeding

86. _____ fetal death within the uterus

87. _____ one induced by mechanical means or by drugs

88. _____ bleeding with threat of miscarriage

Match the following:

89. retroflexion _____ a. forward bend of uterus

90. condylomata _____ b. toxemia of pregnancy

91. para II _____ c. backward bend of uterus

92. prolapse _____ d. a pregnant woman

93. cystocele _____ e. cervical cancer

94. gravida _____ f. venereal warts

95. rectocele _____ g. woman who has given birth twice

96. eclampsia _____ h. first delivery

97. CIN II _____ i. protrusion of the rectum into the vagina

98. primipara _____ j. descent of uterus from normal position

99. anteflexion _____ k. cervical dysplasia

100. CIS _____ l. pouching of the bladder into the vagina

Medical Record Analyses

MEDICAL RECORD 17.1

Jane Foley has seen her gynecologist, Dr. Phyllis Widetick, yearly for a routine examination and Pap smear. Every year the results have been normal. Jane is generally a healthy, active woman. This year, however, Dr. Widetick's examination and Pap smear found a problem. When the test results were in, Jane returned for additional testing.

Directions

Read Medical Record 17.1 for Ms. Foley (pages 482–483) and answer the following questions. This record is the history and physical report dictated by Dr. Widetick after her examination.

Questions about Medical Record 17.1

Write your answers in the spaces provided.

1. In your own words, not using medical terminology, briefly describe the patient's chief complaint:

    _____

    _____

    _____

2. In your own words, not using medical terminology, briefly describe what a Pap smear is.

    _____

    _____

    _____

3. Explain the result of Ms. Foley's Pap smear.

    _____

    _____

    _____

4. Because of this result, Dr. Widetick used colposcopy for further testing. Translate into nonmedical language what she discovered with this diagnostic procedure.

    _____

    _____

    _____

5. What was the positive finding from the biopsy? Define this in your own words.

    _____

    _____

    _____

6. Ms. Foley underwent all the following procedures. Put these in correct sequence by numbering them 1 to 6 in the order they were performed.

_____ follow-up examination

_____ visualization with colposcope

_____ ultrasound

_____ Pap smear

_____ routine physical examination

_____ Bx

7. The sonogram *definitely* showed what finding?

_____

What were the *possible* findings?

_____

_____

8. In nonmedical language define the two previous surgeries Ms. Foley has had:

_____

_____

_____

9. How many children has Ms. Foley had? _____

10. Mark any of the following abnormal findings from the present physical examination.

    a. enlarged uterus

    b. gross reflexes

    c. eroded cervix

    d. hypertension

    e. enlarged thyroid

    f. mobile right ovarian cyst

11. Define Dr. Widetick's final diagnosis and explain what she will do next to treat Ms. Foley.

_____

_____

_____

CENTRAL MEDICAL CENTER

211 Medical Center Drive • Central City, US 90000-1234 • PHONE: (012) 125-6784 • FAX: (012) 125-9999

TO BE ADMITTED: 9/3/9x

HISTORY

CHIEF COMPLAINT:
Right ovarian cyst.

HISTORY OF PRESENT ILLNESS:
This is a 32-year-old Caucasian female who had a routine examination on June 21, 199x, at which time the examination revealed the right ovary to be approximately two to three times normal size. Otherwise, all was normal. The Papanicolaou smear revealed atypical cells of undetermined significance. The patient returned for a colposcopy, and this revealed what appeared to be squamous epithelial lesions CIN I-II. Biopsies were performed which revealed chronic cervicitis and no evidence of CIN. The patient was placed on Lo-Ovral for two cycles and then was rechecked. The right ovary continued to enlarge and got to the point where it was approximately 4 x 5 cm, floating anteriorly in the pelvis, and was fairly firm to palpation. A pelvic sonogram corroborated the clinical findings in that superior to the right adnexa was a 4 x 5 cm mass, possibly with hemorrhage into either a paraovarian cyst or possibly a dermoid cyst. The patient is to be admitted now for an exploratory laparotomy.

PAST HISTORY:
There is no history of severe medical illnesses. The patient had the usual childhood diseases and has had good health as an adult.

PREVIOUS SURGERY: The patient had a hymenotomy and dilatation and curettage in 199x.

MENSTRUAL HISTORY: Menstrual cycle is 30 days, averaging a four to seven day flow.

OBSTETRICAL HISTORY: The patient is a Gravida 0.

FAMILY HISTORY:
Diabetes in the family. Mother and father are living and well

REVIEW OF SYSTEMS:
Noncontributory.

(continued)

P. Widetick, M.D.
P. Widetick, M.D.

PW:bst
D: 9/1/9x   T: 9/2/9x

HISTORY AND PHYSICAL Page 1	PT. NAME: FOLEY, JANE J. ID NO: IP-751014 ROOM NO: 331 ATT. PHYS: P. WIDETICK, M.D.

Medical Record 17.1.

CENTRAL MEDICAL CENTER

211 Medical Center Drive • Central City, US 90000-1234 • PHONE: (012) 125-6784 • FAX: (012) 125-9999

PHYSICAL EXAMINATION

GENERAL:
The patient is a well-developed, well-nourished Caucasian female who is anxious but in no acute distress.

VITAL SIGNS:
HEIGHT: 5 ft 5 in. WEIGHT: 154 lb. BLOOD PRESSURE: 110/82.

HEENT:
Normal.

NECK:
Supple; the trachea is in the midline. The thyroid is not enlarged.

CHEST:
LUNGS: Clear to percussion and auscultation. HEART: Regular sinus rhythm with no murmur.
BREASTS: Normal to palpation.

ABDOMEN:
Soft and flat. No scars or masses.

PELVIC:
The outlet and vagina are normal. The cervix is moderately eroded. The uterus is normal size and anterior. The left adnexa is negative. The right adnexa has a firm, irregular cystic ovary that is anterior and approximately 5 x 5 cm. This is mobile and nontender.

EXTREMITIES:
Normal. Reflexes are grossly intact.

DIAGNOSIS:
Right ovarian cyst.

PLAN:
The patient is to be admitted for exploratory laparotomy and ovarian cystectomy.

P. Widetick, M.D.
P. Widetick, M.D.

PW:bst
D: 9/1/9x   T: 9/2/9x

HISTORY AND PHYSICAL PAGE 2	PT. NAME: FOLEY, JANE J. ID NO: IP-751014 ROOM NO: 331 ATT. PHYS: P. WIDETICK, M.D.

Medical Record 17.1. *Continued.*

MEDICAL RECORD 17.2

Kathleen Montegrande is pregnant with her first child. She has regularly seen her obstetrician, Dr. Linda Fenton, throughout the pregnancy. The pregnancy has gone well so far, although the fetus is in a breech presentation. She has come for a routine obstetrical examination by Dr. Fenton, which confirms the breech presentation. She then reports to Central Medical Center when labor begins.

Directions

Read Medical Record 17.2 for Ms. Montegrande (pages 487–489) and answer the following questions. The first record is the history and physical examination report dictated by Dr. Fenton after Ms. Montegrande's last routine examination, and before delivery. The second record is the discharge summary dictated from Central Medical Center by Dr. Fenton after Ms. Montegrande had her baby.

Questions about Medical Record 17.2

Write your answers in the spaces provided:

1. Below are medical terms used in these records you have not yet encountered in this text. Underline each where it appears in the record and define below.

   Apgar score _____

   rubella vaccination _____

2. In your own words, not using medical terminology, briefly describe a breech presentation.

   _____

   _____

   _____

3. Which two tests that Dr. Fenton performed confirmed the breech presentation?

   a. sonography

   b. cesarean

   c. amniocentesis

   d. Bx

   e. pelvic examination

   f. colposcopy

   g. Pap smear

4. Mark any possible negative findings included in PMH:

    a. rheumatic fever

    b. closed cervix

    c. heart murmur

    d. mitral valve prolapse

5. Where did the autologous blood come from?

    _____

6. Explain what is important about the possibility of Ms. Montegrande's baby being Rh positive.

    _____

    _____

    _____

7. In your own words, explain what "80% effaced" means.

    _____

    _____

    _____

8. What is the main reason for Dr. Fenton's plan to perform a primary cesarean section?

    _____

    _____

    _____

9. What two occurrences brought Ms. Montegrande to the Central Medical Center on March 6?

    _____

    _____

    _____

10. In your own words, describe the surgery Ms. Montegrande underwent.

_____

_____

_____

11. What kind of suture did Dr. Fenton use to close the incision?

_____

12. Two other doctors were present in the surgical suite with Dr. Fenton:

Dr. Nelson was there to help care for (whom) _____

Dr. O'Brien was there to help care for (whom)_____

13. Mark any of the following surgical complications that occurred.

a. uterine hemorrhage

b. postop fever

c. cervical erosion

d. all of the above

e. none of the above

CENTRAL MEDICAL CENTER

211 Medical Center Drive • Central City, US 90000-1234 • PHONE: (012) 125-6784 • FAX: (012) 125-9999

HISTORY

HISTORY OF PRESENT ILLNESS:

The patient is a 31-year-old female, Gravida I Para 0, whose estimated date of confinement is March 8, 199x. The patient has had a relatively normal pregnancy with normal blood pressures and approximately a 53-pound weight gain during her pregnancy. The infant has been noted to be in a breech position since mid December 199x and has remained in that position without any change. This position was confirmed by ultrasound and pelvic examination within the past few days. This patient is scheduled at this time to have a primary cesarean section because of the breech presentation. There is a small amount of amniotic fluid; and external version, I believe, would be injudicious at this time.

PAST MEDICAL HISTORY:

MEDICAL: Entirely negative except for possible mitral valve prolapse in this patient. She has never had any rheumatic fever and has had no other heart disease. She has had no high blood pressure, diabetes, thyroid trouble, varicose veins, or epilepsy. She has never had a blood transfusion. The patient specifically had requested to have one unit of autologous blood drawn earlier in her pregnancy which is available. The patient is Rh negative, and she is not immune to rubella; therefore, she will need a RhoGAM shot if her baby is Rh positive and will need a rubella vaccination before leaving the hospital. The patient was given RhoGAM in our office on December 18, 199x.

Her additional past medical history is noncontributory.

(continued)

L. Fenton, M.D.
L. Fenton, M.D.

LF:pn

D: 3/4/9x
T: 3/5/9x

HISTORY AND PHYSICAL Page 1	PT. NAME: MONTEGRANDE,KATHLEEN L. ID NO: IP-692580 ROOM NO: 377 ADM. DATE: March 8, 19xx ATT. PHYS: L. FENTON, M.D.

Medical Record 17.2.

CENTRAL MEDICAL CENTER

211 Medical Center Drive • Central City, US 90000-1234 • PHONE: (012) 125-6784 • FAX: (012) 125-9999

PHYSICAL EXAMINATION

HEENT:
Essentially normal.

NECK:
The thyroid is not enlarged. There is no lymphadenopathy in the neck or supraclavicular region.

CHEST:
Clear to percussion and auscultation.

CARDIAC: There are no murmurs or irregularities. There are no heaves, thrills, or thrusts.

BREASTS: Examination fails to reveal any masses.

ABDOMEN:
The uterus measures 42 cm by tape measurement. The infant is still in a breech position.

PELVIC:
The cervix is closed, approximately 80% effaced, and soft.

IMPRESSION:
TERM BREECH PREGNANCY IN PRIMIGRAVIDA FEMALE WHO IS RH NEGATIVE.

PLAN:
Primary cesarean section. I have explained the pros and cons of surgery and the possible alternatives. The patient and her husband do understand and have accepted the risks. The patient has one unit of autologous blood available, and she is in need of a rubella immunization prior to discharge from the hospital.

L. Fenton, M.D.

LF:pn

D: 3/4/9x
T: 3/5/9x

HISTORY AND PHYSICAL Page 2	PT. NAME: MONTEGRANDE,KATHLEEN L. ID NO: IP-692580 ROOM NO: 377 ADM. DATE: March 8, 199x ATT. PHYS: L. FENTON, M.D.

Medical Record 17.2. *Continued.*

CENTRAL MEDICAL CENTER

211 Medical Center Drive • Central City, US 90000-1234 • PHONE: (012) 125-6784 • FAX: (012) 125-9999

DISCHARGE SUMMARY

DATE OF ADMISSION: March 6, 199x   **DATE OF DISCHARGE:** March 9, 199x

SUMMARY:
Mrs. Montegrande was scheduled to be admitted to this facility on March 8, 199x, because of a primiparous breech presentation and came in on March 6, 199x, at 0345 hours with a history of spontaneous rupture of the membranes and labor. She is a 31-year-old Gravida I Para 0 Abortus 0 with an EDC of March 8, 199x, and spontaneous ruptured membranes at approximately 0200 hours with onset of contractions probably before that, with a breech presentation confirmed on ultrasound. The cervix is posterior, 3 cm, and soft. There is some meconium staining. The patient was therefore set up for a primary cesarean section. The patient was taken to the operating room where the primary cesarean section was accomplished; and she was delivered out of a frank breech presentation of a 7 lb 8 oz male infant, Apgars 9 and 9, with Dr. O'Brien, the pediatrician, in attendance. The assistant surgeon was Dr. Nelson.

The patient and infant are discharged on this date to home with full instructions; the patient will take Tylenol Double Strength for pain and will be seen in the office in two weeks for staple removal. She is to call if she has any problems with excessive bleeding or fever.

FINAL DIAGNOSIS:
PREGNANCY, UTERINE, DELIVERED.

COMPLICATIONS:
Primiparous breech.

TREATMENT RENDERED:
Low cesarean section.

L. Fenton, M.D.

LF:ti

D: 3/9/9x
T: 3/10/9x

DISCHARGE SUMMARY	PT. NAME:	MONTEGRANDE, KATHLEEN L.
	ID NO:	IP-692580
	ROOM NO:	377
	ATT. PHYS.	L. FENTON, M.D.

Medical Record 17.2. *Continued.*

MEDICAL RECORD 17.3

Carla Woodward has been healthy all her life but is bothered by the unbalanced shape of her breasts. Finally, at age 23, she has chosen to see Dr. Karen McNeil, a plastic surgeon recommended by her personal physician.

Directions

Read Medical Record 17.3 for Ms. Woodward (page 492) and answer the following questions. This record is the consultation report dictated by Dr. McNeil after meeting with and examining Ms. Woodward.

Questions about Medical Record 17.3

Write your answers in the spaces provided:

1. Below are medical terms used in this record you have not yet encountered in this text. Underline each where it appears in the record and define below.

   saline-filled _____

   silicone walled _____

2. In your own words, not using medical terminology, describe Ms. Woodward's chief complaint.

   _____

   _____

   _____

3. Summarize the two past surgeries Ms. Woodward has had. For each, identify the primary body system involved.

   _____

   _____

   _____

4. Ms. Woodward told Dr. McNeil that she has never had a mammogram, a diagnostic procedure used primarily for what purpose?

   _____

   _____

   _____

5. Dr. McNeil's physical examination focuses on Ms. Woodward's breasts. Describe the findings related to the breasts (first give the medical term for the finding, then define it).

Medical Finding   Definition

Left breast _____   _____

_____   _____

Right breast_____   _____

_____   _____

6. In your own words, not using medical language, describe the surgery Dr. McNeil has proposed to Ms. Woodward.

_____

_____

_____

CENTRAL MEDICAL GROUP, INC.

Department of Plastic Surgery

201 Medical Center Drive • Central City, US 90000-1234 • PHONE: (012) 125-8888 • FAX: (012) 125-3434

INITIAL CONSULTATION

PATIENT: WOODWARD, Carla S.

DATE: October 2, 199x

HPI: This is a 23-year-old white female in general good health who has significant bilateral breast asymmetry with macromastia on the left breast and deformity and hypoplasia of the right breast. The patient denies having had any other problems except that her right thumb is shorter than her left thumb.

PMH: A left inguinal herniorrhaphy at age 15 and a laminectomy on March 1, 199x, for treatment of a ruptured disc. The rest of her history is unremarkable.

MEDS: Vicodin 2-3 q d for the past seven months secondary to her surgery.

ALLERGIES: None.

SH: The patient denies history of smoking or alcohol use and has never had a mammogram.

PE: The patient has a sternal nipple-notch distance of 27 cm on the left side and 22 cm on the right side. There are no breast masses or nipple discharge noted. The right breast is atrophic in the medial half of the breast, and the entire breast is hypoplastic. The left breast is large and ptotic. The patient reports being approximately an A-B cup on the right side and a C-D cup on the left side. She feels the right side is much too small and deformed, and the left side is too big.

PLAN: The patient would do well with a left breast reduction and a right breast augmentation/reconstruction of the deformity and atrophy. The risks and benefits of this surgery were discussed with the patient along with the risks and benefits of saline-filled, silicone-wall implants. The patient will think about our discussion today and contact me with a date.

K. McNeil, M.D.

KM:mar

D: 10/2/9x
T: 10/3/9x

Medical Record 17.3.

APPENDIX A

Glossary of Prefixes, Suffixes, and Combining Forms

Term Component to English

a- .... without
ab- .... away from
abdomin/o .... abdomen
-ac .... pertaining to
acous/o .... hearing
acr/o .... extremity or topmost
-acusis .... hearing condition
ad- .... to, toward, or near
aden/o .... gland
adip/o .... fat
adren/o .... adrenal gland
aer/o .... air or gas
-al .... pertaining to
albumin/o .... protein
-algia .... pain
alveol/o .... alveolus (air sac)
ambi- .... both
an- .... without
an/o .... anus
andr/o .... male
angi/o .... vessel
ankyl/o .... crooked or stiff
ante- .... before
anti- .... against or opposed to
aort/o .... aorta
appendic/o .... appendix
aque/o .... water
-ar .... pertaining to
-arche .... beginning
arteri/o .... artery
arthr/o .... joint
articul/o .... joint
-ary .... pertaining to
-ase .... enzyme
-asthenia .... weakness
ather/o .... fat
-ation .... process
atri/o .... atrium
audi/o .... hearing

aur/i .... ear
bacteri/o .... bacteria
balan/o .... glans penis
bi- .... two or both
bil/i .... bile
-blast .... germ or bud
blast/o .... germ or bud
blephar/o .... eyelid
brachi/o .... arm
brady- .... slow
bronch/o............. bronchus (airway)
bronchiol/o .... bronchiole (little airway)
bucc/o .... cheek
capn/o .... carbon dioxide
carb/o .... carbon dioxide
carcin/o .... cancer
cardi/o .... heart
-cele .... pouching or hernia
celi/o .... abdomen
-centesis .... puncture for aspiration
cephal/o .... head
cerebell/o .... cerebellum (little brain)
cerebr/o .... brain
cerumin/o .... wax
cervic/o .... neck or cervix
cheil/o .... lip
chol/e .... bile
choledoch/o .... common bile duct
chondr/o .... cartilage (gristle)
chrom/o .... color
chyl/o .... juice
circum- .... around
col/o .... colon
colon/o .... colon
colp/o .... vagina (sheath)
con- .... together or with
conjunctiv/o ...... conjunctiva (to join together)

contra- .... against or opposed to
corne/o .... cornea
coron/o .... circle or crown
cost/o .... rib
crani/o .... skull
crin/o .... to secrete
cutane/o .... skin
cyan/o .... blue
cyst/o .... bladder or sac
cyt/o .... cell
dacry/o .... tear
dactyl/o .... digit (finger or toe)
de- .... from, down, or not
dent/i .... teeth
derm/o .... skin
dermat/o .... skin
-desis .... binding
dextr/o .... right, or on the right side
dia- .... across or through
diaphor/o .... profuse sweat
dips/o .... thirst
dis- .... separate from or apart
duoden/o .... duodenum
-dynia .... pain
dys- .... painful, difficult, or faulty
-e .... noun marker
e- .... out or away
-eal .... pertaining to
ec- .... out or away
-ectasis .... expansion or dilation
ecto- .... outside
-ectomy .... excision (removal)
-emesis .... vomiting

-emia .... blood condition
en- .... within
encephal/o .... brain
endo- .... within
enter/o .... small intestine
epi- .... upon
epididym/o .... epididymis
episi/o .... vulva (covering)
erythr/o .... red
esophag/o .... esophagus
esthesi/o .... sensation
eu- .... good or normal
ex- .... out or away
exo- .... outside
extra- .... outside
fasci/o .... fascia (a band)
femor/o .... femur
fibr/o .... fiber
gangli/o .... ganglion (knot)
gastr/o .... stomach
-gen .... origin or production
-genesis .... origin or production
-genic .... origin or production
gingiv/o .... gums
gli/o .... glue
glomerul/o .... glomerulus (little ball)
gloss/o .... tongue
glott/o .... opening
gluc/o .... sugar
glyc/o .... sugar
glycos/o .... sugar
gnos/o .... knowing
-gram .... record
-graph .... instrument for recording
-graphy .... process of recording
gynec/o .... woman
hem/o .... blood
hemat/o .... blood
hemi- .... half

493

hepat/o,
hepatic/o .... liver
herni/o .... hernia
hidr/o .... sweat
hist/o .... tissue
histi/o .... tissue
hormon/o .... hormone
(an urging
on)
hydr/o .... water
hyper- .... above or
excessive
hypo- .... below or
deficient
hyster/o .... uterus
-ia .... condition of
-iasis .... formation of
or presence
of
-iatrics .... treatment
-iatry .... treatment
-ic .... pertaining
to
-icle .... small
ile/o .... ileum
immun/o .... safe
infra- .... below or
under
inguin/o .... groin
inter- .... between
intra- .... within
ir/o .... iris (colored
circle)
irid/o .... iris (colored
circle)
-ism .... condition of
iso- .... equal, like
-ist .... one who
specializes
in
-itis .... inflammation
-ium .... structure or
tissue
jejun/o .... jejunum
(empty)
kerat/o .... hard or
cornea
ket/o .... ketone
bodies
keton/o .... ketone
bodies
kinesi/o .... movement
kyph/o .... humped
lacrim/o .... tear
lact/o .... milk
lapar/o .... abdomen
laryng/o .... larynx
(voice box)

lei/o .... smooth
-lepsy .... seizure
leuc/o .... white
leuk/o .... white
lingu/o .... tongue
lip/o .... fat
lith/o .... stone or
calculus
lob/o .... lobe (a
portion)
-logist .... one who
specialized
in the study
or treatment
of
-logy .... study of
lord/o .... bent
lumb/o .... loin (lower
back)
lymph/o .... clear fluid
-lysis .... breaking
down or
dissolution
macr/o .... large or long
-malacia .... softening
mamm/o .... breast
mast/o .... breast
meat/o .... opening
-megaly .... enlargement
melan/o .... black
men/o .... menstruation
mening/o .... meninges
(membrane)
meningi/o .... meninges
(membrane)
meso- .... middle
meta- .... beyond,
after, or
change
-meter .... instrument
for
measuring
metr/o .... uterus
-metry .... process of
measuring
micro- .... small
mono- .... one
morph/o .... form
multi- .... many
muscul/o .... muscle
my/o .... muscle
myc/o .... fungus
myel/o .... bone
marrow or
spinal cord
myos/o .... muscle
myring/o .... eardrum

narc/o .... stupor
nas/o .... nose
nat/i .... birth
necr/o .... death
neo- .... new
nephr/o .... kidney
neur/o .... nerve
ocul/o .... eye
-oid .... resembling
-ole .... small
olig/o .... few or
deficient
-oma .... tumor
onych/o .... nail
oophor/o .... ovary
ophthalm/o .... eye
-opia .... condition of
vision
opt/o .... eye
orch/o .... testis (testicle)
orchi/o................ testis (testicle)
orchid/o.............. testis (testicle)
or/o .... mouth
orth/o .... straight,
normal, or
correct
-osis .... condition or
increase
oste/o .... bone
ot/o .... ear
-ous .... pertaining
to
ovari/o .... ovary
ov/i .... egg
ov/o .... egg
ox/o .... oxygen
pachy- .... thick
pan- .... all
pancreat/o .... pancreas
para- .... alongside of
or abnormal
-paresis .... slight
paralysis
patell/o .... knee cap
path/o .... disease
pector/o .... chest
ped/o .... child or foot
pelv/i, pelv/o .... hip bone
-penia .... abnormal
reduction
per- .... through
peri- .... around
perine/o .... perineum
peritone/o .... peritoneum
-pexy .... suspension
or fixation
phac/o .... lens (lentil)

phag/o .... eat or
swallow
phak/o .... lens (lentil)
pharyng/o .... pharynx
(throat)
phas/o .... speech
-phil .... attraction
for
-philia .... attraction
for
phleb/o .... vein
phob/o .... exaggerated
fear or
sensitivity
phon/o .... voice or
speech
phot/o .... light
phren/o .... diaphragm
(also mind)
plas/o .... formation
-plasia................. formation
-plasty .... surgical
repair or
reconstruction
-plegia .... paralysis
pleur/o .... pleura
-pnea .... breathing
pneum/o .... air or lung
pneumon/o .... air or lung
pod/o .... foot
-poiesis .... formation
poly- .... many
post- .... after or
behind
pre- .... before
presby/o .... old age
pro- .... before
proct/o .... rectum
prostat/o .... prostate
psych/o .... mind
-ptosis .... falling or
downward
displacement
pulmon/o .... lung
purpur/o .... purple
py/o .... pus
pyel/o .... basin
pylor/o .... pylorus
(gatekeeper)
quadr/i .... four
radi/o .... radius (a
bone of the
forearm);
radiation
(especially
x-ray)

re- .... again or back
rect/o .... rectum
ren/o .... kidney
reticul/o .... a net
retro- .... backward or behind
rhabd/o .... rod shaped or striated (skeletal)
rhin/o .... nose
-rrhage .... to burst forth
-rrhagia .... to burst forth
-rrhaphy .... suture
-rrhea .... discharge
-rrhexis .... rupture
salping/o .... uterine (fallopian) tube; also eustachian tube
sarc/o .... flesh
schiz/o .... split, division
scler/o .... hard or sclera
scoli/o .... twisted
-scope .... instrument for examination
-scopy .... examination
seb/o .... sebum (oil)
semi- .... half
sial/o .... saliva
sigmoid/o .... sigmoid colon
sinistr/o .... left, or on the left side
sinus/o .... hollow (cavity)
somat/o .... body
somn/o .... sleep
son/o .... sound
-spasm .... involuntary contraction
sperm/o .... sperm (seed)
spermat/o .... sperm (seed)
sphygm/o .... pulse
spin/o .... spine (thorn)
spir/o .... breathing
splen/o .... spleen
spondyl/o .... vertebra
squam/o .... scale

-stasis .... stop or stand
steat/o .... fat
sten/o .... narrow
stere/o .... three dimensional or solid
stern/o .... sternum (breastbone)
steth/o .... chest
stomat/o .... mouth
-stomy .... creation of an opening
sub- .... below or under
super- .... above or excessive
supra- .... above or excessive
sym- .... together or with
syn- .... together or with
tachy- .... fast
tax/o .... order or coordination
ten/o .... tendon (to stretch)
tend/o .... tendon (to stretch)
tendin/o .... tendon (to stretch)
test/o .... testis (testicle)
thalam/o .... thalamus (a room)
thorac/o .... chest
thromb/o .... clot
thym/o .... thymus gland
thyr/o .... thyroid gland (shield)
-tic .... pertaining to
toc/o .... labor or birth
tom/o .... to cut
-tomy .... incision
ton/o .... tone or tension
tonsill/o .... tonsil (almond)
top/o .... place
tox/o .... poison
toxic/o .... poison
trache/o .... trachea (windpipe)

trans- .... across or through
tri- .... three
trich/o .... hair
-tripsy .... crushing
troph/o .... nourishment or development
tympan/o .... eardrum
-ula, -ule .... small
uln/o .... ulna (a bone of the forearm)
ultra- .... beyond or excessive
uni- .... one
ur/o .... urine
ureter/o .... ureter
urethr/o .... urethra
urin/o .... urine
uter/o .... uterus
vagin/o .... vagina (sheath)
varic/o .... swollen or twisted vein
vas/o .... vessel
vascul/o .... vessel
ven/o .... vein
ventricul/o .... ventricle (belly or pouch)
vertebr/o .... vertebra
vesic/o .... bladder or sac
vesicul/o .... bladder or sac
vitre/o .... glassy
vulv/o .... vulva (covering)
xanth/o .... yellow
xer/o .... dry
-y .... condition or process of

English to Term Component
abdomen............. abdomin/o, celi/o, lapar/o
abnormal .... -para-
abnormal reduction.......... -penia
above .... hyper-, super-, supra-
across .... dia-, trans-
adrenal gland...... adren/o

after .... post-, meta-
again .... re-
against .... anti-, contra-
air.......................... aer/o, pneum/o, pneumon/o
air sac .... alveol/o
airway .... bronch/o, bronchi/o
all .... pan-
alongside of .... para-
alveolus............... alveol/o
anus .... an/o
aorta .... aort/o
apart .... dis-
appendix............. appendic/o
arm .... brachi/o
around................. circum-, peri-
artery................... arteri/o
atrium.................. atri/o
attraction for .... -phil, -philia
away .... e-, ec-, ex-
away from .... ab-
back .... re-
backward .... retro-
bacteria............... bacteri/o
basin .... pyel/o
before .... ante-, pre-, pro-
beginning............ -arche
behind .... post-, retro-
below .... hypo-, infra-, sub-
bent...................... lord/o
between............... inter-
beyond .... meta-, ultra-
bile .... bil/i, chol/e
bile duct.............. choledoch/o
binding................ -desis
birth .... nat/i, toc/o
black .... melan/o
bladder................ cyst/o, vesic/o, vesicul/o
blood .... hem/o, hemat/o,
blood condition .. -emia
blue,....................... cyan/o
body .... somat/o
bone..................... oste/o
bone marrow....... myel/o
both...................... ambi-, bi-
brain .... cerebr/o, encephal/o
breaking down .. -lysis

breast	mamm/o, mast/o
breathing	-pnea, spir/o
bronchus	bronch/o, bronchi/o
bud	-blast, blast/o
burst forth	-rrhage, -rrhagia
calculus	lith/o
cancer	carcin/o
carbon dioxide	capn/o, carb/o
cartilage	chondr/o
cavity (sinus)	atri/o, sin/o
cell	cyt/o
cerebellum	cerebell/o
cerebrum	cerebr/o
cervix	cervic/o
change	meta-
cheek	bucc/o
chest	pectoro, steth/o, thorac/o
child	ped/o
circle	coron/o
clear fluid	lymph/o
clot	thromb/o
colon	col/o, colon/o
colon, sigmoid	sigmoid/o
color	chrom/o
colored circle	irid/o, ir/o
condition	-osis
condition of	-ia, -ism, ium, -y
contraction, involuntary	-spasm
coordination	tax/o
cornea	corne/o, kerat/o
correct	ortho-
creation of an opening	-stomy
crooked	ankyl/o
crown	coron/o
crushing	-tripsy
to cut	tom/o
death	necr/o
deficient	hypo-, olig/o
development	troph/o
diaphragm	phren/o
difficult	dys-

digit (finger or toe)	dactyl/o
dilation or expansion	-ectasis
discharge	-rrhea
disease	path/o
dissolution	-lysis
division	schiz/o
down	de-
downward displacement	-ptosis
dry	xer/o
duodenum	duoden/o
ear	aur/i, ot/o
eardrum	myring/o, tympan/o
eat, swallow	phag/o
egg	ov/i, ov/o
enlargement	-megaly
enzyme	-ase
epididymis	epididym/o
equal	iso-
esophagus	esophag/o
eustachian tube	salping/o
examination	-scopy
excessive	hyper-, super-, supra-, ultra-
excision (removal)	-ectomy
expansion or dilation	-ectasis
extremity	acr/o
eye	ocul/o, ophthalm/o, opt/o
eyelid	blephar/o
falling	-ptosis
fallopian tube	salping/o
fascia	fasci/o
fast	tachy-
fat	adip/o, ather/o, lip/o, steat/o
faulty	dys-
fear, exaggerated	phob/o
femur	femor/o
few	olig/o
fiber	fibr/o
fixation	-pexy
flesh	sarc/o
foot	pod/o, ped/o
form	morph/o

formation	-plasia, plas/o, -poiesis
formation of	-iasis
four	quadri-
from	de-
fungus	myc/o
ganglion	gangli/o
gas	aer/o
germ or bud	-blast, blast/o
gland	aden/o
glans penis	balan/o
glassy	vitre/o
glomerulus	glomerul/o
glue	gli/o
good	eu-
groin	inguin/o
gums	gingiv/o
hair	trich/o
half	hemi-, semi-
hard	kerat/o, scler/o
head	cephal/o
hearing	acous/o, audi/o
hearing condition	-acusis
heart	cardio/o
hernia	-cele, herni/o
hip bone	pelv/i, pelv/o
hormone	hormon/o
humped	kyph/o
ileum	ile/o
incision	-tomy
increase	-osis
inflammation	-itis
instrument for examination	-scope
instrument for measuring	-meter
instrument for recording	-graph
jejunum (empty)	jejun/o
joint	arthr/o, articul/o
juice	chyl/o
ketone bodies	ket/o, keton/o
kidney	nephr/o, ren/o
kneecap	patell/o
knowing	gnos/o

labor	toc/o
large	macr/o
larynx	laryng/o
left or on left side	sinistr/o
lens	phac/o, phak/o
light	phot/o
like	iso-
lip	cheil/o
liver	hepat/o, hepatic/o
lobe	lob/o
loin (lower back)	lumb/o
long	macr/o
lung	pneum/o, pneumon/o, pulmon/o
male	andr/o
many	multi-, poly-
measuring, instrument for	-meter
measuring, process of	metry
meninges	mening/o, meningi/o
menstruation	men/o
milk	lact/o
mind	psych/o, phren/o
mouth	or/o, stomat/o
movement	kinesi/o
muscle	muscul/o, my/o, myos/o
nail	onych/o
narrow	sten/o
near	ad-
neck	cervic/o
nerve	neur/o
net	reticul/o
new	neo-
normal	eu-, ortho-
nose	nas/o, rhin/o
not	de-
nourishment	troph/o
oil	seb/o
old age	presby/o
one	mono-, uni-
one who specializes in	-ist

one who specializes in the study or treatment of..... -logist
opening............... glott/o, meat/o
opening, creation of...................... -stomy
opposed to........... anti-, contra-
order.................... tax/o
origin.................. -gen, -genesis, -genic
out....................... e-, ec-, ex-
outside............... ecto-, exo-, extra-
ovary................... oophor/o, ovari/o
oxygen.................. ox/o
pain...................... -algia, -dynia
painful................. dys-
pancreas.............. pancreat/o
paralysis............... -plegia
paralysis, slight... -paresis
perineum............. perine/o
peritoneum.......... peritone/o
pertaining to........ -ac, -al, -ar, -ary, -eal, -ic, -ous, -tic
pharyn/x............. pharyng/o
place..................... top/o
pleura.................. pleur/o
poison.................. tox/o, toxic/o
portion................ lob/o
pouching.............. -cele
presence of.......... -iasis
process................ -ation
process of............ -y
production.......... -gen, -genic, -genesis
prostate............... prostat/o
protein.................. albumin/o
pulse..................... sphygm/o
puncture for aspiration.......... -centesis
purple.................. purpur/o
pus....................... py/o
pylorus................. pylor/o
radius.................. radi/o
record.................. -gram
recording, process of......... -graphy

rectum................. proct/o, rect/o
red........................ erythr/o
resembling........... -oid
reticulum............ reticul/o
rib........................ cost/o
right or on the right side .... dextr/o
rod shaped........... rhabd/o
rupture................. -rrhexis
sac........................ cyst/o, vesic/o, vesicul/o
safe...................... immun/o
saliva................... sial/o
scale..................... squam/o
sclera................... scler/o
sebum................... seb/o
secrete.................. crin/o
seizure................. -lepsy
sensation.............. esthesi/o
sensitivity, exaggerated..... phob/o
separate from....... dis-
sigmoid colon..... sigmoid/o
sinus.................... sinus/o
skeletal................ rhabd/o
skin...................... cutane/o, derm/o, dermat/o
skull.................... crani/o
sleep.................... somn/o
slow..................... brady-
small.................... -icle, micro-, -ole, -ula, -ule
small intestine..... enter/o
smooth................. lei/o
softening.............. -malacia
sound................... son/o
specializes, one who................... -ist
speech.................. phas/o, phon/o
sperm................... sperm/o, spermat/o
spinal cord........... myel/o
spine.................... spin/o
spleen.................. splen/o
split..................... schiz/o
sternum................ stern/o
stiff...................... ankyl/o
stomach................ gastr/o
stone.................... lith/o
stop or stand....... -stasis
straight................ orth/o
striated................ rhabd/o

structure.............. -ium
study of................ -logy
study of, one who specializes in.... -logist
stupor.................. narc/o
sugar.................... gluc/o, glyc/o, glycos/o
surgical repair or reconstruction.. -plasty
suspension.......... -pexy
suture................... -rrhaphy
swallow............... phag/o
sweat................... hidr/o
sweat, profuse..... diaphor/o
tear...................... dacry/o, lacrim/o
teeth................... dent/i
tendon................. ten/o, tend/o, tendin/o
tension................. ton/o
testis (testicle)..... orch/o, orchi/o, orchid/o, test/o
thalamus.............. thalam/o
thick.................... pachy-
thirst................... dips/o
three.................... tri-
three dimensional or solid............ stere/o
throat................... pharyng/o
through............... dia-, per-, trans-
thymus gland...... thym/o
thyroid gland...... thyr/o
tissue................... hist/o, -ium
to or toward....... ad-
together.............. con-, sym-, syn-
tone..................... ton/o
tongue................. gloss/o, lingu/o
tonsil................... tonsill/o
topmost................ acr/o
trachea................ trache/o
treatment............ -iatrics, -iatry
treatment, one who specializes in..... -logist
tumor.................. -oma
twisted................ scoli/o
two...................... bi-
ulna..................... uln/o
under................... infra-, sub-
upon.................... epi-
ureter................... ureter/o

urethra.................. urethr/o
urine.................... ur/o, urin/o
uterine tube......... salping/o
uterus.................. hyster/o, metr/o, uter/o
vagina.................. colp/o, vagin/o
vein...................... phleb/o, ven/o
vein, swollen or twisted............ varic/o
ventricle.............. ventricul/o
vertebra............... vertebr/o, spondyl/o
vessel................... angi/o, vas/o, vascul/o
vision, condition of..... -opia
voice.................... phon/o
voice box............. laryng/o
vomiting.............. -emesis
vulva................... vulv/o, episi/o
water................... aque/o, hydr/o
wax...................... cerumin/o
weakness............ -asthenia
white................... leuc/o, leuk/o
windpipe............. trache/o
with..................... con-, sym-, syn-
within.................. en-, endo-, intra-
without................ a-, an-
woman................ gynec/o
yellow.................. xanth/o

APPENDIX B

Abbreviations and Symbols

a	before	CAT	computerized axial tomography	EIA	enzyme immunoassay
A	anterior; assessment	CBC	complete blood count	EKG	electrocardiogram
A&P	auscultation and percussion	cc	cubic centimeter	EMG	electromyogram
A&W	alive and well	CC	chief complaint; cardiac catheterization	ENT	ear, nose, throat
AB	abortion			ER	emergency room
ABG	arterial blood gas	CCU	coronary (cardiac) care unit	ERCP	endoscopic retrograde cholangiopancreatography
a.c.	before meals	CHF	congestive heart failure		
ACE	angiotensin-converting enzyme	CIN	cervical intraepithelial neoplasia	ESR	erythrocyte sedimentation rate
ACP	American College of Physicians	CIS	carcinoma in situ	ESWL	extracorporeal shock wave lithotripsy
		cm	centimeter		
ACS	American College of Surgeons	CNS	central nervous system	ETOH	ethyl alcohol
		CO	cardiac output	F	Fahrenheit
ACTH	adrenocorticotrophic hormone	c/o	complains of	F.A.C.P.	fellow of the American College of Physicians
		COPD	chronic obstructive pulmonary disease		
AD	right ear			F.A.C.S.	fellow of the American College of Surgeons
ad lib.	as desired	CP	cerebral palsy; chest pain		
AIDS	acquired immunodeficiency syndrome	CPD	cephalopelvic disproportion	FBS	fasting blood sugar
		CPR	cardiopulmonary resuscitation	FH	family history
alb	albumin			fl oz	fluid ounce
a.m.	morning	CSF	cerebrospinal fluid	FS	frozen section
AMBS	American Board of Medical Specialists	CT	computed tomography	FSH	follicle-stimulating hormone
		cu mm	cubic millimeter	Fx	fracture
amt	amount	CVA	cerebrovascular accident	g	gram
ANS	autonomic nervous system	CVS	chorionic villus sampling	GERD	gastroesophageal reflux disease
AP	anterior posterior	CXR	chest x-ray		
aq	water	d	day	GH	growth hormone
AS	left ear	D&C	dilation and curettage	GI	gastrointestinal
ASD	atrial septal defect	DC, D/C	discharge; discontinue	gm	gram
ASHD	arteriosclerotic heart disease	D.C.	doctor of chiropractic medicine	gr	grain
				gt	drop
AU	both ears			gtt	drops
AV	atrioventricular	D.D.S.	doctor of dental surgery	GTT	glucose tolerance test
Ⓑ	bilateral	DJD	degenerative joint disease	GYN	gynecology
BCP	biochemistry panel	D.O.	doctor of osteopathic medicine	h	hour
b.i.d.	twice a day			H&P	history and physical
BM	black male; bowel movement	D.P.M.	doctor of podiatric medicine	HBV	hepatitis B virus
BP	blood pressure	dr	dram	HCT or	
BPH	benign prostatic hypertrophy/hyperplasia	DRE	digital rectal examination	Hct	hematocrit
		DTR	deep tendon reflex	HD	Huntington's disease
BRP	bathroom privileges	DVT	deep vein thrombosis	HEENT	head, eyes, ears, nose, throat
BS	blood sugar	Dx	diagnosis	HGB or	
BUN	blood urea nitrogen	ECG	electrocardiogram	Hgb	hemoglobin
Bx	biopsy	ECHO	echocardiogram	HIV	human immunodeficiency virus
c	with	ECU	emergency care unit		
C	Celsius; centigrade	EDC	estimated date of confinement	HPI	history of present illness
C&S	culture and sensitivity			HPV	human papilloma virus
CABG	coronary artery bypass graft	EEG	electroencephalogram	HRT	hormone replacement therapy
CAD	coronary artery disease	EGD	esophagogastroduodenoscopy	h.s.	bedtime (hour of sleep)
cap	capsule				

HSV-1	herpes simplex virus Type 1
HSV-2	herpes simplex virus Type 2
Ht	height
HTN	hypertension
Hx	history
I&D	incision and drainage
ICD	implantable cardioverter defibrillator
ICU	intensive care unit
ID	intradermal
IDDM	insulin-dependent diabetes mellitus
IM	intramuscular
IMP	impression
IOL	intraocular lens implant
IP	inpatient
IUD	intrauterine device
IV	intravenous
IVP	intravenous pyelogram
kg	kilogram
KUB	kidney, ureter, bladder
L	left, liter
L&W	living and well
lb	pound
LEEP	loop electrosurgical excision procedure
LH	luteinizing hormone
LLETZ	loop electrosurgical excision procedure
LLQ	left lower quadrant
LP	lumbar puncture
LTB	laryngotracheobronchitis
LUQ	left upper quadrant
ⓜ	murmur
m	meter
MCH	mean corpuscular (cell) hemoglobin
MCHC	mean corpuscular (cell) hemoglobin concentration
MCV	mean corpuscular (cell) volume
MD	muscular dystrophy; medical doctor
mg	milligram
MI	myocardial infarction
ml, mL	milliliter
mm	millimeter
MRA	magnetic resonance angiography
MRI	magnetic resonance imaging
MS	multiple sclerosis; musculoskeletal
MSH	melanocyte-stimulating hormone
MVP	mitral valve prolapse
NCV	nerve conduction velocity
NG	nasogastric

NIDDM	non–insulin-dependent diabetes mellitus
NKA	no known allergy
NKDA	no known drug allergy
noc.	night
NPO	nothing by mouth
NSR	normal sinus rhythm
O	objective
OB	obstetrics
OD	right eye; doctor of optometry
OH	occupational history
OP	outpatient
OR	operating room
ORIF	open reduction, internal fixation
OS	left eye
OU	both eyes
oz	ounce
p	after
P	plan; posterior; pulse
PA	posterior anterior
PaCO$_2$	arterial partial pressure of carbon dioxide
PaO$_2$	arterial partial pressure of oxygen
PAP	Papanicolaou test (smear)
PAR	postanesthetic recovery
p.c .	after meals
PDA	patent ductus arteriosus
PE	physical examination
PEFR	peak expiratory flow rate
per	by
PERRLA	pupils equal, round, and reactive to light and accommodation
PET	positron emission tomography
PF	peak flow
PFT	pulmonary function testing
PH	past history
Ph.D.	doctor of philosophy
PI	present illness
PID	pelvic inflammatory disease
PIH	pregnancy induced hypertension
p.m.	afternoon
PMH	past medical history
PNS	peripheral nervous system
p.o.	by mouth
post op	postoperation
PPBS	postprandial blood sugar
PR	per rectum
pre op	preoperation
p.r.n.	as needed
PSA	prostate-specific antigen
PSG	polysomnography
pt	patient

PT	physical therapy; prothrombin time
PTCA	percutaneous transluminal coronary angioplasty
PTH	parathyroid hormone
PTT	partial thromboplastin time
PV	per vagina
PVC	premature ventricular contraction
Px	physical examination
q	every
qd	every day
qh	every hour
q2h	every two hours
q.i.d.	four times a day
q.n.s	quantity not sufficient
q.o.d.	every other day
q.s.	quantity sufficient
qt	quart
R	right; respiration
RBC	red blood cell; red blood count
RIA	radioimmunoassay
RLQ	right lower quadrant
R/O	rule out
ROM	range of motion
ROS	review of symptoms
RP	retrograde pyelogram
RRR	regular rate and rhythm
RTC	return to clinic
RTO	return to office
RUQ	right upper quadrant
Rx	recipe; take thou
s	without
S	subjective
SA	sinoatrial
SC	subcutaneous
SH	social history
Sig:	instruction to patient
SLE	systemic lupus erythematosus
SMA	sequential multiple analyzer
SOB	shortness of breath
SPECT	single photon emission computed tomography
SpGr	specific gravity
SQ	subcutaneous
SR	systems review
ss	one-half
STAT	immediately
STD	sexually transmitted disease
suppos	suppository
SV	stroke volume
Sx	symptom
T	temperature
T&A	tonsillectomy and adenoidectomy
tab	tablet
TAB	therapeutic abortion
TB	tuberculosis

TB	tuberculosis	UTI	urinary tract infection	°	degree or hour
TEDS	thrombo-embolic disease stockings	VC	vital capacity	↑	increased; above
		VCU	voiding cystourethrogram	↓	decreased; below
TEE	transesophageal echocardiogram	VS	vital signs	Ø	none or negative
		VSD	ventricular septal defect		standing
TIA	transient ischemic attack	V_T	tidal volume		sitting
t.i.d.	three times a day	w.a.	while awake		lying
TM	tympanic membrane	WBC	white blood cell, white blood count	×	times or for
TPR	temperature, pulse, respiration			>	greater than
Tr	treatment	WDWN	well developed, well nourished	<	less than
TSH	thyroid-stimulating hormone	wk	week		one
TURP	transurethral resection of the prostate	WNL	within normal limits		two
		wt	weight		three
TV	tidal volume	y.o.	year old		four
Tx	treatment; traction	yr	year	I, II, III,	
UA	urinalysis	♀	female	IV, V, VI,	
UCHD	usual childhood diseases	♂	male	VII, VIII,	
URI	upper respiratory infection	#	number or pound	IX, X	uppercase Roman numerals 1–10

APPENDIX C

Commonly Prescribed Drugs

The following is an alphabetical index of commonly prescribed drugs (trade and generic) excerpted from the listings of new and refill prescriptions dispensed in the United States in 1994. Trade (brand) names are uppercase, and generic names are lowercase. Common drug classifications for each are provided.

Name	Classification
Accupril (quinapril hydrochloride)	antihypertensive; angiotensin-converting enzyme (ACE) inhibitor
acetaminophen and codeine	analgesic, antipyretic
Adalat (nifedipine)	antianginal; calcium channel blocker
Advil (ibuprofen)	analgesic; nonsteroidal anti-inflammatory (NSAID)
albuterol	bronchodilator
alprazolam	antianxiety
Altase (ramipril)	antihypertensive; angiotensin-converting enzyme (ACE) inhibitor
Ambien (zolpidem tartrate)	hypnotic; sedative
amitriptyline hydrochloride	antidepressant
amoxicillin trihydrate	antibiotic
Amoxil (amoxicillin trihydrate)	antibiotic
ampicillin	antibiotic
atenolol	antianginal; beta-adrenergic blocker
Ativan (lorazepam)	antianxiety; hypnotic; sedative
Atrovent (ipratropium bromide)	bronchodilator
Augmentin (amoxicillin/clavulanic acid)	antibiotic
Axid (nizatidine)	antiulcer; histamine-2 antagonist
Azmacort (triamcinolone)	anti-inflammatory; corticosteroid
Bactroban (mupirocin)	antibiotic
Beconase AQ (beclomethasone dipropionate)	anti-inflammatory; corticosteroid
Beepen-VK (penicillin v potassium)	antibiotic
Biaxin (clarithromycin)	antibiotic
Bumex (bumetanide)	diuretic
BuSpar (buspirone hydrochloride)	antianxiety
Calan SR (verapamil hydrochloride)	antianginal; antiarrhythmic; calcium channel blocker

Name	Classification
Capoten (captopril)	antihypertensive; angiotensin-converting enzyme (ACE) inhibitor
Carafate (sucralfate)	gastrointestinal agent
Cardizem CD (diltiazem hydrochloride)	antianginal; calcium channel blocker
Cardec DM (carbinoxamine, pseudoephedrine, and dextromethorphan)	antihistamine/decongestant combination; antitussive
Cardura (doxazosin mesylate)	antihypertensive; alpha-adrenergic blocker
carisoprodate/carisoprodol	skeletal muscle relaxant
Ceclor (cefaclor)	antibiotic
Ceftin (cefuroxime)	antibiotic
Cefzil (cefprozil)	antibiotic
cephalexin	antibiotic
Cipro (ciprofloxacin hydrochloride)	antibiotic
Claritin (loratadine)	antihistamine
Compazine (prochlorperazine)	antiemetic; antipsychotic
Contuss XT (guaifenesin and phenylpropanolamine)	decongestant; expectorant
Cotrim (cotrimoxazole)	antibiotic
Coumadin (warfarin sodium)	anticoagulant
cyclobenzaprine hydrochloride	skeletal muscle relaxant
Cycrin (medroxyprogesterone acetate)	progestin; contraceptive
Darvocet-N 100 (propoxyphene and acetaminophen)	analgesic, narcotic; antipyretic
Daypro (oxaprozin)	nonsteroidal anti-inflammatory (NSAID)
Deltasone (prednisone)	anti-inflammatory; corticosteroid
Demulen 1/35-28 (ethinyl estradiol and ethynodiol diacetate)	oral contraceptive

Name	Classification
Depakote (valproic and derivatives)	anticonvulsant
Desogen (ethinyl estradiol and desogestrel)	oral contraceptive
DiaBeta (glyburide)	antidiabetic; hypoglycemic
diazepam	antianxiety agent; anticonvulsant; sedative
dicyclomine hydrochloride	antispasmodic
Diflucan (fluconazole)	antifungal
Dilacor (diltiazem hydrochloride)	antianginal; calcium channel blocker
Dilantin (phenytoin)	anticonvulsant; antiarrhythmic
doxycycline	antibiotic
Duricef (cefadroxil monohydrate)	antibiotic
Dyazide (hydrochlorothiazide and triamterene)	diuretic
DynaCirc (isradipine)	antihypertensive; calcium channel blocker
E.E.S. (erythromycin)	antibiotic
Elocon (mometasone furoate)	anti-inflammatory; corticosteroid; antipruritic
E-Mycin 333 (erythromycin)	antibiotic
Entex LA (guaifenesin and phenylpropanolamine)	decongestant; expectorant
Ery-Tab (erythromycin)	antibiotic
Erythrocin (erythromycin)	antibiotic
erythromycin	antibiotic
Estrace (estradiol)	estrogen derivative
Estraderm (estradiol)	estrogen derivative
ferrous sulfate	iron salt
Fiorinal (butalbital compound and codeine)	analgesic, narcotic; barbiturate
Floxin (ofloxacin)	antibiotic
furosemide	diuretic
gemfibrozil	antilipemic
Glucotrol (glipizide)	antidiabetic; hypoglycemic
glyburide	antidiabetic; hypoglycemic
Glynase Prestab (glyburide)	antidiabetic; hypoglycemic
guaifenesin and phenylpropanolamine	decongestant; expectorant
Hismanal (astemizole)	antihistamine
Humulin (insulin preparation)	antidiabetic
hydrochlorothiazide	diuretic
hydrocodone and acetaminophen	analgesic, narcotic; antipyretic
hydrocortisone	anti-inflammatory; corticosteroid
Hytrin (terazosin)	antihypertensive; alpha-adrenergic blocking agent
ibuprofen	analgesic; nonsteroidal anti-inflammatory (NSAID)

Name	Classification
Imitrex (sumatriptan succinate)	antimigraine agent
Intal (cromolyn sodium)	antihistamine; asthma prophylactic
iodinated glycerol and dextromethorphan	antitussive; expectorant
isosorbide dinitrate	antianginal; coronary vasodilator
K-Dur (potassium chloride)	potassium salt; electrolyte supplement
Klonopin (clonazepam)	anticonvulsant
Klor-Con 10 (potassium chloride)	potassium salt; electrolyte supplement
Lanoxin (digoxin)	cardiotonic; antiarrhythmic
Lasix (furosemide)	diuretic
Levoxyl (levothyroxine sodium)	thyroid product
Lodine (etodolac)	analgesic, nonsteroidal anti-inflammatory (NSAID)
Loestrin-FE 1.5/30 (ethinyl estradiol and norethindrone)	oral contraceptive
Lo/Ovral-28 (ethinyl estradiol)	oral contraceptive
Lopressor (metoprolol)	antihypertensive; antianginal; beta-adrenergic blocker
Lorabid (loracarbef)	antibiotic
lorazepam	antianxiety; hypnotic; sedative
Lorcet Plus (hydrocodone and acetaminophen)	analgesic, narcotic; antipyretic
Lotrisone (betamethasone dipropionate and clotrimazole)	antifungal
Lozol (indapamide)	diuretic
Macrobid (nitrofurantoin)	antibiotic
meclizine hydrochloride	antiemetic; antihistamine
medroxyprogesterone acetate	progestin; contraceptive
Mevacor (lovastatin)	antilipemic
methylphenidate hydrochloride	central nervous system stimulant
methylprednisolone	anti-inflammatory; corticosteroid
metoprolol	antihypertensive; antianginal; beta-adrenergic blocker
metronidazole	antibiotic
Micro-K 10 (potassium chloride)	potassium salt; electrolyte supplement
Micronase (glyburide)	antidiabetic; hypoglycemic
Motrin (ibuprofen)	analgesic; nonsteroidal anti-inflammatory (NSAID)
Naprosyn (naproxen)	analgesic, nonsteroidal anti-inflammatory (NSAID)
naproxen	analgesic, nonsteroidal anti-inflammatory (NSAID)
Nasacort (triamcinolone)	anti-inflammatory; corticosteroid
neomycin and polymyxin b	antibiotic
Nitro-Dur (nitroglycerin)	antianginal; coronary vasodilator

Name	Classification
Nitrostat (nitroglycerin)	antianginal; coronary vasodilator
Nizoral (ketoconazole)	antifungal
Nolvadex (tamoxifen citrate)	antineoplastic agent
nortriptyline hydrochloride	antidepressant
Norvasc (amlodipine)	antihypertensive; antianginal; calcium channel blocker
Novolin (insulin preparation)	antidiabetic
nystatin	antifungal
Ogen (estropipate)	estrogen derivative
Ortho-Cept 28 (ethinyl estradiol and desogestrel)	oral contraceptive
Ortho-Novum 1/35-28 (ethinyl estradiol and norethindrone)	oral contraceptive
Ortho-Novum 7/7/7-28 (ethinyl estradiol and norethindrone)	oral contraceptive
Oruvail (ketoprofen)	analgesic; nonsteroidal anti-inflammatory (NSAID)
Paxil (paroxetine)	antidepressant
Penicillin VK (penicillin v potassium)	antibiotic
Pen-Vee K (penicillin v potassium)	antibiotic
Pepcid (famotidine)	antiulcer; histamine-2 antagonist
Percocet (oxycodone and acetaminophen)	analgesic, narcotic; antipyretic
Peridex (chlorhexidine gluconate)	antibiotic
Phenergan (promethazine hydrochloride)	antiemetic; antihistamine; sedative
phenobarbital	anticonvulsant; hypnotic; sedative
potassium chloride	potassium salt; electrolyte supplement
Pravachol (pravastatin sodium)	antilipemic
prednisone	anti-inflammatory; corticosteroid
Premarin (conjugated estrogens)	estrogen derivative
Prilosec (omeprazole)	gastric acid secretion inhibitor
Principen (ampicillin)	antibiotic
Prinivil (lisinopril)	antihypertensive; angiotensin-converting enzyme (ACE) inhibitor
Procardia XL (nifedipine)	antianginal; calcium channel blocker
promethazine and codeine	antihistamine; antitussive
Propacet (propoxyphene and acetaminophen)	analgesic, narcotic; antipyretic
propoxyphene	analgesic, narcotic
propoxyphene and acetaminophen	analgesic, narcotic; antipyretic
Propulsid (cisapride)	antiemetic
Proventil (albuterol)	bronchodilator

Name	Classification
Provera (medroxyprogesterone acetate)	contraceptive; progestin
Prozac (fluoxetine hydrochloride)	antidepressant
Relafen (nabumetone)	nonsteroidal anti-inflammatory (NSAID)
Retin-A (tretinoin)	acne product
Ritalin (methylphenidate hydrochloride)	central nervous system stimulant
Roxicet (oxycodone and acetaminophen)	analgesic, narcotic; antipyretic
Seldane (terfenadine)	antihistamine
Seldane-D (terfenadine and pseudoephedrine)	antihistamine/decongestant
Slo-bid (theophylline)	antiasthmatic; bronchodilator
Sumycin (tetracycline)	antibiotic; acne product
Suprax (cefixime)	antibiotic
Synthroid (levothyroxine sodium)	thyroid product
Tagamet (cimetidine)	antiulcer; histamine-2 antagonist
Tegretol (carbamazepine)	anticonvulsant; miscellaneous
temazepam	hypnotic; sedative
Tenormin (atenolol)	antianginal; beta-adrenergic blocker
Terazol (terconazole)	vaginal antifungal
tetracycline	antibiotic
Theo-Dur (theophylline)	antiasthmatic; bronchodilator
thyroid	thyroid product
Timoptic (timolol maleate)	ophthalmic beta-adrenergic blocker; antiglaucoma
TobraDex (tobramycin and dexamethasone)	ophthalmic antibiotic
Toradol (ketorolac tromethamine)	analgesic; nonsteroidal anti-inflammatory (NSAID)
trazodone hydrochloride	antidepressant
Trental (pentoxifylline)	blood viscosity reducer agent
triamcinolone	anti-inflammatory; corticosteroid
triamtereme and hydrochlorothiazide (HCTZ)	diuretic
Tri-Levlen 28 (ethinyl estradiol and levonorgestrel)	oral contraceptive
trimethoprim-sulfamethoxazole	antibiotic
Trimox (amoxicillin trihydrate)	antibiotic
Triphasil (ethinyl estradiol and levonorgestrel)	oral contraceptive
Tussionex (hydrocodone and chlorpheniramine)	antitussive
Tylenol with Codeine (acetaminophen and codeine)	analgesic, narcotic, antipyretic

Name	Classification	Name	Classification
Valium (diazepam)	antianxiety; anticonvulsant; sedative	Verelan (verapamil hydrochloride)	antianginal; antiarrhythmic; calcium channel blocker
Vancenase AQ (beclomethasone dipropionate)	anti-inflammatory; corticosteroid	Vicodin (hydrocodone and acetaminophen)	analgesic, narcotic; antipyretic
Vanceril (beclomethasone dipropionate)	anti-inflammatory; corticosteroid	Voltaren (diclofenac sodium)	analgesic; nonsteroidal anti-inflammatory (NSAID)
Vantin (cefpodoxime proxetil)	antibiotic	Xanax (aprazolam)	antianxiety agent
		Zantac (ranitidine hydrochloride)	antiulcer; histamine-2 antagonist
Vasotec (enalapril)	antihypertensive; angiotensin-converting enzyme (ACE) inhibitor	Zestril (lisinopril)	antihypertensive; angiotensin-converting enzyme (ACE) inhibitor
Veetids (penicillin v potassium)	antibiotic	Zithromax (azithromycin dihydrate)	antibiotic
Ventolin (albuterol)	bronchodilator	Zocor (simvastatin)	antilipemic
verapamil hydrochloride	antianginal; antiarrhythmic; calcium channel blocker	Zoloft (sertraline hydrochloride)	antidepressant
		Zovirax (acyclovir)	antiviral

References

Quick Look Drug Book 1994. Baltimore: Williams & Wilkins, 1994.

Simonsen LLaP. Top 200 drugs. Rx prices still moderating as managed care grows. Pharmacy Times 1995; Apr: 17.

APPENDIX D

Answers to Practice Exercises

CHAPTER 1 (Practice Exercises begin on page 7)
1. personal commitment
2. answers will vary
3. a. act immediately to focus on goals
   b. don't try to take on too much at once
   c. divide materials into smaller, more manageable portions
   d. celebrate progress along the way and look forward to future benefits for learning (note: class discussion will bring out other good ideas)
4. promotes possibility thinking and self-confidence that lead to success
5. answers will vary
6. a. organize study area and find a comfortable place
   b. listen to enjoyable music while studying
   c. replace negative self-talk with "can do" affirmatives
   d. think positively and visualize myself as a successful learner
7. stress reduction and mental stamina
8. see it, say it, write it
9. Make a 3×5 card for each prefix, suffix, and combining form listed in Chapter 2. Write each component on the front and its meaning on the back. Include a sample word.
10. a. draw pictures of word components
    b. listen to audiotapes
    c. make up songs or rhymes
    d. find a person or group to study with

CHAPTER 2 (Practice Exercises begin on page 28)
1. laparo/tomy — abdomen/incision
2. cephal/algia — head/pain
3. neo/plasia — new/formation
4. hydro/philia — water/attraction for
5. patho/psycho/logy — disease/mind/study of
6. inter/fibr/al — between/fiber/pertaining to
7. pyo/genesis — pus/origin or production
8. pachy/cephal/y — thick/head/condition or process of
9. ultra/sono/graphy — beyond or excessive/sound/process of recording
10. melano/cyt/oma — black/cell/tumor
11. gastro/pexy — stomach/suspension or fixation
12. exo/card/ia — outside/heart/condition of
13. cephalo/metry — head/process of measuring
14. peri/aden/itis — around/gland/inflammation
15. pan/cyto/penia — all/cell/abnormal reduction
16. endo/tox/emia — within/poison/blood condition
17. carcin/oma — cancer/tumor
18. intra/gastr/ic — within/stomach/pertaining to
19. cyan/osis — blue/condition or increase
20. meta/morph/osis — beyond, after, or *change/form/ *condition or increase
21. abdomino/centesis — abdomen/puncture for aspiration
22. erythro/poiesis — red/formation
23. litho/tripsy — stone/crushing
24. eu/phon/ia — good or normal voice or speech/condition of
25. hemo/dia/lysis — blood/across or through/breaking down or dissolution
26. hyper/troph/ic — above or *excessive/nourishment or *development/pertaining to
27. cyto/rrhexis — cell/rupture
28. vaso/spasm — vessel/involuntary contraction
29. pod/iatry — foot/treatment
30. leuko/rrhea — white/discharge
31. tachy/card/ia — fast/heart/condition of
32. poly/phob/ia — many/exaggerated fear/condition of
33. dys/phon/ic — painful, difficult, or faulty/voice or speech/pertaining to
34. hemi/gastr/ectomy — half/stomach/excision (removal)
35. fibr/oid — fiber/resembling
36. gastro/ptosis — stomach/falling or downward displacement
37. angio/megaly — vessel/enlargement
38. ecto/genic — outside/origin or production
39. macro/cephal/ous — *large or long/head/pertaining to
40. adeno/malacia — gland/softening
41. cardio/graph — heart/instrument for recording
42. epi/gastro/cele — upon/stomach/pouching or hernia
43. hypo/lip/iasis — below or deficient/fat/formation of or presence of

44. uro/logist   urine/one who specializes in study or treatment of
45. sub/scler/al   below or under/hard/pertaining to
46. gastro/stomy   stomach/creation of an opening
47. necro/scopy   death/examination
48. acro/dynia   extremity/pain
49. ped/iatrics   *child or foot/treatment
50. pre/or/al   before/mouth/pertaining to
51. micro/scope   small/instrument for examination
52. oligo/ur/ia   few or deficient/urine/condition of
53. gastro/rrhaphy   stomach/suture
54. aero/meter   air or gas/instrument for measuring
55. ortho/ped/ic   straight normal, or correct/foot or child/pertaining to
56. syn/desis   together or with/binding
57. angi/ectasis   vessel/expansion or dilation
58. pod/algia   foot/pain
59. son/ar   sound/pertaining to
60. epi/gastr/ium   upon/stomach/structure or tissue

*Preferred answer.

Prefixes in parentheses have the same meaning, although they are not used in the term.

61. supranasal = above the nose (super-, hyper-)
62. disjointed = separated from joint
63. reproduce = make again
64. preoperative = before surgery (pro-, ante-)
65. postpartum = after labor
66. dehydrated = not watered
67. monomorphic = pertaining to one form (uni-)
68. transdermal = across or through the skin (dia-)
69. superacute = excessively severe (hyper-, supra-)
70. infraumbilical = below or under the navel (hypo-, sub-)
71. seminormal = half normal (hemi-)
72. exhalation = breathe out (e-, ec-)
73. retroversion = to turn backward
74. extracranial = outside the skull (ecto-, exo-)
75. paramedic = alongside of the doctor
76. anteflexion = bend before (pre-, pro-)
77. dysphonia = difficult voice
78. abduction = to turn away from
79. prophylaxis = to guard before (pre-, ante-)
80. polyarthritis = inflammation of many joints (multi-)
81. bradycardia = slow heart
82. circumvascular = around a blood vessel (peri-)
83. contraindicated = against or opposed to being indicated (anti-)
84. adduction = to turn toward or near
85. congenital = born with (syn-, sym-)
86. postcardial = behind the heart (retro-)
87. anaerobic = pertaining to life without air

88. bisexual = pertaining to both sexes (ambi-)
89. antigenic = against origin (contra-)
90. symphysis = growing together (syn-, con-)
91. acellular = pertaining to without cells (an-)
92. polyneuralgia
93. acromegaly
94. gastroenterostomy
95. erythrocytopenia
96. angiectasis
97. abdominocentesis
98. postcardial
99. cephalodynia
100. endarteritis
101. microtia

102–113.
lumpectomy
ileostomy
pericardiectomy
thoracostomy
cardiocentesis
hepatotomy
lithotripsy
colostomy
cervicoplasty
hysteropexy
arthrodesis
herniorrhaphy
114. endoscopies
115. fungi
116. specula
117. ampullae
118. bacteria
119. stomata
120. psychosis
121. phenomenon
122. macula
123. condyloma
124. index
125. bronchus

CHAPTER 3 (Practice Exercises begin on page 43)

1. onco/logy   tumor or mass/study of
2. immuno/logist   safe/one who specializes in the study or treatment of
3. oto/rhino/laryngo/logy   ear/nose/voice box/study of
4. opto/metry   eye/process of measuring
5. procto/logist   rectum/one who specializes in the study or treatment of
6. gyneco/logy   woman/study of
7. patho/logy   disease/study of
8. ortho/ped/ic   straight, normal, or correct/foot/pertaining to

9. uro/logist   urine/one who specializes in the study or treatment of

10. ped/iatric   *child or foot/treatment

11. neuro/logy   nerve/study of

12. psycho/logist   mind/one who specializes in the study or treatment of

13. osteo/pathy   bone/disease

14. ophthalmo/logy   eye/study of

15. obstetr/ic   midwife/pertaining to

16. an/esthesio/logy   without/sensation/study of

17. cardio/logy   heart/study of

18. dermato/logy   skin/study of

19. geronto/logy   old age/study of

20. endo/crino/logist   within/to secrete/one who specializes in the study or treatment of

21. nephro/logist   kidney/one who specializes in the study or treatment of

22. gastro/entero/logy   stomach/intestine/study of

23. hemato/logist   blood/one who specializes in the study or treatment of

24. chiro/pract/ic   hand/to practice/pertaining to

25. ger/iatric   old age/treatment

26. i
27. k
28. o
29. f
30. m
31. n
32. e
33. b
34. d
35. h
36. g
37. l
38. a
39. j
40. c
41. obstetrics/gynecology
42. doctor of dental surgery
43. ear, nose, throat
44. American Board of Medical Specialists
45. doctor of optometry
46. fellow of the American College of Surgeons
47. American College of Physicians
48. doctor of chiropractic
49. doctor of podiatric medicine
50. doctor of osteopathy
51. gynecologist
52. otorhinolaryngologist
53. urologist

54. c
55. a
56. e
57. g
58. f
59. b
60. d

CHAPTER 4 (Practice Exercises begin on page 82)
1. chief complaint
2. occupational history
3. per rectum
4. bathroom privileges
5. postanesthetic recovery
6. past history
7. discontinue or discharge
8. instructions to patient
9. emergency room
10. intensive care unit
11. rule out
12. nothing by mouth
13. living and well
14. blood pressure
15. both ears
16. symptom
17. vital signs
18. review of systems
19. patient
20. right eye
21. subcutaneous
22. history and physical
23. treatment or traction
24. diagnosis
25. present illness
26. d
27. e
28. g
29. a
30. j
31. i
32. b
33. c
34. f
35. h
36. d
37. h
38. f
39. i
40. g
41. j
42. b
43. c
44. a
45. e
46. vital signs every hour for four hours, then every two hours
47. one four times a day, after meals and at bedtime

---

*Preferred answer.

48. two and one-half grains of aspirin (acetylsalicylic acid) every day
49. five grains per rectum every four hours as needed if temperature greater than 101 degrees
50. one every other day in the morning
51. two drops in both eyes three times a day for seven days
52. two capsules immediately, then one every six hours
53. tab †̄ t.i.d. × 7 d or †̄ tab t.i.d. × 7 d
54. suppos †̄ PV h.s. or †̄ suppos PV h.s.
55. gr s̄s̄ b.i.d. or s̄s̄ gr b.i.d.
56. †̄ or †̈ p.o. q 3–4 h p.r.n.
57. gtt †̈ AS q 3 h or †̈ gtt AS q 3 h
58. cap †̄ b.i.d. a.m. and p.m. or †̄ cap b.i.d. a.m. and p.m.
59. †̈ STAT, then †̄ q 6 h
60. 30 mg p.o. h.s. p.r.n.
61. 0100
62. 1430
63. 2400
64. 1300
65. 1900

CHAPTER 5 (Practice Exercises begin on page 105)

1. pachy/onych/ia — thick/nail/condition of
2. kerato/myc/osis — hard/fungus/condition or increase
3. dermato/logist — skin/one who specializes in treatment of
4. histo/troph/ic — tissue/nourishment or development/pertaining to
5. hyper/onych/ia — above or excessive/nail/condition of
6. leuko/trich/ia — white/hair/condition of
7. kerat/osis — hard/condition or increase
8. pachy/dermat/osis — thick/skin/condition or increase
9. epi/dermis — upon/skin
10. lip/oma — fat/tumor
11. sub/cutane/ous — below or under/skin/pertaining to
12. an/hidr/osis — without/sweat/condition or increase
13. histo/dia/lysis — tissue/across or through/breaking down or dissolution
14. dys/plas/ia — painful, difficult or faulty/formation/condition of
15. xantho/derma — yellow/skin
16. dys/plas/tic — painful, difficult or faulty/formation/pertaining to
17. pachy/dermato/cele — thick/skin/pouching or hernia
18. erythro/dermat/itis — red/skin/inflammation
19. histo/tox/ic — tissue/poison/pertaining to
20. melano/cyt/e — black/cell/noun marker

21. xer/osis — dry/condition or increase
22. purpur/ic — purple/pertaining to
23. squam/ous — scale/pertaining to
24. sebo/rrhea — sebum (oil)/discharge
25. steato/lysis — fat/breaking down or dissolution
26. gangrene
27. autograft
28. ecchymosis
29. pruritus
30. carbuncle
31. tinea
32. urticaria
33. heterograft
34. pediculosis pubis
35. furuncle
36. macule or macula
37. scale
38. pediculosis capitis
39. alopecia
40. herpes simplex virus Type 1
41. histology
42. erythema
43. comedo
44. cicatrix
45. fissure
46. diaphoresis
47. biopsy
48. eruption
49. keloid
50. melanoma
51. seborrhea
52. pachyderma
53. excoriation
54. leukoderma
55. frozen section
56. erythroderma
57. keratoderma
58. seborrheic keratoses
59. lipoma or steatoma
60. xanthoderma
61. mycosis
62. hypodermic
63. cherry angioma
64. xeroderma
65. rubella
66. varicella
67. rubeola
68. f
69. i
70. c
71. h
72. d
73. g
74. a
75. j

76. b
77. e
78. herpes simplex virus Type 2
79. biopsy
80. frozen section
81. incision and drainage
82. keratoses
83. ecchymoses
84. bullae
85. maculae
86. nevi
87. c
88. d
89. g
90. h
91. i
92. l
93. j
94. m
95. n
96. k
97. a
98. f
99. b
100. e

CHAPTER 6 (Practice Exercises begin on page 147)

1. hemi/pelv/ectomy   half/hip bone/excision (removal)
2. arthr/itis   joint/inflammation
3. myo/fasci/al   muscle/fascia (a band)/pertaining to
4. arthro/path/y   joint/disease/condition or process of
5. spondylo/lysis   vertebra/breaking down or
                            dissolution
6. osteo/genic   bone/origin or production
7. chondr/ectomy   cartilage/excision (removal)
8. myo/necr/osis   muscle/death/condition or increase
9. spondylo/syn/desis vertebra/together or with/binding
10. peri/oste/itis   around/bone/inflammation
11. leio/myo/sarc/oma   smooth/muscle/flesh/tumor
12. myelo/cyt/e   bone marrow/cell/noun marker
13. costo/tomy   rib/incision
14. spondylo/malacia   vertebra/softening
15. osteo/arthr/itis   bone/joint/inflammation
16. inter/cost/al   between/rib/pertaining to
17. orth/osis   straight, normal, correct/condition
                            or increase
18. cranio/tomy   skull/incision
19. myo/ton/ia   muscle/tone/condition of
20. kyph/osis   humped/condition or increase

21. crani/ectomy   skull/excision (removal)
22. arthro/desis   joint/binding
23. osteo/plasty   bone/surgical repair or reconstruction
24. fibro/my/algia   fiber/muscle/pain
25. rhabdo/my/oma   rod shaped or striated (skeletal)/
                            muscle/tumor
26. arthro/gram   joint/record
27. intra/articul/ar   within/joint/pertaining to
28. lord/osis   bent/condition or increase
29. syn/dactyl/ism   together or with/digit/condition of
30. teno/myo/tomy   tendon/muscle/incision
31. cervico/brachi/al   neck/arm/pertaining to
32. hypo/ton/ia   below or deficient/tone/condition of
33. arthro/scopy   joint/examination
34. lumbo/dynia   loin (lower back)/pain
35. thorac/ic   chest/pertaining to
36. oste/algia   bone/pain
37. costo/vertebr/al   rib/vertebra/pertaining to
38. scoliosis
39. arthralgia or arthrodynia
40. osteoma
41. myoma
42. crepitation or crepitus
43. ostealgia or osteodynia
44. arthrogram
45. sagittal
46. osteoplasty
47. coronal or frontal
48. atrophy
49. rhabdomyoma
50. electromyogram
51. leiomyoma
52. traction
53. flaccid
54. horizontal recumbent, or supine
55. myeloma
56. gouty arthritis
57. transverse
58. pronation
59. ankylosis
60. subluxation
61. proximal
62. prone
63. prosthesis
64. bone scan
65. superior (cephalic)
66. dorsiflexion
67. open reduction internal fixation of a fracture (ORIF)
68. rickets
69. sonography
70. radiologist
71. rigor, rigidity

72. inter<u>cost</u>al
73. rhab<u>do</u>myosarcoma
74. hyper<u>troph</u>y
75. myo<u>rrhaphy</u>
76. spondylosyn<u>desis</u>
77. <u>leio</u>myoma
78. osteo<u>malacia</u>
79. <u>spondylo</u>listhesis
80. arthro<u>gram</u>
81. <u>osteo</u>tomy
82. epiphys<u>itis</u>
83. <u>cervic</u>al
84. bone <u>necrosis</u>
85. <u>chondroma</u>
86. arthro<u>centesis</u>
87. c
88. d
89. a
90. b
91. f
92. e
93. computed tomography
94. physical therapy
95. traction or treatment
96. range of motion
97. fracture (broken bone)

CHAPTER 7 (Practice Exercises begin on page 185)

1. angio/graphy — <u>vessel/process of recording</u>
2. varic/osis — <u>swollen or twisted vein/condition or increase</u>
3. pector/al — <u>chest/pertaining to</u>
4. vaso/spasm — <u>vessel/involuntary contraction</u>
5. ven/ous — <u>vein/pertaining to</u>
6. aorto/coron/ary — <u>aorta/circle or crown/pertaining to</u>
7. thrombo/phleb/itis — <u>clot/vein/inflammation</u>
8. arterio/scler/osis — <u>artery/hard/condition or increase</u>
9. vasculo/path/y — <u>vessel/disease/condition or process of</u>
10. athero/genesis — <u>fat/origin or production</u>
11. cardio/myo/lip/osis — <u>heart/muscle/fat/condition or increase</u>
12. atri/al — <u>atrium/pertaining to</u>
13. stetho/scope — <u>chest/instrument for examination</u>
14. arterio/rrhexis — <u>artery/rupture</u>
15. myo/card/ium — <u>muscle/heart/structure or tissue</u>
16. aorto/plasty — <u>aorta/surgical repair or reconstruction</u>
17. sphygm/oid — <u>pulse/resembling</u>
18. veno/stomy — <u>vein/creation of an opening</u>
19. arterio/sten/osis — <u>artery/narrow/condition or increase</u>
20. arterio/tomy — <u>artery/incision</u>
21. thrombo/poiesis — <u>clot/formation</u>

22. cardio/aort/ic — <u>heart/aorta/pertaining to</u>
23. ventriculo/gram — <u>ventricle (belly or pouch)/record</u>
24. angio/dys/troph/ia — <u>vessel/painful, difficult, or faulty/ nourishment or development/ condition of</u>
25. phleb/itis — <u>vein/inflammation</u>
26. thrombo/philia — <u>clot/attraction for</u>
27. angio/plasty — <u>vessel/surgical repair or reconstruction</u>
28. veno/stasis — <u>vein/stop or stand</u>
29. end/arter/ectomy — <u>within/artery/excision</u>
30. cardio/tox/ic — <u>heart/poison/pertaining to</u>
31. arterio/gram — <u>artery/record</u>
32. ather/ectomy — <u>fat/excision</u>
33. thrombo/lysis — <u>clot/breaking down or dissolution</u>
34. aorto/rrhaphy — <u>aorta/suture</u>
35. cardi/ac — <u>heart/pertaining to</u>
36. h
37. o
38. n
39. i
40. g
41. j
42. a
43. c
44. l
45. e
46. m
47. d
48. k
49. f
50. b
51. congenital anomalies
52. arteriosclerosis
53. arrhythmia
54. cardiomyopathy
55. anastomosis
56. gallop
57. echocardiogram
58. cor pulmonale
59. coronary angiogram
60. stress electrocardiogram
61. premature ventricular contraction
62. patent ductus arteriosus
63. arteriosclerotic heart disease
64. implantable cardioverter defibrillator
65. congestive heart failure
66. coronary artery disease
67. hypertension
68. mitral valve prolapse
69. magnetic resonance angiography
70. ventricular septal defect
71. e

72. h
73. b
74. a
75. j
76. c
77. i
78. d
79. f
80. g

CHAPTER 8 (Practice Exercises begin on page 214)

1. erythro/blast/osis   red/germ or bud/condition or increase
2. chylo/poiesis   juice/formation
3. hemo/cyto/meter   blood/cell/instrument for measuring
4. spleno/rrhagia   spleen/to burst forth
5. lymph/aden/itis   clear fluid/gland/inflammation
6. erythro/chrom/ia   red/color/condition of
7. reticulo/cyt/osis   a net/cell/condition or increase
8. thymo/path/y   thymus gland/disease /condition or process of
9. leuko/cyt/ic   white/cell/pertaining to
10. lymph/angio/gram   clear fluid/vessel/record
11. spleno/malacia   spleen/softening
12. erythro/cyto/rrhexis   red/cell/rupture
13. reticul/ar   a net/pertaining to
14. lymph/oid   clear fluid/resembling
15. pro/myelo/cyt/e   before/bone marrow or spinal cord/ cell/noun marker
16. meta/myelo/cyt/e   beyond, after, or change/bone marrow or spinal cord/cell/ noun marker
17. chromo/phil/ic   color/attraction for/pertaining to
18. leuko/cyto/penia   white/cell/abnormal reduction
19. splen/ectomy   spleen/excision (removal)
20. immuno/log/ic   safe/study/pertaining to
21. chylo/rrhea   juice/discharge
22. hemo/dia/lysis   blood/across or through/breaking down or dissolution
23. lymph/oma   clear fluid/tumor
24. cyto/morpho/logy   cell/form/study of
25. hemo/lysis   blood/breaking down or dissolution
26. lymph/aden/ectomy   clear fluid/gland/excision (removal)
27. meta/stasis   beyond, after, or change/stop or stand
28. an/emia   without/blood condition
29. spleno/megaly   spleen/enlargement
30. immuno/tox/ic   safe/poison/pertaining to
31. mean corpuscular (cell) volume (MCV)
32. mean corpuscular (cell) hemoglobin (MCH)
33. mean corpuscular (cell) hemoglobin concentration (MCHC)
34. white blood count, WBC
35. hemoglobin, HGB or Hgb
36. hematocrit, HCT or Hct
37. differential count
38. prothrombin time
39. erythrocyte sedimentation rate
40. partial thromboplastin time
41. complete blood count
42. l
43. j
44. k
45. g
46. c
47. e
48. f
49. b
50. d
51. i
52. h
53. a
54. neutropenia
55. autologous blood
56. immunosuppression
57. crossmatching
58. acquired immunodeficiency syndrome, AIDS
59. plasmapheresis
60. homologous blood

CHAPTER 9 (Practice Exercises begin on page 245)

1. broncho/stomy   bronchus (airway)/creation of an opening
2. tracheo/py/osis   trachea (windpipe)/pus/condition or increase
3. hyper/pnea   above or excessive/breathing
4. thora/centesis   chest/puncture for aspiration
5. rhino/sten/osis   nose/narrow/condition or increase
6. hyp/ox/ia   below or deficient/oxygen/ condition of
7. sinus/itis   sinus (cavity)/inflammation
8. hyp/ox/emia   below or deficient/oxygen/blood condition
9. pleur/itis   pleura/inflammation
10. hyper/carb/ia   above or excessive/carbon dioxide/ condition of
11. tracheo/tomy   trachea (windpipe)/incision
12. dys/phon/ia   painful, difficult, or faulty/voice or speech/condition of
13. broncho/scope   bronchus (airway)/instrument for examination

14. oro/pharyng/eal   mouth/pharynx (throat)/pertaining to

15. hypo/pnea   below or deficient/breathing

16. pneumon/ectomy   air or lung/excision

17. rhino/rrhea   nose/discharge

18. thoraco/stomy   chest/creation of an opening

19. eu/pnea   normal/breathing

20. tonsill/ectomy   tonsil (almond)/excision

21. pharyng/itis   pharynx (throat)/inflammation

22. broncho/spasm   bronchus (airway)/involuntary
                            contraction

23. laryngo/sten/osis   larynx (voice box)/narrow/condition
                            or increase

24. tracheo/bronch/itis   trachea (windpipe)/bronchus
                            (airway)/ inflammation

25. rhino/phon/ia   nose/voice or speech/condition of

26. phreno/ptosis   diaphragm/downward displacement

27. peri/pleur/al   around/pleura/pertaining to

28. stetho/scope   chest/instrument for examination

29. rhino/scler/oma   nose/hard/tumor

30. pneumon/ic   air or lung/pertaining to

31. broncho/rrhea   bronchus (airway)/discharge

32. naso/pharyngo/scopy   nose/pharynx (throat)/examination

33. bronchi/ectasis   bronchus (airway)/expansion or
                            dilation

34. rhin/itis   nose/inflammation

35. sinuso/tomy   sinus (cavity)/incision

36. lob/ectomy   lobe (a portion/excision (removal)

38. pector/al   chest/pertaining to

39. rhino/plasty   nose/surgical repair or reconstruction

40. alveol/itis   alveolus (air sac)/inflammation

41. pneumothorax

42. empyema or pyothorax

43. hemothorax

44. auscultation

45. bronchoscope

46. expectoration

47. pleurisy or pleuritis

48. percussion

49. hypoventilation

50. thoracentesis

51. nuclear medicine

52. dysphonia

53. laryngitis

54. hypoxia

55. emphysema

56. epistaxis

57. bronchogenic carcinoma

58. coryza

59. atelectasis

60. sputum

61. stridor

62. pulmonary embolism

63. tracheostomy

64. asthma

65. hyperventilation

66. pneumocystis pneumonia

67. chronic obstructive pulmonary disease

68. pneumoconiosis

69. bronchiectasis

70. thoracoplasty

71. pneumonitis

72. spirometry

73. eupnea

74. bradypnea

75. dyspnea

76. orthopnea

77. apnea

78. tachypnea

79. peak expiratory flow rate

80. vital capacity

81. tuberculosis

82. cardiopulmonary resuscitation

83. chronic obstructive pulmonary disease

84. partial pressure of carbon dioxide

85. upper respiratory infection

86. tidal volume

87. pulmonary function testing

88. CXR

89. ABG

90. T&A

91. e

92. h

93. g

94. f

95. i

96. j

97. d

98. c

99. b

100. a

CHAPTER 10 (Practice Exercises begin on page 285)

1. gangli/oma   ganglion (knot)/tumor

2. neuro/genic   nerve/origin or production

3. encephalo/cele   brain/pouching or hernia

4. dys/tax/ia   painful, difficult, or faulty/order or
                          coordination/condition of

5. ventricul/itis   ventricle (belly or pouch)/inflammation

6. myelo/rrhaphy   *spinal cord or bone marrow/suture

7. esthesio/neur/osis   sensation/nerve/condition or
                          increase

8. cerebr/al angio/gram brain/pertaining to vessel/record

*Preferred answer.

9. spondylo/syn/desis   vertebra/together or with/binding

10. hemi/plegia   half/paralysis

11. cranio/tomy   skull/incision

12. topo/an/esthes/ia   place/without/sensation/condition of

13. neuro/gli/al   nerve/glue/pertaining to

14. neuro/cyto/lysis   nerve/cell/break down or dissolution

15. somni/pathy   sleep/disease

16. myelo/pathy   *spinal cord or bone marrow/disease

17. hydro/cephal/ic   water/head/pertaining to

18. poly/neur/itis   many/nerve/inflammation

19. neur/algia   nerve/pain

20. encephal/itis   brain/inflammation

21. para/somn/ia   alongside of or *abnormal/sleep/ condition of

22. narco/lepsy   stupor/seizure

23. stereo/tax/y   solid or three dimensional/order or coordination/condition or process of

24. hemi/paresis   half/ slight paralysis

25. neur/asthenia   nerve/weakness

26. gli/oma   glue/tumor

27. intra/crani/al   within/skull/pertaining to

28. a/phas/ic   without/speech/pertaining to

29. a/gnos/ia   without/knowing/condition of

30. cerebro/spin/al   brain/spine (thorn)/pertaining to

31. myelogram
32. meningitis
33. discectomy
34. atopognosis
35. Parkinson's disease
36. Babinski's sign or reflex
37. paresthesia
38. coma
39. convulsion
40. spina bifida
41. astereognosis
42. electroencephalogram
43. spondylosyndesis
44. craniectomy
45. cerebral atherosclerosis
46. hyperesthesia
47. dysphasia
48. analgesia
49. i
50. h
51. j
52. a
53. f
54. g
55. e
56. b

57. c
58. d
59. computed tomography
60. magnetic resonance imaging
61. nerve conduction velocity
62. positron emission tomography
63. multiple sclerosis
64. central nervous system
65. cerebral palsy
66. transient ischemic attack
67. electroencephalogram
68. deep tendon reflexes
69. single photon emission computed tomography
70. polysomnography
71. autonomic nervous system
72. peripheral nervous system
73. cerebrospinal fluid
74. magnetic resonance angiography
75. cerebrovascular accident

CHAPTER 11 (Practice Exercises begin on page 312)

1. hypo/para/thyroid/ism   below or deficient/*alongside of or abnormal/ thyroid gland (shield)/ condition of

2. aden/itis   gland/inflammation

3. hyper/glyc/emia   above or excessive/sugar/blood condition

4. thyro/toxic/osis   thyroid gland (shield)/poison/ condition or increase

5. poly/dips/ia   many/thirst/condition of

6. hormon/al   hormone (an urging on)/pertaining to

7. ket/osis   ketone bodies/condition or increase

8. poly/ur/ia   many/urine/condition of

9. endo/crin/e   within/to secrete/noun marker

10. thyro/ptosis   thyroid gland (shield)/falling or downward displacement

11. thym/oma   thymus gland/tumor

12. acro/megaly   *extremity or topmost/enlargement

13. andr/oid   male/resembling

14. adreno/troph/ic   adrenal gland/nourishment or development/pertaining to

15. pancreato/genic   pancreas/origin or production
16. myxedema
17. cretinism
18. hyperthyroidism or thyrotoxicosis
19. Cushing's syndrome
20. acromegaly
21. goiter
22. exophthalmos or exophthalmus
23. pituitary dwarfism
24. hypokalemia
25. thyroid uptake and image

*Preferred answer.

26. gigantism or pituitary gigantism
27. e
28. h
29. j
30. f
31. c
32. i
33. b
34. g
35. a
36. d
37. poly<u>dip</u>sia
38. <u>hyper</u>secretion
39. <u>hypo</u>glycemia
40. glucos<u>uria</u>
41. <u>hypo</u>secretion
42. <u>hyper</u>glycemia
43. <u>son</u>ography
44. blood sugar
45. insulin-dependent diabetes mellitus
46. fasting blood sugar
47. computed tomography
48. postprandial blood sugar
49. glucose tolerance test
50. non–insulin-dependent diabetes mellitus

CHAPTER 12 (Practice Exercises begin on page 338)

1. blepharo/ptosis — eyelid/falling or downward displacement
2. irido/tomy — iris (colored circle)/incision
3. ophthalmo/logy — eye/study of
4. vitr/ectomy — glassy/excision (removal)
5. dacryo/cyst/itis — tear/bladder or *sac/inflammation
6. lacrim/al — tear/pertaining to
7. corneo/scler/al — cornea/hard or *sclera/pertaining to
8. kerato/tomy — hard or *cornea/incision
9. blepharo/plasty — eyelid/surgical repair or reconstruction
10. dacryo/cysto/ rhino/stomy — tear/bladder or sac/nose/creation of an opening
11. photo/phob/ia — light/exaggerated fear or *sensitivity/ condition of
12. opt/ic/al — eye/pertaining to/pertaining to
13. sclero/malacia — hard or *sclera/softening
14. ocul/ar — eye/pertaining to
15. sclero/stomy — hard or *sclera/creation of an opening
16. b
17. d
18. a
19. e
20. c
21. <u>kerat</u>itis

22. <u>photo</u>phobia
23. dacryo<u>cyst</u>ectomy
24. <u>ex</u>ophthalmos
25. <u>blepharo</u>chalasis or <u>dermato</u>chalasis
26. inward turn of rim of the eyelid
27. double vision
28. instrument to measure intraocular pressure
29. outward turn of rim of the eyelid
30. blind spot in vision
31. conjunctivitis
32. blepharitis
33. asthenopia
34. mydriatic
35. aphakia
36. hordeolum
37. cataract
38. macular degeneration
39. blepharospasm
40. nystagmus

CHAPTER 13 (Practice Exercises begin on page 354)

1. aer/ot/itis — air or gas/ear/inflammation
2. oto/scler/osis — ear/hard/condition or increase
3. myringo/plasty — eardrum/surgical repair or reconstruction
4. acous/tic — hearing/pertaining to
5. tympano/tomy — eardrum/incision
6. cerumino/lysis — wax/breaking down or dissolution
7. salpingo/scope — eustachian tube/instrument for examination
8. oto/pyo/rrhea — ear/pus/discharge
9. audio/metry — hearing/process of measuring
10. tympano/centesis — eardrum/puncture for aspiration
11. oto/dynia — ear/pain
12. audio/genic — hearing/origin
13. myring/ectomy — eardrum/excision (removal)
14. cerumin/al — wax/pertaining to
15. tympan/itis — eardrum/inflammation
16. otos<u>cler</u>osis
17. aero<u>tit</u>is media
18. <u>audio</u>logist
19. <u>myringo</u>tomy
20. <u>oto</u>scope
21. labyrinthitis
22. vertigo
23. otorrhagia
24. paracusis
25. presbycusis
26. tinnitus
27. stapedectomy
28. cerumen impaction
29. otalgia
30. audiology

---

*Preferred answer.

CHAPTER 14 (Practice Exercises begin on page 386)

1.	gastro/genic	stomach/origin or production
2.	gingivo/gloss/itis	gum/tongue/inflammation
3.	stomat/algia	mouth/pain
4.	procto/logy	rectum/study of
5.	hemat/emesis	blood/vomiting
6.	cheilo/stomato/plasty	lip/mouth/surgical repair or reconstruction
7.	entero/cele	small intestine/pouching or hernia
8.	hyper/emesis	above or excessive/vomiting
9.	chole/cyst/ectomy	bile/bladder or sac/excision (removal)
10.	gastr/ectasis	stomach/expansion or dilation
11.	cheilo/phag/ia	lip/eat or swallow/condition of
12.	glosso/spasm	tongue/involuntary contraction
13.	gastro/esophag/itis	stomach/esophagus/inflammation
14.	recto/sigmoid/al	rectum/sigmoid colon/pertaining to
15.	choledocho/jejuno/stomy	common bile duct/jejunum/creation of an opening
16.	dys/phag/ia	painful, difficult, or faulty/eat or swallow/condition of
17.	laparo/scopy	abdomen/examination
18.	chole/cysto/gram	bile/bladder or sac/record
19.	glosso/pathy	tongue/disease
20.	oro/lingu/al	mouth/tongue/pertaining to
21.	ceilo/gastro/tomy	abdomen/stomach/incision
22.	pancreato/duodeno/stomy	pancreas/duodenum/creation of an opening
23.	colo/enter/itis	colon/small intestine/inflammation
24.	ano/scope	anus/instrument to examine
25.	sigmoido/scopy	sigmoid colon/examination
26.	hepato/tox/ic	liver/poison/pertaining to
27.	bucc/al	cheek/pertaining to
28.	sialo/rrhea	saliva/discharge
29.	pylor/ectomy	pylorus (gatekeeper)/excision (removal)
30.	hernio/plasty	hernia/surgical repair or reconstruction
31.	retro/periton/eal	backward or behind/peritoneum/pertaining to
32.	abdomino/centesis	abdomen/puncture for aspiration
33.	steato/lysis	fat/breaking down or dissolution
34.	ileo/rrhaphy	ileum/suture
35.	dent/algia	tooth/pain
36.	gastritis	

37. anorexia
38. aphagia
39. buccal
40. flatulence
41. hernia
42. melena
43. eructation
44. anoscope or proctoscope
45. colitis
46. barium swallow
47. ascites
48. cholecystitis
49. steatorrhea
50. diverticulitis
51. gastric ulcer
52. hepatomegaly
53. ankyloglossia
54. hemigastrectomy
55. appendicitis
56. cheilorrhaphy
57. cholelithotripsy
58. stomatoplasty
59. cholangiogram
60. hyperbilirubinemia
61. gastric resection
62. diverticulosis
63. inguinal regions
64. hypochondriac regions
65. epigastric region
66. hypogastric region
67. lumbar regions
68. umbilical region
69. right upper quadrant (RUQ)
70. left upper quadrant (LUQ)
71. right lower quadrant (RLQ)
72. left lower quadrant (LLQ)
73. m
74. f
75. d
76. h
77. k
78. g
79. j
80. i
81. l
82. b
83. e
84. a
85. c
86. laparoscope
87. anoscope or proctoscope
88. gastroscope
89. sigmoidoscope or colonoscope
90. peritoneoscope
91. esophagoscope

92. incarcerated
93. excisional biopsy
94. nasogastric tube
95. endoscopic retrograde cholangiopancreatography
96. gastroesophageal reflux disease
97. left upper quadrant
98. gastrointestinal
99. magnetic resonance imaging
100. esophagogastroduodenoscopy

CHAPTER 15 (Practice Exercises begin on page 419)

1. py/ur/ia — pus/urine/condition of
2. cyst/itis — bladder or sac/inflammation
3. nephro/megaly — kidney/enlargement
4. vesico/stomy — bladder or sac/creation of an opening
5. urethro/cyst/itis — urethra/bladder or sac/inflammation
6. nephro/ptosis — kidney/falling or downward displacement
7. poly/dips/ia — many/thirst/condition of
8. glomerulo/scler/osis — glomerulus (little ball)/hard/condition or increase
9. pyo/nephr/itis — pus/kidney/inflammation
10. dys/ur/ia — painful, difficult, or faulty/urine/condition of
11. vesico/tomy — bladder or sac/incision
12. glycos/ur/ia — sugar/urine/condition of
13. meat/al — opening/pertaining to
14. pyelo/nephr/osis — basin/kidney/condition or increase
15. cyst/ectomy — bladder/excision (removal)
16. uro/logist — urine/one who specializes in the study or treatment of
17. reno/gram — kidney/record
18. urethro/sten/osis — urethra/narrow/condition or increase
19. uro/stomy — urine/creation of an opening
20. urethro/pexy — urethra/suspension or fixation
21. nephro/hyper/trophy — kidney/above or excessive/nourishment or development
22. trans/urethr/al — across or through/urethra/pertaining to
23. uretero/litho/tomy — ureter/stone/incision
24. ket/osis — ketone bodies/condition or increase
25. meato/rrhaphy — opening/suture
26. bacter/oid — bacteria/resembling
27. reno/pathy — kidney/disease
28. hydro/nephr/osis — water/kidney/condition or increase

29. cystitis
30. nocturia
31. enuresis
32. nephrorrhaphy
33. nephrosis
34. albuminuria or proteinuria
35. urethral stenosis
36. nephrotomy
37. renal or kidney biopsy
38. urinalysis
39. cystoscopy
40. urethral stenosis
41. extracorporeal shock wave lithotripsy
42. resectoscope
43. oliguria
44. dysuria
45. pyuria
46. hematuria
47. anuresis
48. enuresis
49. stress incontinence
50. occult blood
51. RP
52. renal Bx or kidney Bx
53. UA
54. h
55. d
56. g
57. e
58. a
59. b
60. f
61. c
62. culture and sensitivity
63. voiding cystourethrogram
64. albumin or protein
65. intravenous pyelogram
66. extracorporeal shock wave lithotripsy
67. kidney, ureters, bladder
68. specific gravity
69. urinary tract infection
70. retrograde pyelogram

CHAPTER 16 (Practice Exercises begin on page 438)

1. oligo/sperm/ia — few or deficient/sperm (seed)/condition of
2. perine/al — perineum/pertaining to
3. orchi/algia — testis or testicle/pain
4. balano/rrhagia — glans penis/to burst forth
5. prostato/dynia — prostate/pain
6. orchid/ectomy — testis or testicle/excision (removal)
7. an/orch/ism — without/testis or testicle/condition of
8. vas/ectomy — vessel/excision (removal)
9. a/sperm/ia — without/sperm (seed)/condition of
10. prostat/itis — prostate/inflammation

11. balan/itis   glans penis/inflammation
12. orchio/plasty   testis or testicle/surgical repair or reconstruction
13. hydro/cele   water/pouching or hernia
14. epididym/ectomy   epididymis/excision (removal)
15. vaso/vaso/stomy   vessel/vessel/creation of an opening
16. anorchism
17. balanitis
18. impotence
19. varicocele
20. seminoma
21. azoospermia
22. oligospermia
23. orchiopexy
24. resectoscope
25. benign prostatic hypertrophy/hyperplasia
26. hydrocele
27. vasectomy
28. Peyronie's disease
29. circumcision
30. cryptorchism
31. digital rectal exam
32. endorectal or transrectal sonogram of prostate
33. glans penis
34. aspermia
35. c
36. d
37. f
38. e
39. a
40. b
41. prostate specific antigen
42. benign prostatic hypertrophy/hyperplasia
43. transurethral resection of the prostate
44. digital rectal exam
45. biopsy

CHAPTER 17 (Practice Exercises begin on page 475)

1. vulv/itis   vulva/inflammation
2. masto/ptosis   breast/falling or downward displacement
3. vagin/osis   vagina/condition or increase
4. toco/lysis   labor or birth/breaking down or dissolution
5. salpingo/tomy   uterine (fallopian) tube/incision
6. mammo/troph/ic   breast/nourishment or development/ pertaining to
7. episio/rrhaphy   vulva/suture
8. trans/vagin/al   across or through/vagina/ pertaining to
9. hystero/rrhexis   uterus/rupture

10. gyneco/logy   woman/study of
11. colpo/scopy   vagina/examination
12. meno/stasis   menstruation/*stop or stand
13. hyper/plasia   above or *excessive/formation
14. mammo/gram   breast/record
15. metro/malacia   uterus/softening
16. ovario/centesis   ovary/puncture for aspiration
17. men/arche   menstruation/beginning
18. poly/mast/ia   many/breast/condition of
19. pyo/salping/itis   pus/uterine tube/inflammation
20. oophoro/stomy   ovary/creation of an opening
21. oligo/meno/rrhea   few or *deficient/menstruation/ discharge
22. vagin/itis   vagina/inflammation
23. masto/tomy   breast/incision
24. dys/toc/ia   painful, *difficult or faulty/labor or birth/condition of
25. gyneco/logist   woman/one who specializes in study or treatment of
26. hyster/ectomy   uterus/excision
27. colpo/cyst/itis   vagina/bladder or sac/inflammation
28. episio/tomy   vulva/incision
29. colpo/rrhaphy   vagina/suture
30. hystero/spasm   uterus/involuntary contraction
31. ovario/cele   ovary/pouching or hernia
32. vulv/ectomy   vulva/excision
33. lacto/genesis   milk/origin or production
34. endo/metr/itis   within/uterus/inflammation
35. salpingo/lysis   uterine (fallopian) tube/*breaking down or dissolution
36. mast/ectomy   breast/excision (removal)
37. pelvi/meter   pelvic cavity/instrument for measuring
38. ov/oid   egg/resembling
39. adeno/carcin/oma   gland/cancer/tumor
40. intrauterine device
41. human papilloma virus
42. chorionic villus sampling
43. dilation and curettage
44. hepatitis B virus
45. estimated date of confinement
46. herpes simplex virus
47. sexually transmitted virus
48. therapeutic abortion
49. hormone replacement therapy
50. i
51. f
52. e
53. g

*Preferred answer.

54. h
55. b
56. d
57. j
58. c
59. a
60. fibrocystic breasts
61. vesicovaginal fistula
62. tubal ligation
63. polymastia
64. syphilis
65. hysterosalpingogram
66. Papanicolaou smear (Pap)
67. endometriosis
68. rectovaginal fistula
69. colporrhaphy—posterior repair
70. menopause
71. dysmenorrhea
72. amenorrhea
73. oligomenorrhea
74. menorrhagia
75. metrorrhagia
76. gynecomastia
77. amastia
78. hypomastia or micromastia; augmentation mammoplasty
79. hypermastia or macromastia; reduction mammoplasty
80. mastopexy
81. mastectomy
82. lumpectomy
83. spontaneous abortion
84. habitual abortion
85. incomplete abortion
86. missed abortion
87. therapeutic abortion
88. threatened abortion
89. c
90. f
91. g
92. j
93. l
94. d
95. i
96. b
97. k
98. h
99. a
100. e

FIGURE CREDIT LIST

Figure 1.1. Redrawn from Bliss EC. Getting things done. New York: Bantam, 1976:67.

Figure 3.1. From Sheldon H. Boyd's introduction to the study of disease, 11th ed. Philadelphia: Lea & Febiger, 1992:35.

Figure 3.2. From Hotel Dieu Museum, Beaune, France.

Figure 3.3. From Sheldon H. Boyd's introduction to the study of disease, 11th ed. Philadelphia: Lea & Febiger, 1992:580.

Unnumbered figure page 57. Courtesy of Welch Allyn, Inc., Skaneateles Falls, NY.

Color Plate 3. Squamous cell carcinomas and basal cell carcinomas. Reprinted with permission of Skin Cancer Foundation, New York, NY. Figures 1–4. Courtesy of American Cancer Society, Atlanta, GA.

Color Plate 4. Primary lesions. Courtesy of American Academy of Dermatology, Schamburg, IL. Petechia, syphilitic chancre, chancroid. Courtesy of LJ Underwood and RD Underwood, Mission Viejo, CA. Condylomata. From Micha JP. Genital warts: treatable warning of cancer. Belle Mead NJ: Excerpta Medica, p. 31. HSV-2. Patient Care 1990; Apr 30:85.

Color Plate 7. CT of skull. Courtesy of West Coast Radiology Center, Santa Ana, CA.

Color Plate 8. From Yochum TR, Rowe LJ. Essentials of skeletal radiology. 1987;1:xxvii.

Color Plate 11. Echocardiogram. Courtesy of Orange Coast College, Costa Mesa, CA.

Color Plate 12. PTCA. Courtesy of Medtronic Interventional Vascular, San Diego, CA.

Color Plate 13. Doppler color flow. Courtesy of Hoag Memorial Hospital Presbyterian, Newport Beach, CA.

Color Plate 14. Color flow Doppler. Courtesy of Acuson Corp., Mt. View, CA.

Color Plate 15. White blood cells and red blood cells. Wintrobe's clinical hematology, 9th ed. Philadelphia: Lea & Febiger, 1993. Platelets. Courtesy of Mosby's medical nursing and allied health dictionary, 4th ed. St. Louis: Mosby Yearbook, 1994:1230.

Color Plate 18. Courtesy of Temple University Health Sciences Center, Philadelphia, PA.

Color Plate 19. From Haines DL. Neuroanatomy: an atlas of structures, sections, and systems, 4th ed. Baltimore: Williams & Wilkins, 1995:29.

Color Plate 20. From Haines DL. Neuroanatomy: an atlas of structures, sections, and systems, 4th ed. Baltimore: Williams & Wilkins, 1995:131, 237.

Color Plate 22. EEG. Courtesy of Orange Coast College, Costa Mesa, CA. PET scans. Courtesy of Newport Diagnostic Center, Newport Beach, CA.

Color Plate 25. Courtesy of Welch Allen, Inc. Skaneateles Falls, NY.

Color Plate 26. Courtesy of Welch Allen, Inc. Skaneateles Falls, NY.

Color Plate 28. Redrawn from poster created by Reed & Carnrick, Kenilworth, NJ. Endoscope and fiberoptics. Courtesy of Olympus America, Inc., Lake Success, NY. Photographs. Courtesy of Mission Hospital Regional Medical Center, Mission Viejo, CA.

Color Plate 31. Cervical colposcopy. Courtesy of American Society for Colposcopy and Cervical Pathology, Washington, DC.

Color Plate 32. Sperm and ovum. Courtesy of Lucinda Veeck, New York, NY.

Figure 5.3. Courtesy of Laurence J and Richard D Underwood, Mission Viejo, CA.

Figure 5.4. Courtesy of Laurence J and Richard D Underwood, Mission Viejo, CA.

Figure 5.5. Courtesy of Laurence J and Richard D Underwood, Mission Viejo, CA.

Figure 5.6. From Georgiade GS, Georgiade NG, Riefkohl R, Barwick WJ. Textbook of plastic, maxillofacial, and reconstructive surgery, 2nd ed. Baltimore: Williams & Wilkins, 1992.

Figure 5.7. Courtesy of Laurence J and Richard D Underwood, Mission Viejo, CA.

Figure 5.9. Courtesy of Laurence J and Richard D Underwood, Mission Viejo, CA.

Figure 5.10. Courtesy of Ellman International, Hewlett, NY (Randolph Waldman, M.D., photographer).

Figure 5.12. Courtesy of Ellman International, Hewlett, NY (Randolph Waldman, M.D., photographer).

Figure 6.6. From Malone TR, ed. Hand and wrist injuries and treatment. Baltimore: Williams & Wilkins, 1989:5.

Figure 6.8. Harris JH Jr, Harris WH, Novelline RA. The radiology of emergency medicine, 3rd ed. Baltimore: Williams & Wilkins, 1993:440, 467.

Figure 6.9. Courtesy of Orange Coast College Radiologic Technology Program.

Figure 6.13. Courtesy of Orange Coast College Radiologic Technology Program.

Figure 6.15. Inset courtesy of Mission Regional Imaging, Mission Viejo, CA. **B.** Courtesy of General Electric Medical Systems, Milwaukee, WI.

Figure 6.16. Courtesy of Hoag Memorial Presbyterian Hospital, Newport Beach, CA.

Figure 6.17. Courtesy of Deutsches Roentgen-Museum, Remscheid-Lennep, Germany.

Figure 6.18. Inset and **B.** Courtesy of Orange Coast College. **C.** General Electric Medical Systems, Milwaukee, WI.

Figure 6.19. Courtesy of General Electric Medical Systems, Milwaukee, WI.

Figure 6.20. Inset courtesy of Coherent Medical, Inc., Palo Alto, CA.

Figure 6.22. From MacEwen GD, Kasser JR, Heinrich, SD. Pediatric fractures: a practical assessment and treatment. Baltimore: Williams & Wilkins, 1993:167.

Figure 6.23. From First aid responding to emergencies. St Louis: Mosby-Year Book, 1991.

Figure 6.24. From Prentice WE. Therapeutic modalities in sports medicine. St Louis: Times Mirror/Mosby, 1986:194.

Figure 6.25. Courtesy of Smith & Nephew Systems, Inc., Memphis, TN.

Figure 6.26. Courtesy of Camp International, Jackson, MI.

Figure 6.27. From Buchanan LE, Nawoczenski DA, eds. Spinal cord injury: concepts and management. Baltimore: Williams & Wilkins, 1987:151.

Figure 6.28. Courtesy RGP Prosthetic Research Center, San Diego, CA.

Figure 7.7. From Sheldon H. Boyd's introduction to the study of disease, 11th ed. Philadelphia: Lea & Febiger, 1992:309.

Figure 7.14. From Sheldon H. Boyd's introduction to the study of disease, 11th ed. Philadelphia: Lea & Febiger, 1992:90.

Figure 7.15. From Willms J. Physical diagnosis: bedside evaluation of diagnosis and function. Baltimore: Williams & Wilkins, 1994.

Figure 7.16B. Courtesy of Burdick Corporation, Milton, WI.

Figure 7.17. Courtesy of Burdick Corporation, Milton, WI.

Figure 7.18. From Heupler F. Ergonovine maleate provocative test for coronary arterial spasm. Am J Cardiol 1978;41:631–640.

Figure 7.19. B. Courtesy of Mallinckrodt Medical, St. Louis, MO. **C.** Courtesy of General Electric Medical Systems, Milwaukee, WI.

Figure 7.20. Courtesy of Acuson Corporation, Mt. View, CA.

Figure 7.21. Courtesy of Acuson Corporation, Mt. View, CA.

Figure 7.23. From Sheldon H. Boyd's introduction to the study of disease, 11th ed. Philadelphia: Lea & Febiger, 1992.

Figure 7.25. Courtesy of Hewlett-Packard, McMinniville, OR.

Figure 7.26. A. Redrawn from About your pacemaker. Sylmar, CA: Siemens Pacesetter, p. 18. **B.** Courtesy of Philips Medical Systems, Shelton, CT.

Figure 8.2. From Lee GR, et al. Wintrobe's clinical hematology, 9th ed. Philadelphia: Lea & Febiger, 1993;1:793.

Figure 8.3. From Lee GR, et al. Wintrobe's clinical hematology, 9th ed. Philadelphia: Lea & Febiger, 1993;1:758.

Figure 8.4. From Bonewit-West K. Clinical procedures for medical assistants, 4th ed. Philadelphia: Saunders, 1995:360.

Figure 8.7. Courtesy of Orange Coast College Radiologic Technology Program.

Figure 9.8. From Sheldon H. Boyd's introduction to the study of disease, 11th ed. Philadelphia: Lea & Febiger, 1992:340.

Figure 9.10. Sheldon H. Boyd's introduction to the study of disease, 11th ed. Philadelphia: Lea & Febiger, 1992:344.

Figure 9.11. A. Courtesy of General Electric Medical Systems, Milwaukee, WI. **B** and **C.** Courtesy of Felix Wang, M.D., University of California Irvine.

Figure 9.12B. Courtesy of SensorMedics, Yorba Linda, CA.

Figure 9.13. Courtesy of HealthScan Products, Cedar Grove, NJ.

Figure 9.14. Courtesy of Felix Wang, M.D., University of California Irvine.

Figure 9.17. Courtesy of Sherwood Medical Industries, St. Louis, MO.

Figure 9.18. Courtesy of Siemens Medical Systems, Inc., Electromedical Group, Danvers, MA.

Figure 10.6. Courtesy of Orange Coast College Neurodiagnostic Technology Program.

Figure 10.8. From Moore KL, Agur AMR. Essential clinical anatomy. Baltimore: Williams & Wilkins, 1996:366.

Figure 10.9. Courtesy of Mission Regional Imaging, Mission Viejo, CA.

Figure 10.10. From Sheldon H. Boyd's introduction to the study of disease, 11th ed. Philadelphia: Lea & Febiger, 1992:533.

Figure 10.11. From Salter RB. Textbook of disorders and injuries of the musculoskeletal system. Baltimore: Williams & Wilkins, 1983:135.

Figure 10.12. Courtesy of Cadwell Laboratories, Inc., Knee Wick, WA.

Figure 10.13. Courtesy of Cadwell Laboratories, Inc., Knee Wick, WA.

Figure 10.14. Courtesy of SensorMedics.

Figure 10.15. Courtesy of General Electric Medical Systems, Milwaukee, WI.

Figure 10.16. Courtesy of Hoag Memorial Presbyterian Hospital, Newport Beach, CA.

Figure 10.17. Courtesy of General Electric Medical Systems, Milwaukee, WI.

Figure 10.19. Courtesy of Acuson Corporation, Mt. View, CA.

Figure 10.21. Courtesy of Carl Zeiss, Inc.

Figure 10.23. Courtesy of Philips Medical Systems, Shelton, CT.

Figure 10.24. Courtesy of Radionics, Burlington, MA.

Figure 11.2. Courtesy of Novo Nordisk Pharmaceuticals Inc.

Figure 11.3. From Sheldon H. Boyd's introduction to the study of disease, 11th ed. Philadelphia: Lea & Febiger, 1992:479.

Figure 11.4. From National Portrait Galley, Smithsonian Institution, Washington DC.

Figure 11.5. Sheldon H. Boyd's introduction to the study of disease, 11th ed. Philadelphia: Lea & Febiger, 1992:640.

Figure 11.6. From Drimmer F. Born different: the amazing stories of some very special people. New York: Macmillan, 1988.

Figure 11.7. Sheldon H. Boyd's introduction to the study of disease, 11th ed. Philadelphia: Lea & Febiger, 1992:481.

Figure 11.9. A. Courtesy of Boehringer Mannheim, Indianapolis, IN. **B.** From Zakus SM. Clinical procedures for medical assistants, 3rd ed. St. Louis: Mosby-Year Book, 1995.

Figure 11.10. Courtesy of Felix Wang, M.D., University of California Irvine).

Figure 12.4. Courtesy of Ellman International, Hewlett, NY (Robert Baran, M.D., photographer).

Figure 12.5. Courtesy of Jackie Moody, Irvine, CA.

Figure 12.6. From Coles WH. Ophthalmology: a diagnostic text. Baltimore: Williams & Wilkins, 1989:203, 205.

Figure 12.7. From Coles WH. Ophthalmology: a diagnostic text. Baltimore: Williams & Wilkins, 1989:347.

Figure 12.9. From Stedman's medical dictionary, 25th ed. Baltimore: Williams & Wilkins, 1990:1578.

Figure 12.10. Courtesy of Nikon, Inc., Melville, NY.

Figure 12.11. Courtesy of Keeler Instruments, Inc., Broomall, PA.

Figure 12.12. Courtesy of Coherent, Medical Inc., Palo Alto, CA.

Figure 12.13. Courtesy of Jackie Moody, Irvine, CA.

Figure 13.2. Courtesy of Welch Allyn, Inc., Skaneateles Falls, NY.

Figure 13.3. Courtesy of Welch Allyn, Inc., Skaneateles Falls, NY.

Figure 13.5. Courtesy of Welch Allyn, Inc., Skaneateles Falls, NY. **B.** Photo courtesy of Dr. Michael Hawke.

Figure 14.5. From West J Med 1981;134:415.

Figure 14.14. From Am Fam Physician 1991;44:827.

Figure 14.15. Courtesy of William Brant, M.D.

Figure 14.17. A. From Brant WE, Helms CA. Fundamentals of diagnostic radiology. Baltimore: Williams & Wilkins, 1994. **B.** Courtesy of Philips Medical Systems, Shelton, CT.

Figure 14.18. A. Courtesy of Acuson Corporation, Mt. View, CA. **B.** Courtesy of Mission Regional Imaging, Mission Viejo, CA.

Figure 15.3. From McClatchey KD. Clinical laboratory medicine. Baltimore: Williams & Wilkins, 1994:536.

Figure 15.4. From McClatchey KD. Clinical laboratory medicine. Baltimore: Williams & Wilkins, 1994:536.

Figure 15.5. From Sheldon H. Boyd's introduction to the study of disease, 11th ed. Philadelphia: Lea & Febiger, 1992:436.

Figure 15.8. Courtesy of Mission Regional Imaging, Mission Viejo, CA.

Figure 15.10. Courtesy of Circon Corporation, Santa Barbara, CA.

Figure 15.11. Courtesy of Circon Corporation, Santa Barbara, CA.

Figure 15.15. Redrawn from art created by MedStone International, Inc., Aliso Viejo, CA.

Figure 17.9. A. Courtesy of General Electric Medical Systems, Milwaukee, WI. **B.** From Brant WE, Helms CA. Fundamentals of diagnostic radiology. Baltimore: Williams & Wilkins, 1994:548.

Figure 17.10. Insets to **B** and **C.** Courtesy of Siemens Medical Systems, Inc., Danvers, MA.

Figure 17.17. Georgiade GS, et al. Textbook of plastic, maxillofacial and reconstructive surgery, 2nd ed. Baltimore: Williams & Wilkins, 1992:853, 863.

Figure 17.18. Georgiade GS, et al. Textbook of plastic, maxillofacial and reconstructive surgery, 2nd ed. Baltimore: Williams & Wilkins, 1992:795.

Figure 17.22. A. Courtesy of Advanced Technology Laboratory, Bothell, WA. **B.** Courtesy of Mission Regional Imaging, Mission Viejo, CA.

INDEX

Page numbers in *italics* denote figures.

Abbreviations and symbols, 498–500
  on history and physical, 48–50
  for medical care facilities, 72
  pharmaceutical, 75–76
  for prescription writing, 78–80
  related to patient care, 72–73
Abdomen. *See also* Gastrointestinal system
  anatomical and clinical divisions of,
    368, *369*
  distention of, *371*
  sites of abdominal pain, *370*
Abdominocentesis, 383
Abduction, 126
Abortifacients, 473
Abortion, 469
  therapeutic, 473
Abruptio placentae, 471
Abscess, 97
Absorption, 365
Accents, 18
Accommodation, 328
Acidosis, 303
Acne, 96, *97*
Acquired immunodeficiency syndrome
  (AIDS), 205
Acromegaly, 305, *305*
Adduction, 126
Adenocarcinoma of breast, 457
Adenoidectomy, 240, 241
Adenoids, 229
Adhesiolysis, 461
Adhesions, pelvic, 455
Adhesiotomy, 461
Adnexa, 451
Adrenal virilism, 304
Adrenalectomy, 311
Adrenocorticotrophic hormone, 301
Aerotitis media, 350
Agnosia, 270
Agranulocytes, 202
Airways, *A18*
Albinism, 96
Albuminuria, 408, 413
Allergy, 39
Allied health care professions, 42
Alopecia, 95
Alveoli, 229
Alzheimer's disease, **270**
Amastia, 457
Amenorrhea, 452
American Board of Medical Specialists
  (ABMS), 36–37

Amniocentesis, 471
Amnioinfusion, 473
Ampulla, rectal, 367
Amputation, 139
Anacusis, 349
Anal fistula, 375, *376*
Anal fistulectomy, 384
Analgesics, 146, 283, 418
Anastomosis
  bowel, 384
  vascular, 179
Anatomical position, 124–126
Anatomical terms, 10
  related to blood, 201–202
  related to cardiovascular system, 160–162
  related to ear, 347–348
  related to endocrine system, 299–302
  related to eye, 325–327
  related to gastrointestinal system, 365–368
  related to integumentary system, 91–92
  related to lymphatic system, 203–204
  related to musculoskeletal system, 120–124
    bones, 120–122
    joints and muscles, 122–124
  related to reproductive system
    female, 450–452
    male, 428–430
  related to respiratory system, 229–230
  related to urinary system, 406–408
Anatomy, A1–A33
  of ear, 346–347, *347*
  of endocrine system, *A24–25, 300*
  of eye, *A26,* 324–325, *325*
  of gastrointestinal system, *366*
  of heart, *A12–A13,* 158–159
  of lymphatic system, *203*
  of reproductive system
    female, *A32, 450*
    male, *A31, 429*
  of respiratory system, *A18, 228*
  skeletal, *A6–A9, 121*
  of skin, *A4, 90,* 90–91
  of urinary system, *A30,* 406–407
Androgens, 300
Anemia, 205–206, *206–207*
Anesthesiologist's report, 57
Anesthesiology, 39
Anesthetics, 104
Aneurysm, 165, *165*
  cerebral, 270
Angina pectoris, 165
Angiograms, 174–175, *176*
Angiography, 174
  cerebral, 279
  fluorescein, 333
  magnetic resonance, 278, *279*

  pulmonary, 240, *240*
  renal, 413
Angioma
  cherry, *A5,* 94
  spider, 94
Angioplasty, percutaneous transluminal
  coronary, *A13,* 181
Angioscopy, 179
Angiotensin-converting enzyme (ACE)
  inhibitors, 184
Anisocytosis, 204
Ankyloglossia, 372
Ankylosis, 129
Anorchism, 430
Anorexia, 370
Anovulation, 452
Antacids, 385
Anterior, 125
Anterior-posterior, 125
Antianginal drugs, 184
Antiarrhythmic drugs, 184
Antibiotics, 104, 243, 337, 353, 418
Antibody, 204
Anticoagulants, 184, 213, 243
Anticonvulsants, 283
Antidepressants, 283
Antidiuretic hormone, 302
Antiemetics, 385
Antifungal agents, 104
Antigen, 204
Antihistamines, 104, 243, 353
Antihypertensive drugs, 184
Antihypoglycemic drugs, 311
Anti-inflammatory drugs, 104, 146, 353
Antipruritics, 104
Antipyretics, 146
Antiseptics, 104
Antispasmodics, 385, 418
Anuresis, 408
Anuria, 408
Anus, 367
Aorta, 161
  coarctation of, 168, *170*
Aortogram, 175
Aphagia, 370
Aphakia, 328
Aphasia, 268
Aplastic anemia, 206
Apnea, 231
  sleep, 275
Apothecary system, 75–76
Appendectomy, 384
Appendicitis, 374
Appendix, vermiform, 367
Aqueous humor, 325
Areola, 451